Nadey Hakim (Ed)

Artificial Organs

Springer

Editor
Nadey Hakim
Renal and Transplant Services
Hammersmith Hospital
London, UK

ISBN 978-1-84882-281-8   e-ISBN 978-1-84882-283-2
DOI 10.1007/978-1-84882-283-2

British Library Cataloguing in Publication Data
A catalogue record for this book is available from the British Library

Library of Congress Control Number: 2009920379

© Springer-Verlag London Limited 2009
Apart from any fair dealing for the purposes of research or private study, or criticism or review, as permitted under the Copyright, Designs and Patents Act 1988, this publication may only be reproduced, stored or transmitted, in any form or by any means, with the prior permission in writing of the publishers, or in the case of reprographic reproduction in accordance with the terms of licenses issued by the Copyright Licensing Agency. Enquiries concerning reproduction outside those terms should be sent to the publishers.

The use of registered names, trademarks, etc., in this publication does not imply, even in the absence of a specific statement, that such names are exempt from the relevant laws and regulations and therefore free for general use. Product liability: The publisher can give no guarantee for information about drug dosage and application thereof contained in this book. In every individual case the respective user must check its accuracy by consulting other pharmaceutical literature.

Printed on acid-free paper

Springer Science+Business Media
springer.com

Foreword

Artificial organs have come a long way since the first dialysis machine, the rotating artificial kidney, was invented in 1944 by Willem Johan Kolff, who is known as the "father of artificial organs". At that time he met stiff resistance from his hospital superiors but his persistence paid off and a million saved lives have been attributed to his first invention. He was indeed the first to mix medicine and engineering. An artificial organ is any machine, device, or other material that is used to replace the functions of a faulty or missing organ or other parts of the human body. Some body parts are more of a challenge than others. The heart has one purpose and it is to pump blood; however, the liver has biochemical and physiological functions which are difficult to simulate. The implantation of an artificial organ is critical because of the patient life dependency on the artificial organ itself. The treatment of choice is organ transplantation, however, transplant candidates face a long waiting time and many die while on the waiting list. In addition there are patients who are excluded from transplantation because of age or presence of other diseases. This book presents an overview of the current state of knowledge of artificial organs including the liver, pancreas, kidney, heart, cochlea, skin, stem cells, composite tissue allograft, and sphincters. It is designed for students interested in the field of organ replacement and bioartificial organs and it promotes an understanding of the designs and materials required for successful implants. It fulfills a useful place in the medical literature. The editors have gathered together experts in a variety of different fields both from the experimental and clinical aspects. Research in the field of artificial organs will lead to a closer relationship between science and technology and provides a stepping stone for the future.

Professor the Lord Darzi of Denham KBE

Contents

1. Management of Multiorgan Failure After Artificial Organ Implantation
   Michael Devile, Parind Patel and Carlos MH Gómez 1

2. Artificial Circulatory Support
   John Mulholland 21

3. The Artificial Kidney
   Christopher Kirwan and Andrew Frankel 39

4. Liver Substitution
   Sambit Sen and Roger Williams 57

5. Glucose Sensors and Insulin Pumps: Prospects for an Artificial Pancreas
   Martin Press 77

6. From Basic Wound Healing to Modern Skin Engineering
   L.C. Andersson, H.C. Nettelblad and G. Kratz 93

7. Artificial Sphincters
   Austin Obichere and Ibnauf Suliman 107

8. Cochlear Implant
   George Fayad and Behrad Elmiyeh 133

9. Stem Cells and Organ Replacement
   *Nataša Levičar, Ioannis Dimarakis, Catherine Flores,
   Evangelia I Prodromidi, Myrtle Y Gordon and Nagy A Habib* 137

10. Composite Tissue Transplantation: A Stage Between Surgical Reconstruction and Cloning
    Earl R. Owen and Nadey S. Hakim 165

Index 179

Contributors

L C Andersson MD Dr med PhD
Consultant Plastic Surgeon
Anelca Clinic
Specialist Clinic for Aesthetic
  and Reconstructive Plastic Surgery
London
UK

Michael Devile BSc MBBS MRCP(UK)
Specialist Trainee Registrar
  in Anaesthesia
Oxford Deanery
Oxfordshire
UK

Ioannis Dimarakis MRCS
Department of Surgical Oncology
  and Technology
Faculty of Medicine
Imperial College London
London
UK

Mr B Elmiyeh MBBS MRCS DO-HNS
Basildon Hospital
Basildon, Essex
UK

Mr G Fayad MD FRCS FICS
Basildon Hospital
Nethermayne
Basildon
Essex
UK

Catherine Flores PhD
Department of Haematology
Faculty of Medicine
Imperial College London
London
UK

Andrew Frankel MBBS MD BSc FR
Consultant Nephrologist
West London Renal and Transplant
  Centre
Imperial College Healthcare NHS Trust
Hammersmith Hospital
London
UK

Carlos MH Gómez LMS FRCA MD
  EDICM
Consultant in Intensive Care Medicine
  and Anaesthesia
St Mary's Hospital
Imperial NHS Trust
London
UK

Myrtle Y Gordon PhD DSc
Department of Haematology
Faculty of Medicine
Imperial College London
London
UK

Nagy A Habib ChM FRCS
Department of Surgical Oncology
  and Technology
Faculty of Medicine
Imperial College London
London
UK

Nadey Hakim KCJSJ, MD, PhD, FRCS,
  FRCSI, FACS, FICS(Hon)
Max Thorek Professor of Surgery
West London Renal and Transplant
  Centre
Imperial College Healthcare NHS Trust
London
UK

Christopher Kirwan MD
Specialist Registrar Renal Medicine
West London Renal and Transplant Centre
Hammersmith Hospitals NHS Trust
London
UK

G Kratz MD
Department of Hand Surgery
Plastic Surgery and Burns
University Hospital Linköping
Linköping
Sweden

Nataša Levičar PhD
Department of Surgical Oncology and Technology
Faculty of Medicine
Imperial College London
London
UK

John Mulholland BEng BSc MSc
Clinical Perfusion Scientist
London Perfusion Science
Westminster
London
UK

HC Nettelblad M.D. PhD
Associate Professor
Anelca Clinic
Specialist Clinic for Aesthetic and Reconstructive Plastic Surgery
London
UK

Mr Austin Obichere MBBS MD FRCS FRCS (Gem)
Consultant Colorectal Surgeon
Department of Surgery
University College London Hospital
London
UK

Professor Earl R Owen AO MBBS (Uni of Syd) MD(Lyon) DSc FRACS FRCS PICS FRCSE
Specialist in Microsurgery, Hand and Infertility Surgery
North Sydney, NSW
Australia

Parind Patel BSc MBBS DMS FRCA EDICM
Consultant in Intensive Care Medicine
Hammersmith Hospital
Imperial NHS Trust
London
UK

Dr Martin Press MA MSc FRCP
Consultant Endocrinologist
Royal Free Hospital
London
UK

Evangelia I Prodromidi PhD MSc
Department of Renal Medicine
Faculty of Medicine
Imperial College London
London
UK

Sambit Sen MD MRCP
Department of Gastroenterology
Luton and Dunstable Hospital
Lewsey Road
Luton, Bedfordshire
UK

Mr Ibnauf Suliman BSc(Hons) BM MRCS(Eng)
Specialist Registrar
South East Thames
London Deanery
London
UK

Roger Williams CBE MD FRCP FRCS FRCPE FRACP FMedSci FRCPI(Hon) FACP(Hon)
Professor of Hepatology and Consultant Physician
The Institute of Hepatology
University College London
London
UK

Management of Multiorgan Failure After Artificial Organ Implantation

Michael Devile, Parind Patel and Carlos MH Gómez

Cardiovascular Failure

The requirements of hemodynamic support in patients with artificial organs follow the same principles as for any other patient. Ultimately the need for such support will arise if the patient is in shock. The key disturbance in shock is the inability of the tissues and cells to obtain and utilize enough oxygen for their aerobic respiratory needs, ultimately resulting in cell death.

Classification

Shock is classified into four types based on the underlying pathophysiological mechanism: hypovolemic, cardiogenic, obstructive, and distributive. (Table 1-1). The patient with artificial organs will have a higher risk of all of the above mechanisms at various stages of the peri and postoperative process and extra vigilance is therefore necessary. The management of shock should nevertheless follow basic critical care principles: re-establishing perfusion to vital organs while treating the underlying condition.

Hypovolemic Shock

This can often present as an emergency (due to massive hemorrhage for instance) or in a more indolent manner leading to slow organ hypoperfusion (due to a mismatch of fluid input and output). Initial resuscitation should consist of restoring intravascular volume, but more importantly reversing the cause (bleeding vessels, coagulopathy, reversing gastrointestinal losses). The choice of fluid should be based on the fluid type that has been lost. For example, blood and blood products should replace blood and crystalloid should be used for vomiting and dehydration. For mild to moderate blood loss similar to that expected in a routine renal transplant crystalloid (2–3 times the lost blood volume) or colloid (1–2 times the lost blood volume) is usually appropriate.

The debate of crystalloids versus colloid has not been resolved; there exists numerous conflicting trials, meta-analysis, and opinions. The crystalloids of choice in resuscitation are normal saline or lactated Ringer's solution because their osmolality is similar to that of the intravascular volume. In large-volume resuscitation, however, excessive normal saline infusion may produce hyperchloremic metabolic acidosis. As the volume of distribution is much larger for crystalloids than for colloids, resuscitation with crystalloids requires more fluid to achieve the same end points and results in more edema. Crystalloids are less expensive. The current choice of colloids includes hydroxyethyl starch, gelatins, and albumin all of which offer more efficient intravascular volume expansion. The administration of hydroxyethyl starch may increase the risk of acute renal failure, although newer preparations appear to be less problematic. Previous concerns of albumin resuscitation leading to increased mortality has recently been dispelled by the SAFE study indicating that albumin administration was safe and as effective as crystalloid. With any fluid there is inevitable dilution of blood (red blood cells) and coagulation factors which needs to be considered.

Table 1-1. Causes of Shock

Type of shock	Signs	Hemodynamic variables	Causes relevant to artificial organs
Hypovolemic	Weak pulse	ˉCVP/PAOP	Massive hemorrhage
	Narrow pulse pressure	ˉCO	Gastrointestinal fluid loss
	Poor peripheral perfusion	↑SVR	Diuresis
Cardiogenic	Pulmonary/peripheral edema	↑CVP/PAOP	Acute coronary syndrome
	Gallop rhythm, arrhythmias, & murmurs	ˉCO	Valvular heart disease/dysrhythmias
	Poor peripheral perfusion	↑SVR	Cardiomyopathy
Obstructive	Distended neck veins	↑CVP/PAOP	Tension pneumothorax
	Poor peripheral perfusion	ˉCO	Cardiac tamponade
	Respiratory failure	↑SVR	Pulmonary embolism
Distributive	Pyrexia	ˉCVP/PAOP	Sepsis/SIRS
	Warm and vasodilated peripheries	↑CO	Anaphylaxis
	Edema	ˉSVR	Acute liver failure

Whatever the fluid, the therapy should be titrated to re-establish normal blood pressure, pulse, cardiac output, and end-organ perfusion.

Cardiogenic Shock

Cardiogenic shock essentially refers to the failing pump. The blood flow to the vital organs and peripheries is decreased due to an intrinsic defect in cardiac function. This can be due to pathology affecting the heart muscle, rhythm, or the valves.

The most common cause, both generally and within transplant medicine and artificial organs, is myocardial ischemia. As in all types of shock, treating must be the priority: in cardiogenic shock this is achieved by reversing the ischemia (with angioplasty, thrombolysis, or emergency coronary artery bypass grafting), correcting the dysrhythmias, or simply supporting the circulation while allowing time for the stunned myocardium to recover while preserving perfusion. The early introduction of such measures has resulted in a significant improvement in ischemia induced cardiogenic shock and mortality.

In terms of hemodynamic support, various inotropic agents exist (Table 1-2) which act via modulation of the sympathetic nervous system either as direct agonists (dobutamine, dopexamine, dopamine, adrenaline) or indirectly by inhibiting phosphodiesterase III (e.g., milrinone). Both mechanisms result in an increase in cAMP, an intracellular modulator of myocardial contractility and arteriolar vasodilation. Often the inotropes, because of the arterial vasodilatory effects or the concurrent systemic inflammatory response syndrome that may occur with cell death, are combined with vasopressors to maintain overall perfusion pressure in general and coronary artery perfusion pressure in particular. Although the use of these agents is thought of as essential to the care of a hemodynamically unstable patient, there is great variability within countries and centers as to the optimum agent. It is also notable that the role of

Table 1-2. Vasoactive Drugs in Sepsis and the Usual Hemodynamic Responses

Drug	Dose	Principal mechanism	Cardiac output	Blood pressure	SVR
Dobutamine	2–20 mcg/kg/min	Beta 1	++	+	+
Dopamine	2–10 mcg/kg/min	Dopamine→Beta 1→Alpha	++	+	+
Dopexamine	0.25–4 mcg/kg/min	Dopamine + Beta 2	++	+/−	−
Epinephrine	0.01–1 mcg/kg/min	Beta 1+ Beta 2 + Alpha	++	+	+
Milrinone	0.3–0.7 mcg/kg/min	Phosphodiesterase inhibitor	+	+/−	−
Norepinephrine	0.01–1 mcg/kg/min	Alpha > beta 1, beta 2	+	++	++
Phenylephrine	0.2–2.5 mcg/kg/min	Alpha	+	++	++
Vasopressin	0.4–0.10 U/min	V1 receptor	+	+	++

sympathetic nervous system stimulation is of questionable benefit in the failing heart where the underlying cause of failure has not been addressed.

Recently Levosimendan, an inotropic agent that acts independently of the sympathetic nervous system by sensitizing the myocardial contractile proteins to calcium has been shown to improve hemodynamics and cardiac output in patients with cardiogenic shock following ACS as well as after coronary bypass surgery. This may prove useful as a pharmacological bridge during myocardial stunning, possibly with fewer (sympathetically mediated) detrimental effects.

Combined with revascularization, mechanical support with IABP counterpulsation improves outcome in patients with cardiogenic shock following acute coronary syndrome. Specific to cardiogenic shock, the use of ventricular assist devices may transiently improve hemodynamics but this has not yet been translated into mortality benefits and presently is reserved as a salvage strategy in centers where it exists and other measures have failed. The same can be said of extracorporeal membrane oxygenation, although both of these techniques are more useful following cardiac transplantation.

It must also be remembered that hypovolemia may also play a significant part in cardiogenic shock, requiring the careful administration of fluid to improve cardiac output via the Frank–Starling principle. Simultaneous monitoring for fluid overload via central venous, pulmonary artery pressures, and signs of pulmonary edema must be undertaken.

Distributive Shock

Distributive shock occurs when peripheral vascular dilatation causes a fall in systemic vascular resistance. As a result cardiac output is often increased but the perfusion of many vital organs is compromised because the blood pressure is too low and the body loses its ability to distribute blood properly

The most common cause is septic shock, but a similar picture can be seen in anaphylaxis and acute adrenal insufficiency. In addition a significant organ reperfusion induced systemic inflammatory response syndrome (SIRS) immediately follows transplantation which can mimic distributive shock. However, newer immunosuppressive agents have dramatically reduced the rates of acute graft rejection over the last decade but instead have exacerbated the problem of post-transplant infections. Although clinical features include warm peripheries bounding pulses, the significant alterations in the microcirculation results in tissue and organ dysfunction. The longer the distributive shock remains the greater the organ failure and mortality. As a result of the persistently high mortality from septic shock, the Surviving Sepsis Guidelines have been acknowledged and implemented across the world. Incorporated within these are the essential themes of early and appropriate administration of antibiotics and early goal directed shock resuscitation. In the initial stage, because of capillary leakage, hypovolemia contributes significantly to the shock. Hence fluid resuscitation should be initiated as in hypovolemic shock. Simultaneously, vasopressor therapy is required to maintain perfusion in the face of life-threatening hypotension, even when hypovolemia has not yet been resolved. Below a certain mean arterial pressure, autoregulation in various vascular beds can be lost and perfusion can become linearly dependent on pressure. A mean arterial pressure of 65 mmHg is generally accepted as a target to preserve tissue perfusion. However, in those who have hypertension, as in many renal transplant patients, autoregulation will occur at a higher point and hence greater MAP will be needed.

Fluids and vasopressors are targeted to hemodynamic variables along with assessment and trends of regional and global perfusion such as urine output, conscious level, acidemia, and blood lactate concentrations.

As shown in Table 1-2 many vasopressors are available. Norepinephrine may have advantages over epinephrine in causing less compromise to the splanchnic circulation and lactatemia. Dopamine may cause unwanted tachycardia and arrhythmias and provides no advantage in preventing renal failure. Concerns also exist about the immunosuppressive effects of dopamine. Vasopressin may be an alternative to norepinephrine or in patients with norepinephrine resistance, although again there is little data to support its routine use and certainly in higher doses cardiac, digital, and splanchnic ischemia have been reported.

To complicate matters, there is significant cardiac dysfunction directly related to sepsis that may require combination therapy with inotropic agents as for cardiogenic shock.

Finally, steroids remain controversial: they probably have significant effects in reversing shock, but long-term side effects such as neuropathy and recurrent infections are thought to be at least in part responsible for the observed lack of mortality benefit.

Obstructive Shock

The treatment of obstructive shock is relatively simple in principle although may prove to be difficult in practice.

Relief of the obstruction is achieved by

- Urgent pericardiocentesis in cardiac tamponade. This is a relatively likely complication following cardiac transplant, but less likely in other solid organs although anticoagulation or coagulopathy that may occur can lead to tamponade.
- Needle thoracostomy followed by formal chest drain in tension pneumothorax. This may occur perioperatively secondary to diaphragmatic damage or as a complication of central venous catheterization or positive pressure ventilation.
- Thrombolysis, pulmonary embolectomy, or surgical removal of a massive pulmonary embolism should be considered in any post-transplant patient presenting with sudden dyspnoea and hypoxia. The condition along with fat embolism is more frequent following lung transplant.

Maintaining a high preload may help with obstructive shock, with fluid resuscitation improving the patient's cardiac output and hypotension temporarily while buying time for definitive intervention.

Conclusion

Shock is one of the most frequent situations encountered in critical care patients. Post-transplant and/or artificial organ insertion shock is associated with poor outcome unless rapidly treated and reversed. In any shocked patient, hemodynamic therapy should be targeted to achievable goals. This includes

- Find and treat the cause: this is the most difficult and yet crucial aspect as the diagnosis of the underlying problem may be difficult to establish. Without addressing the ischemia or hemorrhage the remaining targets would be pointless.
- Establish adequate intravascular volume resuscitation: this is relevant to hypovolemic but also to other forms of shock in order to optimize cardiovascular function.
- Establish an adequate blood pressure: this may require the use of vasopressors and inotropes, often in combination.
- Ensure organ function by targeting the above therapy to maintain and preserve function of all systems and prevent the situation cascading into multi-organ failure.

The challenge is to reverse the patient's deteriorating condition rapidly to achieve an overall successful outcome.

Respiratory Failure

Respiration is the complex process involving ventilation, pulmonary gas exchange, oxygen delivery by the circulation, and oxygen utilization by the tissues for the production of cellular high-energy phosphate. By convention, respiratory failure is used in a clinical context to mean failure of ventilation and/or pulmonary gas exchange.

Respiratory support in a transplant patient may be required immediately postoperatively or at a later occasion for indications similar to that of the general population.

The principle of the management of respiratory failure should begin primarily with the diagnosis and treatment of the underlying pathology, often simultaneously with respiratory support.

Definition

Type 1

This is defined as hypoxemia without hypercapnia, indeed the CO_2 level may be normal or low. It is typically caused by a ventilation/perfusion mismatch; the air flowing in and out of the lungs is not matched with the flow of blood to the lungs.

This type is caused by conditions that affect oxygenation like:

- Parenchymal disease
- Diseases of vasculature and shunts.

Type 2

This is defined as build up of carbon dioxide from energy utilization. The underlying causes include

- Reduced breathing effort (in the fatigued patient)
- Increased resistance to breathing (such as in asthma)
- A decrease in the area of the lung available for gas exchange (such as in emphysema).

There are of course situations in which both mechanisms coexist in varying degrees such as asthmatics who develop chest infections.

Causes of Respiratory Failure

Many of the causes (Table 1-3) have specific treatments. Respiratory support may become necessary due to either continued deterioration of the primary cause or development of acute lung injury. Table 1-4 outlines some factors known to precipitate lung injury.

Mortality from acute respiratory failure is approximately 40%, but rises significantly if associated with failure of other organs.

Management of Respiratory Failure

Treating the underlying cause must be the priority. Ventilation, either non-invasive or invasive, merely supports the respiratory function of the lungs while they are recovering from the primary pathology.

Initial supportive management may consist of supplemental oxygen progressing to non-invasive ventilation. The effectiveness of NIV will depend on the underlying condition and is now considered as a first-line intervention in patients with COPD exacerbation. In acute cardiogenic pulmonary edema, NIV either as continuous positive airway pressure (CPAP) or as Bi-level positive airway pressure (BiPAP) will improve gas exchange, reduce respiratory rate, and the need for intubation. Its use in other causes of respiratory failure (pneumonia, asthma, acute lung disease, and neuromuscular disease) are less well defined, but at the very least may provide time to prepare for intubation or more definitive treatment.

The indications for intubation and mechanical support are also difficult to describe as they depend not only on the degree of hypoxia and/or hypercarbia but also on the clinical observations. These include trends in respiratory rate, use of accessory muscles, ability to cough and talk, and changes in mental state.

Once ventilated, the emphasis should continue with treatment of the predisposing cause of respiratory failure, as well as avoidance of ventilator induced lung injury and ventilator-associated pneumonia. The causes of respiratory failure (Table 1-3) may also lead to acute lung injury directly or as a result of prolonged mechanical ventilation.

Acute Lung Injury

Definition

Acute lung injury and its more severe form, acute respiratory distress syndrome (ARDS) are an inflammatory response of the lung. The insult

Table 1-3. Causes of Respiratory Failure

Pulmonary dysfunction
Asthma
Chronic obstructive pulmonary disease
Pneumonia
Pneumothorax
Hemothorax
Acute lung injury (ALI) or acute respiratory distress syndrome (ARDS)
Cystic fibrosis
Cardiac dysfunction
Pulmonary edema
Valve pathology
Other
Fatigue due to prolonged *tachypnoea* in *metabolic acidosis*
Intoxication with drugs (i.e., *morphine, benzodiazepines*) suppresses respiration.
Coma
Neuromuscular disease

Table 1-4. Precipitating Conditions Relevant to Transplant Medicine

Direct	Indirect
Pneumonia	Massive transfusion
Lung contusion	Sepsis
Aspiration of gastric contents	Pancreatitis
Fat embolism	Cardiopulmonary bypass
Toxic inhalation	Burns
Pulmonary surgery	Bone marrow transplant
Reperfusion injury	Drugs and toxins

may be direct (pulmonary) or indirect (non-pulmonary) and the result is characterized by:
Acute onset
Bilateral infiltrates on chest radiograph
Clinical or measurable absence of left atrial hypertension
Hypoxemia: Pa O2/FiO2 of <40 kPa for ALI and < 26.7 kPa for ARDS

Epidemiology

The reported incidence of ALI is variable. A recent population-based study from Washington showed an incidence of acute lung injury of 78.9 per 100,000 person-years.. The mortality does appear to be declining. In the late 1980s, the reported mortality was around 60–70% (1995). The KCLIP study shows the in-hospital mortality rate for ALI of 38.5% and ARDS of 41%. The incidence of acute lung injury increased with age from 16 per 100,000 person-years for those 15 through 19 years of age to 306 per 100,000 person-years for those 75 through 84 years of age. Mortality increased with age from 24% for patients 15 through 19 years of age to 60% for patients 85 years of age or older. It is estimated that there are 190,600 cases of acute lung injury in the United States which are associated with 74,500 deaths and 3.6 million hospital days.

There is no data regarding the incidence of ALI or ARDS following artificial organ implantation, although it seems likely the incidence is greater as patients are more susceptible to many of the causes, in particular infection and sepsis.

Pathogenesis

The initial insult to the lungs results in an inflammatory response which causes alveolar deposition of fibrin and collagen, pulmonary microthrombi, and acute destruction of the alveolo-capillary membrane leading to increased permeability and widespread inflammatory alveolar exudate.[28] There may follow a fibrotic response characterized by repair and proliferation of fibroblasts and type II pneumocytes.

The consequences of such changes are alveolar edema and collapse, reduced lung compliance, increased venous admixture, and hypoxemia. There is also pulmonary vasoconstriction, which increases alveolar dead space, exacerbates the ventilation-perfusion mismatch and may lead to pulmonary hypertension and increased right ventricular work with consequent failure.

Management

Continuous positive airways pressure (CPAP) may be of benefit in mild cases, however, most patients will require early intubation and mechanical ventilation. Indications include hypoxemic or hypercarbic respiratory failure, acidemia, exhaustion, and reduced or altered consciousness. Profound sedation is usually required for ventilation as struggling or coughing can cause loss of recruited lung and worsening oxygenation. Paralysis may be necessary if sedation alone does not settle the patient.

The aim of ventilation is to improve oxygenation without causing further damage to the lungs. Difficulties arise as some alveoli are normal and open while others are stiff and collapsed. It is therefore necessary to try to open the collapsed alveoli without damaging the normal areas. The main causes of ventilator-induced lung damage are over-distension, alveolar collapse, capillary leak as well as cyclical opening and closing.

Lung Protective Ventilation

"Lung-protective" ventilation strategies use smaller tidal volumes and pressures in an attempt to protect the lung from both overdistension (VILI – "Ventilator Induced Lung Injury") and dampen or prevent the release of inflammatory mediators that may drive the inflammatory response. If respiratory acidosis develops through the use of low tidal volumes, this is often tolerated ("permissive hypercapnia"). The ARDSnet conducted a multicenter, prospective, randomized, controlled trial from 1996 to 1999 to determine whether the use of low tidal volumes would improve clinical outcomes in ARDS. The trial compared "traditional ventilation" (tidal volume of 12 ml/kg of predicted body weight and a plateau airway pressure of <50 cm H_2O) with "low tidal volume" ventilation (tidal volume of 6 ml/kg of predicted body weight and a plateau pressure of <30 cm H_2O). The lower tidal volume group displayed a significantly reduced mortality rate, 31 versus 40%. The debate continues as to whether the low tidal volumes were beneficial or the high tidal volumes were harmful. Nevertheless it appears common practice to ventilate patients on lower tidal volumes (<10 mls/kg).

Fluid Strategy

The management of acutely unwell patients is faced with many dilemmas and ALI is no exception. ALI is characterized by increased pulmonary vascular permeability and some would argue that fluid restriction should decrease alveolar lung edema and improve oxygenation and ventilation. However, this may in turn render the patient hypovolemic, thus reducing cardiac output, oxygen delivery, and organ perfusion. Recent evidence showed restrictive fluid strategy was associated with improved gas exchange and ventilator free days without any detriment to other organs, although without any impact on mortality. Guiding fluid therapy with the use of a pulmonary artery flotation catheter has also shown no benefit in a heterogeneous group of critically ill patients. A simple titration of the least amount of fluid required to maintain general perfusion appears to be the favored strategy at present in ALI patients, particularly with other organ failures.

Positive End Expiratory Pressure

The issue of positive end expiratory pressure (PEEP) is also a source of varying results with large studies showing no benefit but others reporting large beneficial effects on survival and lung physiology. These differences are, in addition to nuances of trial design, probably also reflective of the difficulty in separating PEEP from other ventilatory interventions. There is good evidence to suggest that certain patients with ALI/ARDS have more recruitable lungs and that these certainly are more responsive to PEEP. Current best practice is to set PEEP somewhere above the lower inflection point of the pressure–volume curve and to then perform a PEEP trial in which PEEP is increased so long as there is no corresponding increase in plateau pressure.

PEEP has been applied in ARDS and acute lung injury in an attempt to improve oxygenation and prevent lung shear-stress injury associated with the cyclical opening and closing of collapsed alveoli ("atelectrauma"). In the face of ARDS, most clinicians would apply a PEEP of 5–10 cm H_2O. However, it is important to balance the beneficial effect of PEEP on arterial oxygenation and its adverse effects such as cardiovascular compromise and increased airway pressures and over-distension. The ARDSnet group performed a randomized, controlled trial to determine whether higher levels of PEEP would improve clinical outcomes in patients with ARDS. All patients received mechanical ventilation with a tidal-volume goal of 6 ml/kg of predicted body weight and an end-inspiratory plateau-pressure limit of 30 cm H_2O. Mean PEEP was 8.3 cm H_2O in the lower group and 13.2 cm H_2O in the higher group. There were no significant differences between the groups in the mortality rate or number of ventilator-free days, ICU-free days, or organ-failure free days

Corticosteroids

Corticosteroids have no role in the acute management of ARDS. However, a small trial in only 25 patients (Meduri) suggested a survival benefit if high-dose methylprednisolone is given as a treatment for the later "fibroproliferative" phase. Recently the ARDS Network performed a large multi-center randomized trial to reproduce the previous findings. Although, overall, 60-day mortality was similar between the two groups, methylprednisolone was associated with significantly increased 60- and 180-day mortality rates among patients enrolled at least 14 days after the onset of ARDS. Methylprednisolone therapy increased the number of ventilator-free and shock-free days during the first 28 days, in association with an improvement in oxygenation, with fewer days of vasopressor therapy. When compared with placebo, methylprednisolone did not increase the rate of infectious complications but was associated with a higher rate of neuromuscular weakness. Despite the improvement in cardiopulmonary physiology, the results of this study do not support the routine use of methylprednisolone for persistent ARDS. In addition, starting methylprednisolone therapy more than 2 weeks after the onset of ARDS may increase the risk of death.

Inhaled Pulmonary Vasodilators

Inhaled nitric oxide can selectively vasodilate the pulmonary vascular and reduce pulmonary hypertension, decrease shunting, and improve gas exchange in ARDS. There are no systemic effects because nitric oxide is scavenged rapidly by hemoglobin. However, numerous large clinical trials have failed to demonstrate that the improvements in oxygenation seen in patients treated with nitric oxide translate into improved outcome. Current expert opinion suggests that nitric oxide should not be used routinely but be reserved for patients in whom adequate oxygenation cannot be achieved by lung protective mechanical ventilation and prone positioning.

Inhaled prostacyclin vasodilates the pulmonary bed as effectively as nitric oxide but does not result in the same improvements in oxygenation. Again mortality benefits have not been proven.

Prone Ventilation

The benefits of prone ventilation are explained by an improvement in ventilation perfusion matching, recruitment of atelectasis, and the delivery of more homogenous ventilation to all parts of the lung. Two large randomized trials have compared the effects of prone positioning on mortality from ARDS. In both trials, there was a significant improvement in oxygenation when patients were turned prone. However, this did not translate into improved clinical outcome. The rates of displacement of endotracheal tubes, vascular catheters, and thoracotomy tubes were similar in the two groups in one trial but increased in the prone group in the other trial. Consensus appears to be that prone positioning is only useful in severe ARDS with dependent disease and refractory hypoxemia.

High-Frequency Oscillatory Ventilation

High-frequency oscillatory ventilation (HFOV) is, in theory, a "lung-protective" mode of ventilation. HFOV provides efficient gas exchange by using very low tidal volumes and high respiratory rates. The application of a constant mean airway pressure in HFOV allows the maintenance of alveolar recruitment while avoiding low end-expiratory pressure and high peak pressures. The mean airway pressure generated by HFOV is usually higher than that generated by conventional ventilation (tidal volumes of 10 ml/kg). A randomized controlled comparing HFOV with a conventional ventilation strategy in 148 adults with ARDS confirmed that HFOV is effective and safe and not associated with significant hemodynamic effects. However, there was no significant difference in mortality between the groups. One of the limitations of this (and almost all of the other older studies of ventilation strategy) was that HFOV was not compared with the current gold standard low*-tidal volume approach used by the ARDSnet trial.

Extracorporeal Support

Extracorporeal membrane oxygenation (ECMO) proposes to provide the gas exchange via venovenous bypass while maintaining the lungs at rest. The main advantage is that the lungs are not exposed to injurious ventilatory strategies. Again there have been no advantages demonstrated in randomized clinical trials thus far and the technique is only contemplated in refractory hypoxemia in specialist units. Retrospective single center series reported 67% rate of patients weaned of ECMO with a 52% hospital survival (Hemmila. *Ann Surg.* 04;240:595–607). Results of a prospective controlled study (CESAR Trial) are awaited. Preliminary results suggest a relative risk (survival or severe disability) in favor of ECMO in adults with severe acute respiratory failure of 0.69. Modifying the technique to pumpless extracorporeal carbon dioxide while employing a fully protective lung ventilation strategy may be of benefit where hypercapnia is the major manifestation of ARDS.

In summary, there is good evidence to support the following ventilation strategy: low tidal volumes of 6 ml/kg and plateau pressures not higher than 30 cm H_2O, appropriate PEEP as discussed, target arterial oxygen saturations of 90%, pH above 7.2 and judicious fluid administration.

Disadvantages of Ventilation

Although mechanical ventilation is regarded as life-saving support, there are many potential complications including pneumothorax, airway injury, alveolar damage, and ventilator-associated pneumonia, among others. To tolerate endotracheal intubation patients need to be sedated which in turn has many unwanted effects such as hypotension and gastro-intestinal stasis. Positive pressure ventilation reduces venous return and increases afterload of the right ventricle which in turn may fail and lead to cardiovascular collapse. Patients should be considered for weaning from ventilation at the earliest opportunity

Non-invasive Ventilation (NIV)

This is the use of positive pressure ventilation through specially designed face masks rather than endotracheal tubes. The two most widely used ventilatory modes are continuous positive airway pressure (CPAP) and bilevel positive airway pressure (BiPAP). It is in general less effective in delivery of pressure ventilation than invasive (endotracheal) ventilation but requires less or no sedation and can be administered in properly equipped units outside intensive care.

It is potentially advantageous in cardiogenic pulmonary edema, a condition in which many clinicians find it useful to undertake a" trial of CPAP" accompanied by conventional pharmacological afterload reduction and diuresis. Recently, a meta-analysis pointed to a reduction in the need for endotracheal intubation and mortality in this group of patients.

Some clinicians advocate non-invasive ventilation as a useful tool to facilitate early extubation. Indeed a randomized controlled trial in predominantly medical patients showed reduced length of ventilation, intensive care stay, tracheostomy requirement, and morality in patients receiving NIV.

NIV is widely established as an important component of the treatment of acute exacerbations in chronic obstructive pulmonary disease. Evidence from pooled randomized controlled trials points to improvements in mortality, length of stay, and intubation rate with early introduction of NIV in addition to usual medical treatment. Many groups also use NIV in the treatment of obesity hypoventilation and obstructive sleep apnea syndromes.

NIV in acute lung injury is neither favored by many clinician nor supported by evidence.

Weaning

Withdrawal from mechanical ventilation should be considered at the earliest opportunity, but only if the patient can support there own ventilation and oxygenation. There are several objective parameters to look for when considering withdrawal, but there is no specific criteria that generalizes to all patients. The objective criteria include

- Adequate oxygenation (e.g., 8 kPa on $FIO_2 > 0.4$; PEEP <5–10 cm H_2O; PO_2/FIO_2 >300 mmHg (40 kPa))
- Stable cardiovascular system (e.g., HR <140; stable BP; no (or minimal) pressors or inotropes
- No significant respiratory or metabolic acidosis
- Adequate conscious level (e.g., arousable, GCS >13, obeying commands, no continuous sedative infusions)
- Adequate cough to clear respiratory secretions
- The acute disease process that led to the patient needing mechanical ventilation must also have been reversed or resolved.

Finally, weaning is a complex and disputed area of critical care medicine in which, however, there is evidence of benefit from a multidisciplinary approach, consistency and simplicity, aggressive treatment of infection and heart failure, nutrition, daily weaning trials, and persistence.

Conclusion

The causes of respiratory failure are multiple. Each will have its own specific treatment, but advances in both non-invasive and invasive ventilatory support have had a significant impact on the outcome of such a life-threatening condition. The most notable benefit is time for the diagnosis and treatment of the underlying condition to occur.. ALI or ARDS as a cause of respiratory failure or consequence of the underlying illness and the need for mechanical ventilation also has a dramatic impact on outcome. Despite greater understanding of the cellular and molecular mechanisms, specific therapies do not exist. However, much has been learnt from salvage therapies and the importance of protective ventilation strategies.

Acute Renal Failure

Epidemiology

Acute renal failure (ARF) is a common complication following major surgery. After major surgery, incidences can range from 10% for uncomplicated non-cardiac solid organ transplants and artificial organs to 50% in cardiac transplantation and extracorporeal circulatory support.

Its presence carries a high mortality – ranging from 15% with simple pre-renal azotemia to greater than 60% in those requiring renal replacement therapy (RRT).

The most common etiology of ARF in the critically ill transplant patient is in the context of multi-organ failure. The initial insult is usually pre-renal, with renal hypoperfusion occurring from either vasodilation in severe sepsis or hypovolaemia during the peri and immediate post-operative period, e.g., intra-operative hemorrhage or marked extracellular fluid shifts.

Progression from this initially reversible rise in serum creatinine and urea concentrations leads to acute tubular necrosis (ATN). Pre-renal azotemia and ischemic ATN constitute a continuum of the same pathophysiological processes, and together account for 75% of the cases of acute renal failure. Intrinsic damage from renal disease accounts for around 30% of cases in the post-transplant patient (Table 1-5) and is most likely due to chemical/pharmacological injury. Foremost among these are radiocontrast media, nephrotoxic antibiotics, immunosuppressives, and non-steroidal anti-inflammatory drugs.

Table 1.5. Causes of Acute Renal Failure in the Critically ill Post Transplant Surgery Population [After Cosgrove et al. 2007 *Ann R Coll Surg Engl.* **89**:22–29]

Pre-renal
- Hypotension; sepsis
- Hypovolemia: dehydration, blood loss, acute pancreatitis
- Reduced cardiac output: cardiac tamponade
- Intra-abdominal compartment syndrome

Renal
- Acute tubular necrosis
- Drugs: aminoglycosides, non-steroidal anti-inflammatory drugs, radiographic contrast medium
- Toxins: endotoxins
- Hepatorenal syndrome
- Intra-abdominal compartment syndrome
- Pigment nephropathy (myoglobinuria): drug-induced rhabdomyolysis

Post-renal
- Ureteral obstruction: stones, surgical,
- Bladder dysfunction: surgical
- Urethral obstruction: traumatic/prostatic hypertrophy

Obstructive renal failure is less common (10% approximate incidence) in critically ill patients and may follow complications associated with abdominal surgery.

Establishing the underlying cause of acute renal dysfunction in this group of patients is vitally important for the rapid initiation of effective treatment, maximizing the prospect of reversing any acute renal disease. It is also important for prognostic reasons as mortality in acute tubular necrosis can be as high as 65%, compared with 5–20% for those patients with ARF as part of a multisystem disease.

Risk Factors

The most commonly identified risk factors for the development of renal failure are impaired preoperative renal function. Transplant and artificial organ patients also suffer from other factors known to be associated with renal failure, such as hypertension, hyperlipidemia, atherosclerosis, and diabetes. Patients with pre-existing renal dysfunction are at highest risk of developing postoperative renal failure. Renal dysfunction is particularly common in patients awaiting liver transplantation (and/or receiving artificial liver support) and is well documented as an important determinant of outcome. In these patients, quantification of the severity of renal function is complicated by the impact of hepatorenal dysfunction. This is usually present to some degree by the time these patients require transplantation, even when it has not progressed to the full blown hepatorenal syndrome (HRS). None of the studies of long-term renal function in these patients has factored in the potential impact of post-transplant HRS from poor liver graft function and only a few have segregated patients with recurrent hepatitis C or hepatitis B, who may additionally have hepatitis-associated glomerulonephritis.

The measurement of serum creatinine, however, seems to have a limited ability to identify patients with preoperative renal dysfunction because of its variation with age, sex, and muscle mass. Calculated creatinine clearance as an alternative measure of renal function is probably much better at estimating renal reserve, thereby identifying those at greater risk of needing postoperative renal replacement therapy.

Postoperative renal failure requiring (RRT) seems to increase markedly when creatinine clearance decreases below 60 ml/min, even if the serum creatinine lies in the normal range. Thus, the incorporation of this threshold into the preoperative assessment may help to identify high-risk patients for the early institution of aggressive renal protective therapies, such as volume expansion, use of vasopressors, and/or specific pharmacological therapies.

Age-related predisposition to acute renal failure arises due to a combination of reduced renal reserve, susceptibility to volume depletion, and a reduced ability of the kidney to conserve salt and concentrate urine. Body mass index (BMI) has also been identified as a preoperative predictor of ARF, independent of associated comorbidities such as diabetes and hypertension.

Pathophysiology

Pre-renal Dysfunction and ATN: Renovascular Hemodynamics

Pre-renal disease arises due to either a true hypovolaemia (e.g., acute haemorrhage) or a drop in the effective circulating volume (e.g., fall in cardiac output, widespread systemic vasodilation, or intrarenal vasoconstriction). It arises because, although the normally high renal blood flow exceeds the organ's usual oxygen requirements, only 10% of this passes to the renal medulla, where the P_aO_2 is only 1.2–2.2 kPa. These very metabolically active medullary cells are therefore markedly susceptible to underperfusion and consequent cellular hypoxia.

Autoregulation

Initially the kidney responds by maintaining GFR and renal blood flow to a relatively constant level, through autoregulation. Net filtration pressure and renal perfusion pressure are preserved through an angiotensin II-mediated constriction of the efferent arteriole, accompanied by an intraluminal myogenic compensatory vasodilation of the afferent pre-glomerular arteriole, principally through the paracrine actions of prostaglandins. The net result is maintenance of a near constant renal blood flow within a wide range of mean arterial pressures, from around 60 to 160 mmHg.

Drugs that interfere with this autoregulatory process include antagonists of the renin angiotensin system and cyclo-oxygenase inhibitors such as non-steroidal anti-inflammatory drugs. Another important group of drugs that cause acute constriction of the afferent arteriole after their first postoperative dose is calcineurin inhibitor immunosuppressives (CNI), principally ciclosporin and tacrolimus. These agents cause an acute reduction in renal perfusion by interfering with autoregulation, the effects of which are particularly apparent in situations of hypovolaemia or reduced cardiac output. This is particularly relevant in the immediate postoperative period, where the altered physiological milieu depends on this autoregulatory response.

Postoperative sepsis also directly and specifically interferes with renal hemodynamics through the release of pro-inflammatory cytokines. These interfere with autoregulation through stimulation or antagonism of various mediators, resulting in glomerular endothelial dysfunction and consequent aggravated renal ischemia.

Despite this, pre-renal dysfunction is often reversible if the factors causing the renal hypoperfusion are corrected. The severity and duration of renal ischemia which causes fixed post-ischemic ATN is not well established and variable given different patient characteristics, but there is usually an interval that defines the transition from functional pre-renal to post-ischemic ARF. During this early functional stage, vigilant recognition and aggressive optimization of renal blood flow, through volume expansion and/or cautious systemic vasoconstriction, can restore renal function to normal.

Histological Changes

Histologically, ischemia-induced renal failure in animals includes loss of the proximal tubular brush border, blebbing of apical membranes, and cellular and mitochondrial swelling. With advanced injury, tubular cells detach from the basement membrane and contribute to intraluminal aggregation of cells and proteins leading to tubular obstruction.

It is not clear though, whether this model applies to the critically ill. It has been postulated that in sepsis, cellular malfunction arises through immune-mediated cellular apoptosis. However, post-mortem evidence does not support this, nor do situations where recovery of renal function ensues within days, far quicker than that required for regeneration of renal tubular cells.

An alternative explanation may be that in sepsis cellular energetics are altered due to impaired mitochondrial respiration – a failure of oxygen utilization rather than delivery. This model fits well with the relative paucity of histological tubular changes in septic patients and may account for the occasionally rapid restoration of renal function seen in some critically ill patients.

Renal Optimization After Artificial Organ Implantation

The importance of maintaining adequate hydration and renal perfusion cannot be overstated. The most effective prevention of ARF is stabilization of systemic hemodynamics, optimization of cardiac output and blood pressure and the avoidance of specific risk factors such as nephrotoxic drugs – ensuring meticulous maintenance of immunosuppressive and antibiotic levels. When possible, a CNI should be withheld until renal function has improved, particularly in patients with renal failure from HRS or congestive cardiac failure.

Obstruction to the lower urinary tract should always be excluded and, in postoperative abdominal surgical patients, intra-abdominal hypertension must be considered a contributing factor.

Early recognition and effective management of any acute precipitant can minimize its severity, allowing natural reversal of the pathophysiology. This may include control of surgical bleeding, radiological, or surgical drainage of a septic focus, relief of ureteric and/or urethral obstruction and abdominal decompression to treat abdominal compartment syndrome.

Indeed, the evolution of clinical ATN has been divided, rather arbitrarily, into four stages: (1) initiation, (2) extension, (3) maintenance, and (4) recovery. It is suggested that most of the preventative interventions during ATN should be active during the extension phase.

During the extension and maintenance phases of established ATN, a variety of interventions and drugs have been used either to prevent injury or to hasten recovery of ischemic and/or toxic ATN (e.g., endothelin receptor blockers, growth factors adenosine and adenosine antagonists, nitric oxide synthase inhibitors). Although some of these interventions are effective in altering the course of experimental ATN, all but a few have shown clinical benefit. Unfortunately overall treatments remain largely supportive, with the exception of N-acetylcysteine in radiocontrast-induced renal failure and activated protein C in sepsis. Supportive stabilization of general hemodynamics and optimization of cardiac output are best achieved in critical care with volume expansion, usually followed by vasopressors.

Volume Expansion

Initially volume expansion aimed to achieve supranormal cardiac index values comparable to those shown by survivors and normal values for mixed venous oxygen saturation. More recently, however, less severe organ dysfunction has been demonstrated with early institution of treatment to increase central venous oxygen saturation to 70% or higher as well as avoidance of unnecessarily high increases in cardiac work, especially in individuals observed to have decreased cardiopulmonary reserve.

The importance of volume therapy and hydration may also help to prevent radiocontrast media and amphotericin-induced ATN, as well as drug-induced intrarenal tubular precipitation of crystals following high doses of methotrexate, sulfonamides, or acyclovir.

Vasopressors

When appropriate volume expansion fails to restore adequate mean arterial pressures, vasopressors are indicated. Although there is concern that these may cause intrarenal vasoconstriction and counter any beneficial effects of increased blood pressure, vasopressor administration does improve renal blood flow, especially in patients with sepsis characterized by systemic vasodilation and impaired autoregulation.

Diuretics

Loop diuretics are commonly used in volume control and boast the theoretical benefit of reducing medullary oxygen demand and protecting against ischemic injury. Beyond experimental models, however, renal protection has never been clinically demonstrated. They do not accelerate renal recovery, reduce the need for dialysis, or decrease mortality and although some studies have suggested an increase in mortality, it is likely that they are of no harm or benefit but might be useful in the management of fluid overload. In some patients, they may convert oliguric to non-oliguric renal failure, the latter being associated with a better outcome. It is likely in this situation that patients responding to loop diuretics are characterized by a less severe form of renal failure, rather than a direct beneficial effect of diuretic therapy – offering merely prognostic information rather than definitive treatment. Their use, however, should not delay initiation of renal replacement therapy by producing a "false" diuresis in cases of firmly established dialysis-dependent renal failure.

Renal Replacement Therapy

Physiological Functions of the Kidney and Clinical Measurement

Many renal functions are shared with other organs (e.g., acid–base balance with the lung, calcium regulation with the parathyroid glands, hemoglobin control with the hemopoietic system) and therefore can be monitored. In contrast, other functions are exclusive to the kidney but not routinely measured in the critically ill. There are only two functions routinely measured that are "unique" to the kidney and which are considered clinically important: production of urine and the excretion of water soluble waste products of metabolism. Thus, despite several existing definitions of ARF, which tend to focus on individual factors such as biochemistry, pre-existing renal impairment, nephrotoxic drugs, and pathophysiology, clinicians have focused on the two aspects of renal function that aim to encompass all these common elements: serum creatinine and urine output.

Assessment of Renal Function – the RIFLE Criteria

Urine output and serum creatinine are virtually unique to the kidney and are easily measured. Other biochemical criteria such as raised urea, hyperkalaemia, and acid–base disturbance are more open to influence from extra-renal factors, e.g., gastrointestinal, respiratory, and endocrine disturbances. Limitations of using the serum creatinine rather than creatinine clearance in identifying patients with pre-existing renal disease have already been discussed, as no single creatinine value corresponds to a given GFR in all patients. It is, however, the change in creatinine that is useful in determining the presence of ARF and determining the exact GFR is rarely necessary for clinical purposes. Instead it is important to determine whether renal function is stable or changing and this can usually be determined by monitoring serum creatinine alone.

Urine output is far less specific for renal failure, except when severely reduced or absent; severe ARF can exist despite normal urine output – i.e., non-oliguric ARF. It can also vary depending on factors extrinsic to the kidney, such as post-renal tract obstruction and the use of loop diuretics which, as mentioned above, may convert a non-oliguric ARF to an oliguric renal failure, at the expense of intravascular depletion unless this possibility is recognized and treated.

With this in mind, the *RIFLE* system has formed a new consensus classification from the second International Consensus Conference of the Acute Dialysis Quality Initiative (Table 1-6).

RIFLE stands for *R*isk of renal dysfunction, *I*njury to the kidney, *F*ailure of kidney function, *L*oss of kidney function, and *E*nd stage renal disease.

This is a multilevel classification that helps to stratify and define ARF, where patients can fulfil the criteria through changes in serum creatinine, urine output, or both. It permits the

Table 1-6. The RIFLE Classification for Acute Renal Failure [After Bellomo et al. Acute Renal Failure – Definition, Outcome Measures, Animal Models, Fluid Therapy and Information Technology Needs: the Second International Consensus Conference of the Acute Dialysis Quality Initiative (ADQI) Group. *Crit Care*. 2004;8:R202–12]

	GFR Criteria	Urine output criteria
Risk	Increased creatinine × 1.5 from baseline 25% reduction in GFR	<0.5 ml/kg/h over 6 h
Injury	Increased creatinine × 2 from baseline 50% reduction in GFR	<0.5 ml/kg/h over 12 h
Failure	Increased creatinine × 3 from baseline 75% reduction in GFR	<0.3 ml/kg/h over 24 h
Loss	Persistent ARF. Complete loss of kidney function for >4 weeks	
ESRD	End-stage kidney stage (> 3 months)	

Indications for Renal Replacement Therapy

Common renal and non-renal indications for renal replacement therapy (RRT) after artificial organ implantation are listed in Table 1-7. In the setting of oliguria, fluid overload, deranged electrolytes and acidaemia RRT simplifies fluid and nutritional management and its early use may improve outcome.

However, establishing an extracorporeal circuit is not without risks (bleeding, hypotension, hypothermia, inflammatory response, line infections); in addition, it should not be regarded simply as replacement of all kidney functions. Indeed, other than removal of metabolic waste products, hydrogen ions, fluid balance, and other functions of the kidney are not replaced. ARF requiring RRT in intensive care patients carries a mortality of 40–70% compared with around 10% in similar critically ill patients not requiring RRT. This increased mortality is in fact due to non-renal causes such as bleeding, sepsis, and respiratory failure, suggesting that normal kidney function has additional systemic effects that are not replaced by RRT, the pathological consequences of which are shown in Table 1-8. Thus, ARF carries an independent risk of death, and patients may be dying *"of"* renal failure rather than *"with"* renal failure. The kidney is thought to play a crucial role in inflammation and the evolution of distal organ injury particularly in the context of postoperative sepsis and multi-organ dysfunction (Table 1-9).

Hence if ARF develops, a vicious cycle of cytokine release, dysfunction of distal organs, failure of urinary cytokine clearance, and further distal organ dysfunction ensues. As mentioned, often there exists a window of opportunity between the potentially reversible pre-renal phase and fully established ATN. In those patients at risk of developing ARF either preoperatively or postoperatively, preventative measures should be initiated early to avoid progression of renal dysfunction and its associated poor outcome.

Taking into account the hazards and prognostic implications of RRT, and the possible benefits of its early commencement, there is still no agreed consensus for the optimal point at which to commence filtration. It is hoped, however, that application of the RIFLE criteria may in future aid to the development of specific guidelines.

Table 1-9. Pathophysiological and Immunological Effects of Acute Renal Failure, and Renal Replacement Therapy

The injured kidney: a pro-inflammatory mediator
- Increased release/impaired catabolism and elimination of cytokines
- Activation of immunocompetent cells
- Release of factors promoting distal organ injury

Factors mediated by renal replacement therapies
- Hemodynamic factors
- Loss of nutrients (amino acids/antioxidants)
- Induction of an inflammatory reaction

Table 1-7. Indications for Continuous Renal Replacement Therapy

Renal	Possible non-renal
Uremia	Sepsis
Hyperkalemia	Multiple organ dysfunction syndrome
Metabolic acidosis	Pulmonary edema
Fluid overload	Raised intracranial pressure
	Temperature control

Table 1-8. The Pathological Consequences of Acute Renal Failure

Cardiovascular	Hyperdynamic circulation, cardiomyopathy, pericarditis
Pulmonary	Pulmonary edema, alveolitis, pneumonia, pulmonary hemorrhage
Gastrointestinal	Motility impairment, erosions, ulcerations, hemorrhage, pancreatitis, colitis
Neuromuscular	Neuropathy, myopathy, encephalopathy
Immunological	Impaired humoral and cellular immunity
Hematological	Anemia, thrombocytopenia, bleeding diathesis
Metabolic	Insulin resistance, hyperlipidemia, increased protein catabolism, depletion of antioxidants

Introduction to Renal Replacement Therapy

Renal replacement therapy (RRT) describes a broad spectrum of treatments that ultimately aims to take over fluid control, acid–base balance, and metabolic waste product removal. Treatments involve establishing an extracorporeal circuit via an artery or vein, directing blood flow through a filtration system that removes waste solutes, water and other molecules before being fed back to the patient. This filtration system may be driven by a pressure gradient (hemofiltration) or by a concentration gradient (hemodialysis).

Vascular Access

Most current RRT is veno-venous via a large bore double lumen central venous cannula, with blood flow through the circuit achieved by a peristaltic roller pump. Insertion sites are largely determined by the presence of other central venous catheters already in situ. Subclavian lines have had stenosis rates quoted of up to 90%, which is potentially problematic if formation of an arteriovenous fistula is being considered for long-term renal replacement. The internal jugular permits greater patient mobility but is associated with greater immediate complications. The femoral route is useful for short-term renal replacement but is associated with increased rate of infections.

Anticoagulation

All patients requiring renal replacement therapy need suitable anticoagulation unless there is significant coagulopathy or thrombocytopenia. This is usually in the form of unfractionated heparin, delivered via the extracorporeal circuit rather than systemically to the patient, and is administered upstream of the filter. Prostacyclin is useful in cases of heparin-induced thrombocytopenia and other agents employed include low molecular weight heparin, sodium citrate, and nafamostat mesilate.

Adverse Effects of RRT

The most common complications of RRT are related to the extracorporeal circuit, vascular access, and the consequences of filtration. These are summarized in Table 1-10.

Table 1-10. The Common Complications of RRT

Extracorporeal circuit	Hypothermia, complement activation, hypotension, anemia
Vascular access	Air embolism, clotting and hemorrhage, infection
Consequences of filtration	Electrolyte loss ($\downarrow Na^+$, $\downarrow Ca^{2+}$, $\downarrow Mg^{2+}$, $\downarrow K^+$), arrhythmias, hypovolaemia, metabolic alkalosis, removal of therapeutic drugs

Principle of Hemofiltration

Ultrafiltration is the passage of fluid under pressure across a semi-permeable membrane where solutes are carried along with the fluid by solvent drag (convection). Synthetic biocompatible membranes are made of polyacrylonitrile, polysulfone, polyamide, or cellulose triacetate. These cause minimal complement or leucocyte activation. Fluid balance is maintained by the simultaneous re-infusion of a sterile crystalloid replacement fluid containing essential plasma electrolytes. Replacement fluid can be administered before the filter (pre-dilution) or, more usually, after the filter (post-dilution). Pre-dilution may be useful when high filtration rates are required (10 l/day) or when filter clotting is a problem as it reduces blood viscosity and subsequent clotting in the circuit. However, it may decrease the efficiency of the system as the blood being filtered contains a lower concentration of metabolic waste products.

Hemofiltration is very effective in the removal of fluid and middle-sized molecules. The latter has been suggested as an advantageous feature in the treatment of sepsis, as most of the pro-inflammatory cytokines may be theoretically removed by this technique.

Dialysis is the removal of solutes by diffusion across a semi-permeable membrane down a concentration gradient. The dialysate fluid is of low osmolaltity, and blood and dialysate fluid are circulated in a "counter-current" fashion. However, unlike hemofiltration, no replacement fluid is re-infused. Treatment is intermittent, with large volumes of fluid being dialyzed in a period of a few hours. Blood flow is usually 150–300 ml/min, with dialysis flows at 1000–2000 ml/h.

Continuous Venovenous Hemodiafiltration (CVVHDF)

This is the most popular mode in the ICU and provides solute removal by diffusion and convection simultaneously. It offers high-volume ultrafiltration using replacement fluid, with additional dialysate fluid being passed through the hemofilter in a counter-current fashion to blood flow. This improves the efficiency and solute clearance rate, removing both small and middle molecules.

Optimal Treatment Modalities for RRT

Continuous renal replacement therapy constitutes a diverse range of treatments offering various ways of providing RRT that may influence efficacy and safety. These can be separated into intermittent or continuous modalities.

Intermittent hemodialysis, although widely used in the United States, generates huge osmotic changes, fluid shifts, and consequent hypotension – often to the detriment of renal blood flow, potentially worsening renal ischemia. To compensate, an increase in vasopressor and fluid administration may be required, and the latter can result in greater fluid accumulation than before treatment.

Most physicians intuitively adopt continuous haemofiltration which causes less intravascular volume changes as time is allowed for fluid to re-equilibrate between body compartments. This is likely to be relevant in the postoperative transplant patient, in particular those with vasodilatory shock and capillary leak where sudden, large volume fluid movement between compartments can create life-threatening haemodynamic changes (e.g., sepsis, acute pancreatitis, and hepatic failure). There is, however, limited evidence of the perceived superiority of continuous versus intermittent techniques. It is likely that, in the absence of haemodynamic instability, the two modalities are probably equivalent.

Extracorporeal Inflammatory Mediator Removal

One perceived advantage of haemofiltration in the critically ill is clearance of middle-sized molecules within the range of the various pro-inflammatory cytokines involved in sepsis and the systemic inflammatory response syndrome, not uncommonly seen in postoperative transplant and artificial organ implantation patients.

This theory, however, rests heavily on the assumption that cytokines can be effectively cleared and that the non-specific removal of such mediators is actually beneficial to the patients. Despite numerous studies, there is limited evidence to support this. Some cytokines are removed by haemofilters –albeit in small amounts – largely through adsorption, but the efficiency of this process wanes rapidly, early on in the filter's life span. Given the high turnover of endogenous inflammatory mediators and required high filtration rates to make mediator removal significant, its efficacy is questionable. Nevertheless the theory of middle molecule clearance carries significant weight in the treatment of sepsis and ARF and may have a role to play in the future.

Optimal Dose of Haemofiltration

Higher treatment doses of RRT have been associated with improved survival. In particular critically ill patients with acute renal failure had better outcome at 15 days post-RRT when treated with filtration rates of 35 ml/kg/h when compared with 20 ml/kg/h. Interestingly, a similar study looking at early initiation of high volume haemofiltration (HVHF), compared with the lower dose found no significant difference in mortality. Preliminary experience of early initiation of RRT and HVHF is promising, but prospective randomized comparisons between different timing of RRT seem warranted before one can definitively be recommended over the other.

Choice of Anticoagulation

In the absence of coagulopathy, unfractionated heparin given either intravenously or administered via the extracorporeal circuit is the most common choice of anticoagulation. Only citrate has been shown to be more effective than heparin in terms of filter life and bleeding complications, with some studies showing low molecular weight heparins being associated with an increased risk of hemorrhage, whereas others demonstrate its safe use and longer filter life span.

Table 1-11. Current Best Practice Guidelines of Renal Replacement Therapy in Critical Care

Mode of RRT	CVVHDF/CVVHD
Onset (early/late)	Early
Type of membrane (synthetic/traditional)	Synthetic biocompatible membranes (polyacrylonitrile, polysulfone, polyamide)
Dose of filtration (35/20 ml/kg/h)	≥35 ml/kg/h
Anticoagulation	Unfractionated heparin or sodium citrate
Vascular Access	Internal jugular or *femoral *short-term use only

Current Best Practice Guidelines

In summary, there are many modes, treatments, and doses of renal replacement therapy available. Although current evidence is limited, there are still certain aspects that show more promising preliminary outcomes than others. However, the diversity of worldwide RRT practice is not aligned with best evidence throughout the many different centers, which may contribute to additional morbidity/mortality observed. The current recommended best practice guidelines are summarized in Table 1-11.

References

1. Weil MH, Shubin H. Proposed reclassification of shock states with special reference to distributive defects. *Adv Exp Med Biol*. 1971; 23: 13–23
2. Choi PTL, Yip G, Quinonez LG, Cook DJ. Crystalloids vs. colloids in fluid resuscitation: A systematic review. *Crit Care Med*. 1999;27:200–210
3. Cook D, Guyatt G. Colloid use for fluid resuscitation: Evidence and spin. *Ann Intern Med*. 2001;135:205–208
4. Schierhout G, Roberts I. Fluid resuscitation with colloid or crystalloid solutions in critically ill patients: A systematic review of randomized trials. *BMJ*. 1998;316:961–964
5. Cook D, Guyatt G. Colloid use for fluid resuscitation: Evidence and spin. *Ann Intern Med*. 2001;135:205–208
6. Schortgen F, Lacherade JC, Bruneel F, Cattaneo I, Hemery F, Lemaire F, Brochard L. Effects of hydroxyethyl starch and gelatin on renal function in severe sepsis: a multicentre randomised study. *Lancet*. 2001;357:911–916
7. Sakr Y, Payen D, Reinhart K, Sipmann FS, Zavala E, Bewley J, Marx G, Vincent JL. Effects of hydroxyethyl starch administration on renal function in critically ill patients. *Br J Anaesth*. 2007;98:216–224
8. Finfer S, Bellomo R, Boyce N, French J, Myburgh J, Norton R. SAFE Study Investigators. A comparison of albumin and saline for fluid resuscitation in the intensive care unit. *N Engl J Med*. 2004;350:2247–2256
9. Fang Jing MD a, Mensah George A MD a, Alderman Michael H MD b, Croft Janet B PhD a. Trends in acute myocardial infarction complicated by cardiogenic shock, 1979–2003, United States. *Am Heart J*. December 2006;152(6):1035–1041.
10. Hochman JS, Sleeper LA, Webb JG, et al. Early revascularization in acute myocardial infarction complicated by cardiogenic shock. SHOCK investigators. should we emergently revascularize occluded coronaries for cardiogenic shock. *N Engl J Med*. 1999;341:625–634.
11. Thackray S, Easthaugh J, Freemantle N, Cleland JG. The effectiveness and relative effectiveness of intravenous inotropic drugs acting through the adrenergic pathway in patients with heart failure-a meta-regression analysis. *Eur J Heart Fail*. 2002;4:515–529.
12. Sakr Y, Reinhart K, Vincent JL, et al. Does dopamine administration in shock influence outcome? Results of the Sepsis Occurrence in Acutely Ill Patients (SOAP) Study. *Crit Care Med*. 2006;34:589–597
13. Kohsaka S, Menon V, Lowe AM, et al. Systemic inflammatory response syndrome after acute myocardial infarction complicated by cardiogenic shock. *Arch Intern Med*. 2005;165:1643–1650.
14. Garcia-Gonzalez MJ, Dominguez-Rodriguez A, Ferrer-Hita JJ. Utility of levosimendan, a new calcium sensitizing agent, in the treatment of cardiogenic shock due to myocardial stunning in patients with ST-elevation myocardial infarction: a series of cases. *J Clin Pharmacol*. 2005;45:704–708.
15. Ellger BM, Zahn PK, Van Aken HK, et al. Levosimendan: a promising treatment for myocardial stunning? *Anaesthesia*. 2006;61:61–63.
16. Santa-Cruz RA, Cohen MG, Ohman EM. Aortic counterpulsation: a review of the hemodynamic effects and indications for use. *Catheter Cardiovasc Interv*. 2006;67:68–77.
17. Thiele H, Sick P, Boudriot E, et al. Randomized comparison of intra-aortic balloon support with a percutaneous left ventricular assist device in patients with revascularized acute myocardial infarction complicated by cardiogenic shock. *Eur Heart J*. 2005;26:1276–1283.
18. Chen YS, Yu HY, Huang SC, et al. Experience and result of extracorporeal membrane oxygenation in treating fulminant myocarditis with shock: what mechanical support should be considered first? *J Heart Lung Transplant*. 2005;24:81–87
19. Dharnidharka VR, Stablein DM, Harmon WE. Post-Transplant Infections Now Exceed Acute Rejection as Cause for Hospitalization: A Report of the NAPRTCS. *Am J Transplant*. 2004;4(3):384–389
20. Sakr Y, Dubois MJ, De Backer D, Creteur J Vincent JL. Persistent microcirculatory alterations are associated with organ failure and death in patients with septic shock. *Crit Care Med*. 2004;32(9)1825–31
21. LeDoux D, Astiz ME, Carpati CM, et al: Effects of perfusion pressure on tissue perfusion in septic shock. *Crit Care Med*. 2000;28:2729–2732
22. Dellinger PR, Levy MM, Carlet JM et al. for the International Surviving Sepsis Campaign Guidelines Committee Surviving Sepsis Campaign: International guidelines for management of severe sepsis and septic shock: 2008. *Crit Care Med*. January 2008;36(1):296–327.
23. Regnier B, Rapin M, Gory G, et al. Haemodynamic effects of dopamine in septic shock. *Intensive Care Med*. 1977;3:47–53
24. Bellomo R, Chapman M, Finfer S, et al. Low-dose dopamine in patients with early renal dysfunction: A placebo-controlled randomised trial. Australian and New Zealand Intensive Care Society (ANZICS) Clinical Trials Group. *Lancet*. 2000;356:2139–2143
25. Russell J. Hemodynamic support of sepsis. Vasopressin versus norepinephrine for septic shock. Program and abstracts of the Society of Critical Care Medicine 36th Critical Care Congress. Orlando, Florida; February 17–21, 2007.
26. Dünser MW, Mayr AJ, Tura A, et al. Ischemic skin lesions as a complication of continuous vasopressin infusion in catecholamine-resistant vasodilatory shock: Incidence and risk factors. *Crit Care Med*. 2003;31:1394–1398.
27. Rabuel C, Mebazza A. Septic Shock: a heart story since the 1960s. *Intensive Care Med*. 2006;32(6):799–807.
28. Annane D, Sebille V, Charpentier C, et al. Effect of treatment with low doses of hydrocortisone and fludrocortisone on mortality in patients with septic shock. *JAMA*. 2002;288:862–871

29. Sprung CL, Annane D, Briegel J, et al: Corticosteroid therapy of septic shock (CORTICUS). Abstr. *Am Rev Respir Crit Care Med.* 2007;175:A507
30. Sin DD, McAlister FA, Man SF, Anthonisen NR. Contemporary management of chronic obstructive pulmonary disease: scientific review. *JAMA.* 2003;290:2301–12.
31. Masip J, Roque M, Sanchez B, Fernandez R, Subirana M, Exposito JA. Noninvasive ventilation in acute pulmonary edema: systematic review and meta-analysis. *JAMA.* 294:3124–3130
32. The Acute Respiratory Distress Syndrome Network. Ventilation with lower tidal volumes as compared with traditional tidal volumes for acute lung injury and the acute respiratory distress syndrome. *N Engl J Med.* 2000;342:1301–1308.
33. Ferguson ND, Meade MO, Esteban A et al. Influence of Randomized Trials on usual Clinical Practice. The International Study of Mechanical Ventilation. *Proc Am Thor Soc.* 2006;3:A831
34. National Heart, Lung, and Blood Institute Acute Respiratory Distress Syndrome (ARDS) Clinical Trials Network. Comparison of two fluid-management strategies in acute lung injury. *N Engl J Med.* 2006;354:2564–75.
35. National Heart, Lung, and Blood Institute Acute Respiratory Distress Syndrome (ARDS) Clinical Trials Network. Pulmonary-artery versus central venous catheter to guide treatment of acute lung injury. *N Engl J Med.* 2006;354:2213–24.
36. Derdak S, Mehta S, Stewart TE, et al. High-frequency oscillatory ventilation for acute respiratory distress syndrome in adults. *Am J Respir Crit Care Med.* 2002;166:801–808.
37. The National Heart, Lung and Blood Institute ARDS Clinical Trials Network. Higher versus lower positive end-expiratory pressure in patients with the acute respiratory distress syndrome. *N Engl J Med.* 2004;351:327–336.
38. Griffiths MJ, Evans TW. Inhaled nitric oxide therapy in adults. *N Engl J Med.* 2005;353:2683–95.
39. AdhikariNK, Burns KE, Freidrich JO, Granton JT, Cook DJ, MeadeMO. Effect of nitric oxide on oxygenation and mortality in acute lung injury: systematic review and meta analysis. *BMJ.* 2007;334:779–82.
40. Gattinoni L, Tognoni G, Pesenti A, Taccone P, Mascheroni D, Labarta V, Malacrida R, Di Giulio P, Fumagalli R, Pelosi P, Brazzi L, Latini R, Prone-Supine Study Group. Effect of prone positioning on the survival of patients with acute respiratory failure. *N Engl J Med.* 2001;345: 568-573.
41. Guerin C, Gaillard S, Lemasson S, Ayzac L, Girard R, Beuret P, Palmier B, Le QV, Sirodot M, Rosselli S, Cadiergue V, Sainty JM, Barbe P, Combourieu E, Debatty D, Rouffineau J, Ezingeard E, Millet O, Guelon D, Rodriguez L, Martin O, Renault A, Sibille JP, Kaidomar M. Effects of systematic prone positioning in hypoxemic acute respiratory failure: a randomized controlled trial. *JAMA.* 2004;292:2379–2387.
42. Bein T. Weber F. Philipp A, et al. A new pumpless extracorporeal interventional lung assist in critical hypoxemia/hypercapnia. *Crit Care Med.* 2006;34:1372–77.
43. Meduri GU, Headley AS, Golden E, Carson SJ, Umberger RA, Kelso T, Tolley EA. Effect of prolonged methylprednisolone therapy in unresolving acute respiratory distress syndrome: a randomized controlled trial. *JAMA.* 1998;280:159–165.
44. Steinberg KP, Hudson LD, Goodman RB, Hough CL, Lanken PN, Hyzy R, Thompson BT, Ancukiewicz M. National Heart, Lung, and Blood Institute Acute Respiratory Distress Syndrome (ARDS) Clinical Trials Network. Efficacy and safety of corticosteroids for persistent acute respiratory distress syndrome. *N Engl J Med.* 2006; 354:1671–1684.
45. Winck JC, Azevedo L, Costa-Pereira A, et al. Efficacy and safety of non-invasive ventilation in the treatment of acute cardiogenic pulmonary oedema – a systematic review and meta-analysis. *Crit Care.* 2006;10:R69.
46. Ferrer M, Esquinas A, Arancibia F et al. Noninvasive ventilation during persistent weaning failure. A randomized controlled trial. *Am J Respir Crit Care Med.* 2003;168:70–76.
47. Ram FSF, Picot J, Lightowler J, et al. Non-invasive positive pressure ventilation for treatment of respiratory failure due to exacerbations of chronic obstructive pulmonary disease. *Cochrane Database Syst Rev.* 2004;3:CD004104.
48. Rana S, Jenad H, Gay P et al. Failure of non-invasive ventilation in patients with acute lung injury: observational cohort study. *Crit Care.* 2006;10:R79.
49. MacIntyre NR, Cook DJ, Ely EW Jr, et al. Evidence-based guidelines for weaning and discontinuing ventilatory support: a collective task force facilitated by the American College of Chest Physicians; the American Association for Respiratory Care; and the American College of Critical Care Medicine. *Chest.* 2001;120(6Suppl):375S–395S
50. Boles JM, Bion J, Connors A, et al. Weaning from mechanical ventilation. *Eur Respir J.* 2007;29:1033–56
51. Parikh CR, Sandmaier BM, Rainer F, Blume SK, Sahebi F, Maloney DG, Maris MB, Nieto Y, Edelstein CL, Schrier RW, McSweeney PJ. Acute Renal Failure after Nonmyeloablative Hematopoietic Cell Transplantation *Am Soc Nephrol.* 2004;15:1868–1876.
52. Carmichael P, carmichael AR. acute renal failure in the surgical setting. *ANZ J Surg.* 2003;73(3):144–153.
53. Lameire N, Van Beisen W, Van holder R. Acute renal failure. *Lancet.* 2005;365:417–430.
54. Thakar CV, Arrigain S, Worley S, Yared JP, Paganini EP. A clinical score to predict acute renal failure after cardiac surgery. *J Am Soc Nephrol.* 2005;16:162–168.
55. Wijeysundera DN, Karkouti K, Beattie WS, Rao V, Ivanov J. Improving the identification of patients at risk of postoperative renal failure after cardiac surgery. *Anesthesiology.* 2006;104:65–72.
56. Van den Berghe G, Wouters P, Weekers F, et al. Intensive insulin therapy in the critically ill patients. *N Engl J Med.* 2001;345:1359–1367.
57. Wan L, Bellomo R, Giantomasso DD, Ronco C. The pathogenesis of septic acute renal failure. *Curr Opin Crit Care.* 2003;9:496–502.
58. Warren HS, Suffredini AF, Eichacker PQ, Munford RS. Risks and benefits of activated protein C treatment for severe sepsis. *N Engl J Med.* 2002;347:1027–1030.
59. Krismer AC, Wenzel V, Mayr VD, Voelckel WG, Strohmenger HU, Lurie K, Lindner KH. Arginine vasopressin during cardiopulmonary resuscitation and vasodilatory shock: Current experience and future perspectives. *Curr Opin Crit Care.* 2001;7:157–169.
60. De Vriese S. Prevention and Treatment of Acute Renal Failure in Sepsis. *J Am Soc Nephrol.* 2003;14:792–805.
61. Lameire NH, De Vriese An S, Vanholder R. Prevention and nondialytic treatment of acute renal Failure *Curr Opin Crit Care.* 2003;9(6):481–490.
62. Knaus WA, Wagner DP, Draper EA. The APACHE III prognostic system. Risk predicton of hospital mortality for critically ill hospitalised adults. *Chest.* 1991;1100: 1619–1636.

63. Bellomo R, Ronco C, Kellum JA, Mehta RL, Palevsky P. and the ADQI workgroup. Acute renal failure – definition, outcome measures, animal models, fluid therapy and information technology needs: the Second International Consensus Conference of the Acute Dialysis Quality Initiative (ADQI) Group. *Crit Care.* 2004;8:R202–12.
64. Gettings LG, Reynolds HN, Scalea T, Outcome in posttraumatic acute renal failure when continuous renal replacement therapy is applied early versus late. *Intensive Care Med.* 1999;25:805–13.
65. Wilkinson AH, Cohen DJ. Renal Failure in the Recipients of Nonrenal Solid Organ Transplants *J Am Soc Nephrol.* 1999;10:1136–1144.
66. Metnitz PGH, Krenn CG, Steltzer H, Lang T, Ploder J, Lenz K, Le Gall JR, Druml W. Effect of acute renal failure requiring renal replacement therapy on outcome in critically ill patients. *Critical Care Med.* 2002;30:2051–2058.
67. Levy EM, Viscoli CM, Horwitz RI. The effect of acute renal failure on mortality: a cohort analysis. *JAMA.* 1996;275(19):1489–1494.
68. Petroni KC, Cohen NH. Continuous Renal Replacement Therapy: Anaesthetic Implications *Anesth Analg.* 2002;94:1288–1297.
69. Myers BD, Moran SM. Hemodynamically mediated acute renal failure. *N Engl J Med.* 1986;314:97–105.
70. Van Bommel EFH, Leunissen KML, Weimar W. Continuous renal replacement therapy for critically ill patients: an update. *J Intensive Care Med.* 1994;9:265–80.
71. Druml W. Metabolic aspects of continuous renal replacement therapies. *Kidney Int.* 1999;56:S56–61.
72. Ronco C, Bellomo R, Homel P, Brendolan A, Dan M, Piccinni P, La Greca G. Effects of different doses in continuous veno-venous haemofiltration on outcomes of acute renal failure: a prospective randomised trial. *Lancet.* 2000;356:26–30.
73. Bouman CS, Oudemans-Van Straaten HM, Tijssen JG, Zandstra DF, Kesecioglu J. Effects of early high-volume continuous venovenous hemofiltration on survival and recovery of renal function in intensive care patients with acute renal failure: A prospective, randomized trial. *Crit Care Med.* 2002;30:2205–2211.
74. Reeves JH, Cumming AR, Gallagher L, O'Brien JL, Santamaria JD. A controlled trial of low molecular-weight heparin (dalteparin) versus unfractionated heparin as anticoagulant during continuous venovenous hemodialysis with filtration. *Crit Care Med.* 1999;27: 2224–2228.
75. Langenecker SA, Felfernig M, Werba A, Mueller CM, Chiari A, Zimpfer M. Anticoagulation with prostacyclin and heparin during continuous venovenous hemofiltration. *Crit Care Med.* 1994;22: 1774–1781.
76. Vargas Hein O, von Heymann C, Lipps M, Ziemer S, Ronco C, Neumayer HH, Morgera S, Welte M, Kox WJ, Spies C. Hirudin versus heparin for anticoagulation in continuous renal replacement therapy. *Intensive Care Med.* 2001;27:673–679.

2

Artificial Circulatory Support

John Mulholland

Abstract Extracorporeal cardiopulmonary bypass (CPB) is the most common type of artificial circulatory support. The evolution of cardiac surgery is inextricably linked with the success of cardiopulmonary bypass. It facilitates surgery both on the surface and within the chambers of the heart providing the function of the heart and lungs, giving the blood momentum, and performing gas exchange, respectively. This allows the heart and lungs to be isolated from the patient's systemic circulation. CPB was first used by John Gibbon on the May 6, 1953, to close an atrial septal defect in 18-year-old Cecilia Bavolek. Since then improvements in technology, management and understanding of CPB have significantly contributed to a reduction in patient morbidity and mortality. It has also enabled a shift toward an older more complicated patient population.

This chapter examines the cannulation sites necessary for CPB, their importance, and the options available. The in-depth description of the extracorporeal circuit focuses on the materials used and the properties of the various components. The non-physiological aspects of these components are highlighted and the importance of full patient anticoagulation for extracorporeal support is explained. The roles of the various associated CPB techniques are discussed, including myocardial protection during cross-clamping of the aorta and deep hypothermic arrest. The chapter also gives an insight into many of the acute and long-term complications of CPB and finally gives background information on the support devices allied with cardiac surgery, from intra-aortic balloon counterpulsation to the components of long-term extracorporeal membrane oxygenation (ECMO).

History

The key events in cardiopulmonary bypass history are summarised in Table 2-1. In 1881, Von Schroder developed the method of bubbling air through venous blood thereby aerating the blood. The following year he introduced the first bubble oxygenator. It was 4 years before Von Frey and Gruber introduced the first film oxygenator but all of this was without the ability to control the anticoagulation of the blood. This was made possible in 1916 when McLean isolated heparin. In 1928, Dale and Schuster working at the National Institute for Medical research in Hampstead, England, developed a double perfusion pump intended to carry out whole body perfusion. It did not, but was, however, adopted by Dr. John Gibbon in his first heart–lung machine prototype in 1931.

Gibbon from the Massachusetts General Hospital in Boston conceived the idea of the heart–lung machine for extracorporeal circulation to remove pulmonary emboli from moribund patients. It took him 4 years before the first successful application of the heart–lung machine for extracorporeal circulation – on his cat! The cat survived but it was not until 1939 that the second generation Gibbon heart–lung machine was revealed. It abandoned the Dale–Schuster pumps and incorporated the pump Dr. Michael DeBakey had invented in 1934. Strangely enough it took 10 years before Gibbon utilized protamine to reverse the anticoagulation effects of sodium heparin. During his tenure at Massachusetts General, Gibbon met Thomas Watson, chairman of International Business Machines (IBM) Corporation. Watson, who was fascinated by Gibbon's research, promised to help and by 1949 IBM developed

Table 2-1. Key Events in Cardiopulmonary Bypass History

1628	William Harvey, St. Bartholomew's Hospital, London, presents his theory of the circulatory system. Describes the function of the heart, arteries, and veins. Considered to be one of the greatest advances in medicine
1881	Von Schroder developed the method of bubbling air through venous blood thereby aerating the blood
1916	McLean isolated heparin making controlled anticoagulation possible
1931	Dr. John H. Gibbon, Jr., Massachusetts General Hospital, Boston, conceives the idea of the heart–lung machine for extracorporeal circulation
1935	May 10, Dr. John H. Gibbon, Jr., first successful application of the heart–lung machine for extracorporeal circulation in an animal (cat)
1949	Dr. John H. Gibbon, Jr. uses protamine to reverse the anticoagulation effects of sodium heparin
1953	Dr. John H. Gibbon, Jr., Jefferson Medical College Hospital, Philadelphia. First successful application of extracorporeal circulation in a human, an 18-year-old female with an atrial septal defect

the Gibbon Model 1 heart–lung machine. It consisted of DeBakey Pumps and film oxygenator. For all Gibbons research in the area it was actually Dr. Clarence Dennis who performed the first human open heart surgery cases involving extracorporeal circulation in 1951. The patient did not survive and on June 19 the same year IBM delivered the Gibbon Model 2 heart–lung to Jefferson Medical College Hospital Philadelphia. It was not until 1953 when Dr. Frank F Allbritten designed the left ventricular vent to solve intracardiac air complications that Gibbon performed the first successful application of extracorporeal circulation in a human. It was on the May 6, 1953, at the Jefferson Medical College Hospital, Philadelphia, that Gibbon successfully used the heart–lung machine he had conceived over 22 years previous to provide total heart and lung support for 18-year-old Cecilia Bavolek while he closed a hole in her atrial septum. Since these improvements in technology (see Figure 2-1), management and understanding of cardiopulmonary bypass have significantly contributed to a reduction in patient morbidity and mortality. It has also enabled a shift toward an older more complicated patient population and opened up the possibilities of longer-term support devices.

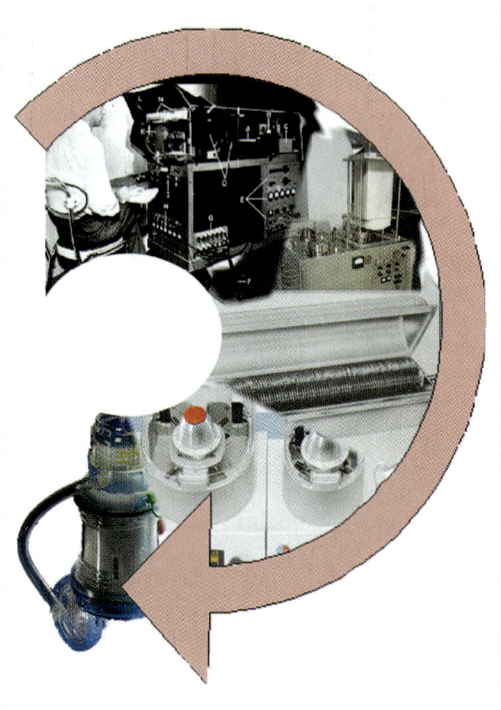

Figure 2-1. Evolution of cardiopulmonary bypass.

Open Heart Surgery

Access to the heart is achieved by median sternotomy and a longitudinal incision in the pericardium. Following cannulation and connection to the CPB circuit (see following sections), blood flow to the heart is stopped by applying a cross-clamp to the ascending aorta. While this facilitates operation on a bloodless field it also stops the blood supply to the myocardium (heart muscle) a situation known as ischemia. The myocardium is protected during this ischemic period using one of the methods outlined in the section on myocardial protection. The required cardiac operation can now be performed.[1]

Coronary Artery Bypass Grafting (CABG)

This involves the use of a suitable conduit to bypass a blockage or multiple blockages in the coronary arteries (see Figure 2-2). The conduit

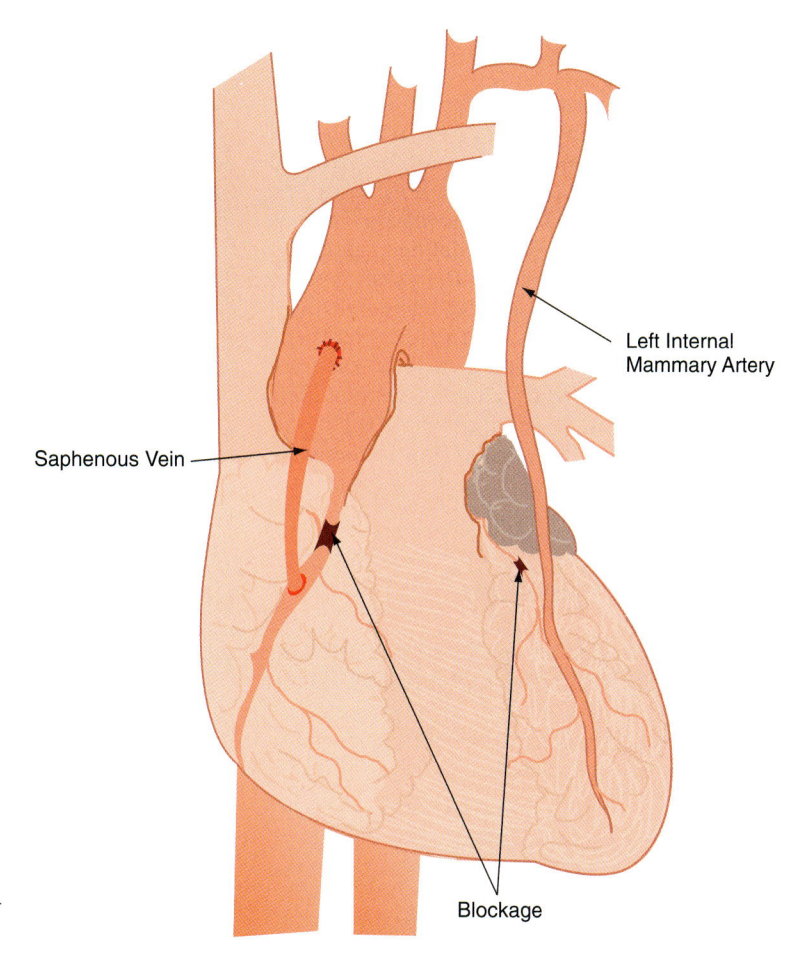

Figure 2-2. Schematic of the Coronary Artery Bypass Operation (CABG).

re-establishes a full blood supply to the area of the myocardium previously compromised by the blockage.

Conduits

- *The internal thoracic artery* – considered to be the most successful conduit in terms of long-term patency and freedom from adverse cardiac events. It is dissected from the underside of the chest wall and has its own blood supply.
- *The long saphenous vein* – this is the most commonly used conduit and is harvested from the medial aspect of the lower limb. Once harvested, side branches are ligated and the vein is used ensuring correct orientation with regards to valves in the vein and the intended blood flow of the bypass graft.
- *The radial artery* – this is a free arterial graft that is harvested from the non-dominant upper limb. Its use and patency rates have increased over the last decade.
- *The short saphenous vein* – usually used if the above conduits are not available but the patency rates are not as good.
- *Others* – other conduits that have been used over the years include the gastroepiploic and inferior epigastric arteries, bovine mammary arteries, and synthetic conduits. All have relatively poor patency rates.

Once the cross-clamp is in place a suitable point in the coronary artery (post blockage) is identified and the distal anastomosis is performed. A longitudinal incision is made in the artery and the anastomosis is made with a single continuous polypropylene suture. Once all of the distal anastomosis are finished the cross-clamp is removed and the top end of the conduit is attached to the aorta using a partial clamp therefore completing the bypass graft.[1]

Valve Operations

Once the cross-clamp is in place the relevant chamber of the heart is opened to provide access to the valve. If the valve cannot be repaired (commonly only certain problems with the mitral valve are repaired), the native valve is removed leaving a clean, defined muscular valve annulus. The prosthetic valve is then fixed in position using sutures that pass through both the muscular annulus and the prosthetic valve sewing ring. Vents are used to keep the operating field (heart chambers) bloodless and the heart must be de-aired before the chamber is closed and the cross-clamp is removed. A schematic of the aortic valve replacement operation is shown in Figure 2-3

Other Cardiac Operations

These include closure of holes in the heart, removal of growths or debris in the heart chambers, and replacement/repair of the aorta. While the operative technique varies the basics of the operation remain the same.

Cannulation for Cardiopulmonary Bypass

Once the patient is anesthetized, the chest is opened via medium sternotomy and the pericardium is lifted to make the heart accessible for cannulation. The objective of cannulation is to facilitate the removal and subsequent return of the patient's entire circulating blood volume, this process will be repeated approximately every 30 s. On the arterial side, the preferred cannulation sites are the aorta, the femoral artery, and sometimes the auxiliary artery.

Isolated right atrial cannulation can be achieved using a wire basket known as a Ross Basket. A two-stage venous cannulae is thought to give better drainage as its tip sits in the inferior vena cava while a second set of holes are positioned in the right atrium. Bi-caval cannulation is used when access to the chambers on the right side of the heart is required. This involves separate cannulae fused to one pipe via a y-connector. The femoral vein is another right-sided cannulation option.

Good cannulation on the arterial side can reduce pressure drops and therefore blood damage, as well as damage to the aorta. On the venous side, good cannulation ensures an empty

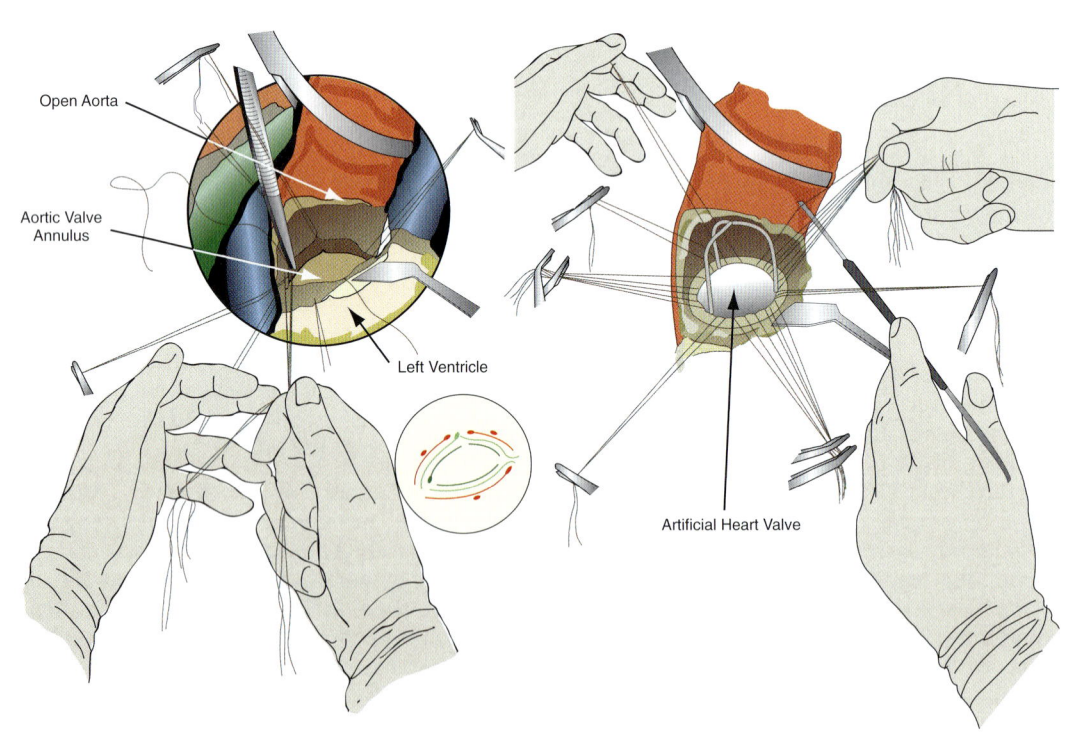

Figure 2-3. Schematic of an Aortic Valve Replacement (AVR).

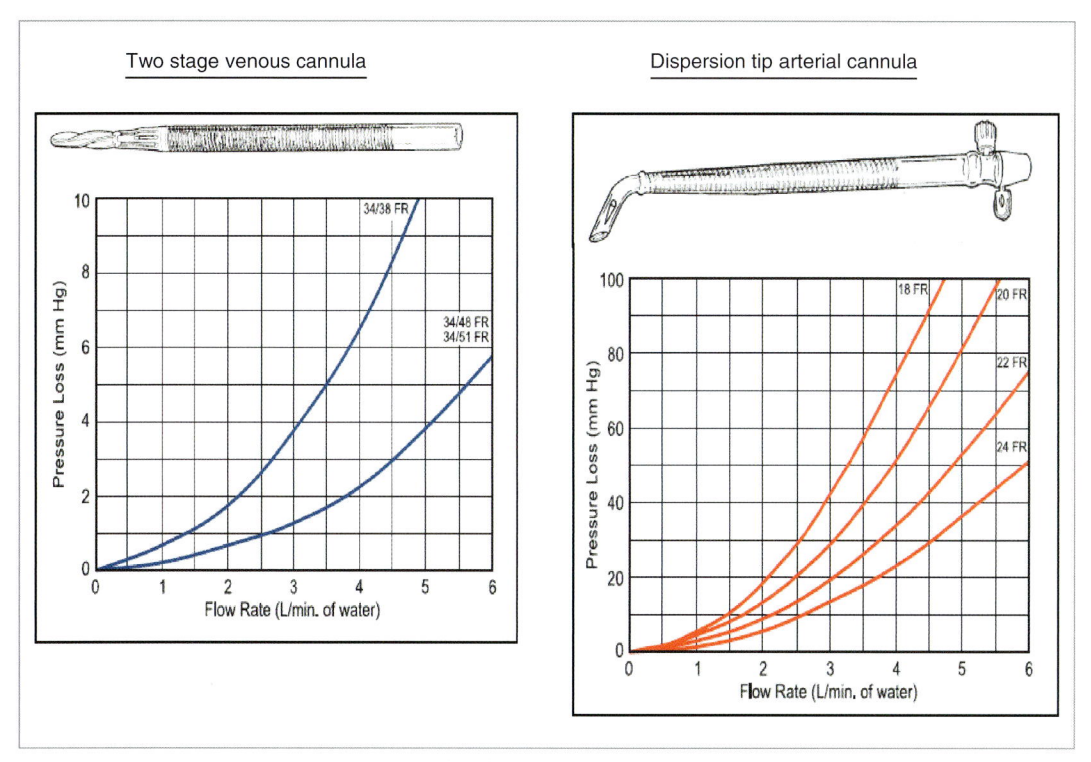

Figure 2-4. Pressure loss vs. flow, for example, high tech venous and arterial cannulae.

heart, which is easier to operate on and reduces the hemodilution caused by fluid addition to maintain a circulating volume.

The ideal cannulae possess a good balance between the lowest possible pressure drop (see Figure 2-4) and a small cross sectional area. A small cross-sectional area, known as the French size, means that smaller holes are required to insert the cannula and that they are less intrusive in the operating field. A low-pressure drop on the arterial side means that higher blood flow rates (artificial cardiac output) can be achieved reducing the risk of blood damage. On the venous side, a low pressure drop will increase the capacity to remove blood from the patient. One of the key design criteria for cannulae is a thin wall. The thinner the wall, the greater the inner diameter and lower the pressure drop to French size ratio. How thin the wall can be is limited by the requirement for structural strength. Figure 2-5 shows how

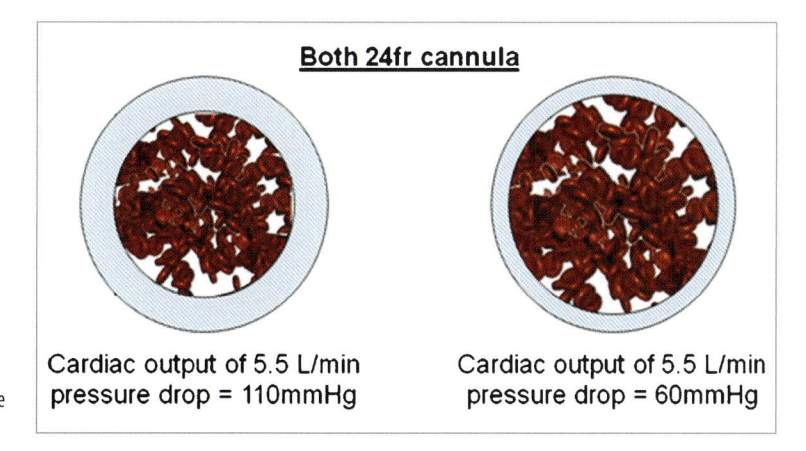

Figure 2-5. The influence of pressure drop on wall thickness.

the wall thickness can effect the pressure drop in two cannulae of the same french size (24fr).

Once cannulation is completed the perfusion team now has access for the removal and supply of blood, the patient can be connected to the CPB circuit. Once the patient's heart and lung support is being provided by the artificial circuit, ventilation of the patient can be stopped.

Summary of the Short-Term CPB Circuit

Figure 2-6 shows the basic components of the CPB circuit. Venous blood drains via gravity from the right atrium through a 0.5 in. polyvinyl chloride (PVC) pipe into the venous reservoir (1,1a). The venous reservoir serves two purposes, the first of which is to filter the blood. This is done in the central column of the reservoir and consists of a porous plastic foam and a polypropylene woven screen (1b). The porous foam presents the blood with a torturous fluid path, removing particulate emboli. The woven polypropylene sheet is designed to remove gaseous microemboli. The combination of the two provides filtration to 40 microns. The second role of the venous reservoir is to act as a capacitance chamber to manage the acute volume shifts experienced during CPB as a result of heart manipulation, shunts, hypothermia and drugs.

The filtered venous blood is then drawn from the reservoir (1c) and pumped toward the heat exchanger and oxygenator block (3). The two types of arterial pump commonly used are a partially occlusive peristaltic roller pump (2a) or a non-occlusive constrained vortex centrifugal pump (2b). The arterial pump is essentially an analogue of the ventricles, providing the blood with momentum. The cardiac output supplied by this pump is calculated using the patients surface area multiplied by a cardiac index ranging

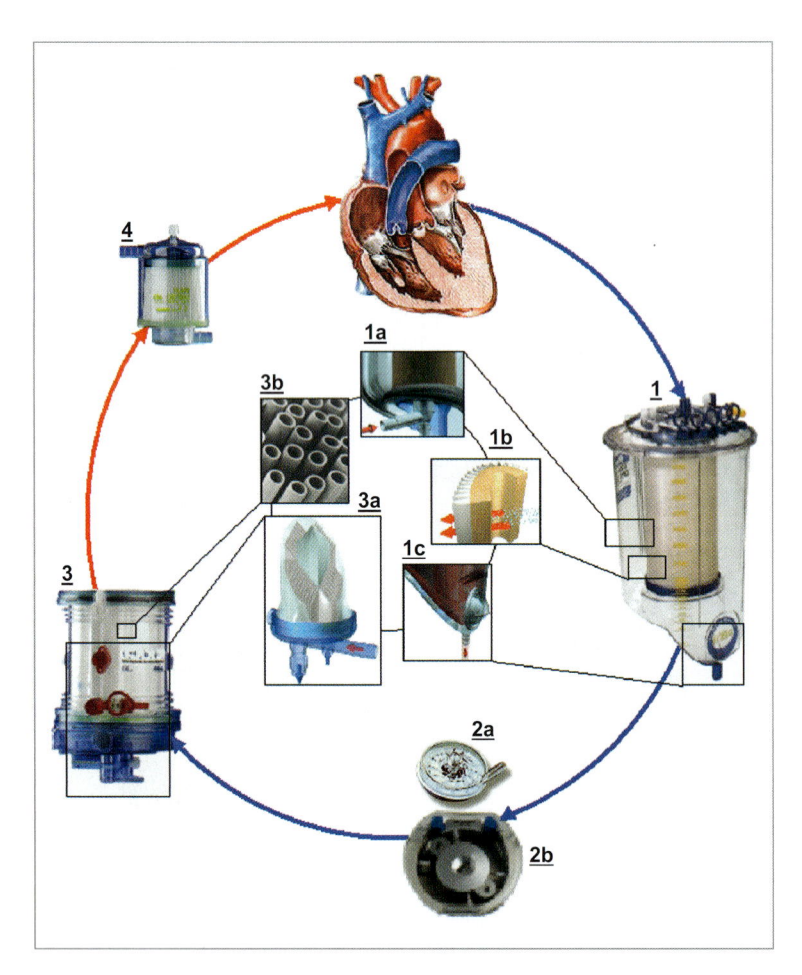

Figure 2-6. Short-term cardiopulmonary bypass circuit.

from 1.8 to 2.4 L/min/m^2, [2]depending on patient temperature. Blood then passes to heat exchanger (3) passing over concertinated plastic-coated aluminium or polypropylene membrane. This membrane separates the blood from temperature-controlled water (controlled by separate heater chiller unit) on the other side (3a). This enables control of the blood temperature and therefore patient temperature. Blood then passes to the oxygenator or gas exchange device (3). This consists of a porous polypropylene membrane arranged in hollow fibers (3b). The tiny holes in the membrane create a virtual blood gas interface but do not allow the passage of fluid. This phenomenon combined with a large surface area (similar concept to the lungs) ensures the efficient addition of oxygen and removal of carbon dioxide. The last component of a standard CPB circuit prior to the aorta is a 40-micron arterial line screen filter (4). This may remove further microemboli and definitely acts as a gross air bubble trap, reducing the risk of patient mortality or morbidity from this source. As with many of the components in the CPB circuit the flow path through this device is from top to bottom, a key characteristic for trapping air.

A Pump to Substitute for the Heart

To successfully substitute for the heart, a pump must meet a number of criteria. It must be capable of delivering up to 7 L/min, be sterile, have a low prime volume and be gentle on the blood's components. Furthermore, it must be affordable and utterly reliable.

The fluid dynamics of blood is complicated by its non-Newtonian character: its viscosity varies with its velocity. Red blood cells change shape becoming more elongated as their velocity increase becoming less viscous. Other notable factors affecting viscosity are temperature – cooled blood is more viscous; and hematocrit – viscosity falls when the concentration of red blood cells falls.

Within the pump, and also throughout the circuit, areas of extreme pressure must be engineered out. Flow of fluid that becomes turbulent produce shear stresses that damage cells, and areas of negative pressure have the ability to drag gas out of solution and thus entrain gas into blood.

The arguments about the advantages of delivering a pulsatile flow are unresolved; Taylor (1989) links improved cerebral perfusion with the delivery of pulsatile flow in prolonged CPB, however, advantages have been difficult to prove and the technique is rarely employed during CPB. The gaining success of pumps providing long-term support is forcing the issue back on to the agenda.

For surgery either a roller pump or the centrifugal pump is utilized to deliver flow during CPB. Outside of the surgery support may also be needed for significantly longer periods of time and other forms of pump might be employed. The longer-term pumps are less frequently used and expensive, with differing cost to benefit ratios.

The Roller Pump

The roller pump (shown in Figure 2-7) is an occlusive, positive displacement pump with a peristaltic action. It delivers a fixed quantity of fluid with each revolution of the rollers in the raceway. The consoles give relatively little flexibility in positioning and the tubing inevitably

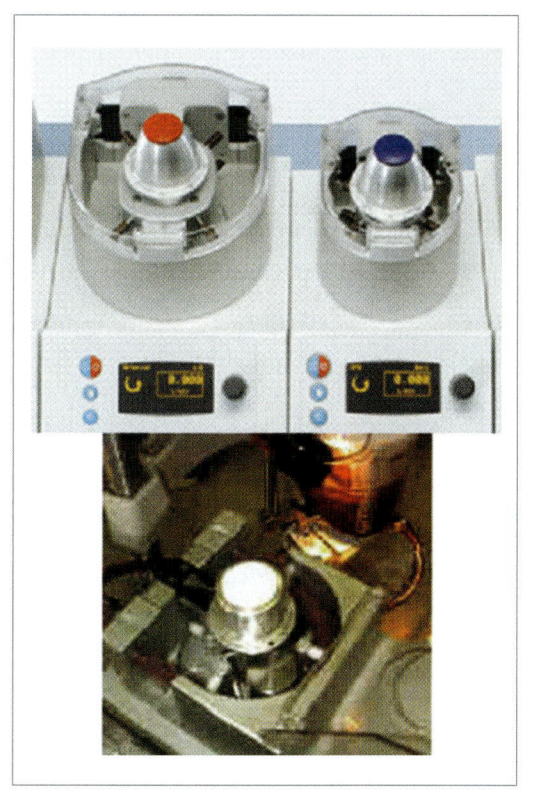

Figure 2-7. The roller pump (peristaltic pump).

suffers from spallation, tubing wear due to the motion of the pumps rollers, shortening the length of their clinical application. Tubing is either PVC or silicone. The roller pump is used for the majority of extracorporeal support internationally being both cheap and highly reliable.

The Centrifugal Pump

Figure 2-8 shows the centrifugal pump (or constrained vortex pump) which is characterized by fluid entering along the axis of its impeller and then emitting in a direction radial (or tangential) to the impellers axis. It is a kinetic pump that adds energy by fluid accelerating past the rotating impeller. It is both pre- and post-load dependent giving it sensitivity to the fluctuating resistance of the patient's vasculature.

The early suggestions that centrifugal pumps reduce heparin consumption and reduce blood damage have not been realized but it is accepted that it will not pump gross air as readily as the roller pump, which is an important safety feature. This is explained by equation $F = mr^2$, where 'F' is the force, 'm' is the mass and 'r' is the radius; air has no mass and therefore will receive no force or momentum in a centrifugal pump.

A magnetic coupling between the impeller and the drive unit provides sterility and a disposable pump head. The centrifugal pump requires little fluid to prime and can be positioned without compromise, allowing the possibility of a shortened circuit. Their Achilles heel is cost: the disposable kit for a roller pump is a length of tubing, whereas for a centrifugal pump it is a relatively sophisticated pump head.

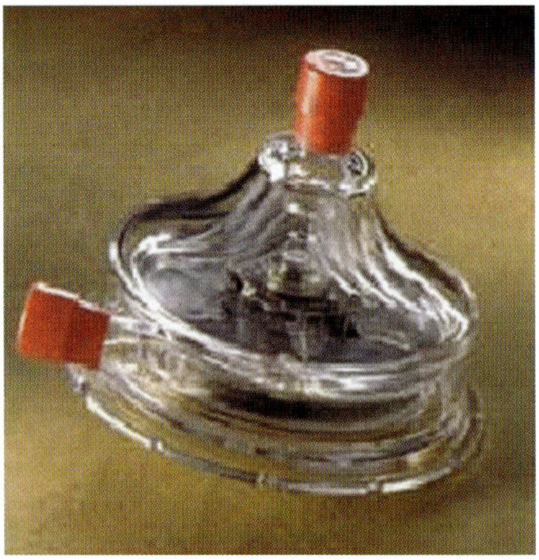

A new generation of centrifugal pumps have entered clinical practice, devoid of bearings and seals. A magnetic field is utilized not only to couple the impeller and the drive unit but also to levitate the impellers within the pump head. Their impressive longevity has earned them prolonged licenses for clinical use.

Replicating the Lungs

The need to not only pump blood but also perform gas exchange in the process brought many challenges. The act of oxygenation and carbon dioxide removal left the blood further damaged and containing multiple gaseous microemboli. The breakthrough of membrane oxygenators resolved a number of the issues generated by the direct gas interface oxygenators. The American Association of Medical Implants (AAMI) sets a minimum time of 8 hours for an oxygenator to perform on bypass, a target achieved by microporous membranes. For prolonged support, true membranes are better suited.

Direct Gas Interface Oxygenators

The direct gas interface oxygenators include screen, rotating disc, and bubble oxygenators all of which have the gas (an oxygen/air mix) in direct contact with the fluid (venous blood). The screen oxygenator shown in Figure 2-9 had 365 working parts and provided oxygen by trickling blood over many vertical sheets. The disc oxygenator shown in Figure 2-10 used discs rotating in a trough of the patient's blood to expose a thin layer of blood to atmospheric oxygen. Bubble oxygenators, a technique first introduced in 1882 by Von Shroder are now rarely, if ever, used in hospitals in Europe and North America. Oxygen bubbles of 3–4 mm in diameter are bubbled through the blood, creating the blood-oxygen interface. To remove these bubbles, the blood is then passed through a de-foaming chamber, a bubble trap, and a filter.

Figure 2-8. Centrifugal pump (constrained vortex).

Artificial Circulatory Support

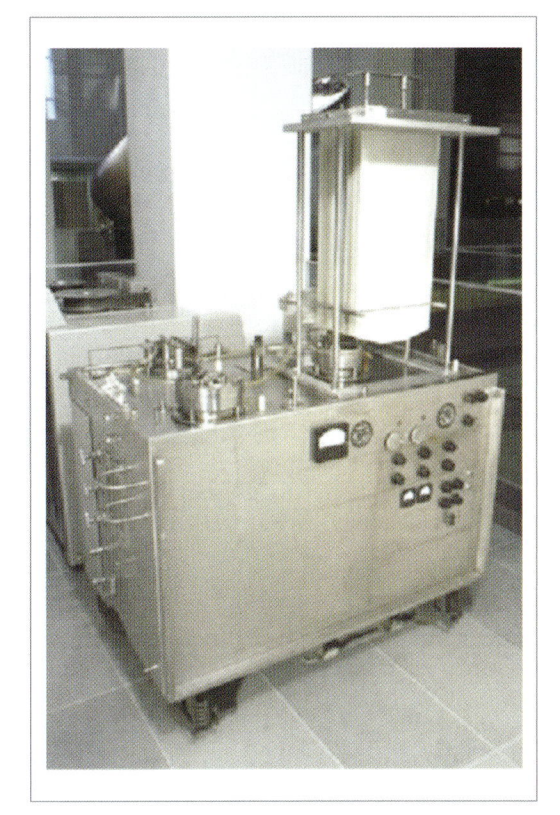

Figure 2-9. Screen oxygenator with 365 working parts.

These suffer from three weaknesses: first, the considerable quantity of microbubbles remaining in the blood postoxygenation; second, the limited amount of gas exchange; and third, the extensive blood–air interface.

Membrane Oxygenators

Microporous Membranes

The widely used hollow fiber microporous oxygenators (Figure 2-11) were first mass produced in the early 1980s. The membrane is created by being drawn longitudinally, with the pores being produced by inducing small ruptures in the tube wall. This makes for a net-like structure with alternating unexpanded regions and small pores.

Sheaves of microporous polypropylene fibers, with diameters between 100 and 200 μm, connect to an inlet and outlet within a cylindrical housing. The gas passes inside the fibers and the blood around the outside. Laminar flow produces a boundary effect that limits the percentage of red blood cells exposed to the membrane. To counter this non-laminar flow is encouraged by manipulating the flow paths through the oxygenator.

Like the lungs the membrane oxygenator presents the blood with a large surface area in order to increase efficiency (commonly between 1.8 and 2.4 m^2). This has resulted in very efficient gas exchange, probably over efficient and therefore future design should move toward reducing the non-physiological surface area of this components and the associated problems.

Seepage through the membrane's micropores is halted primarily due to hydrophilic nature of the polypropylene membrane. Second the blood, on contact with the membrane, deposits a coating of proteins and platelets on the membrane

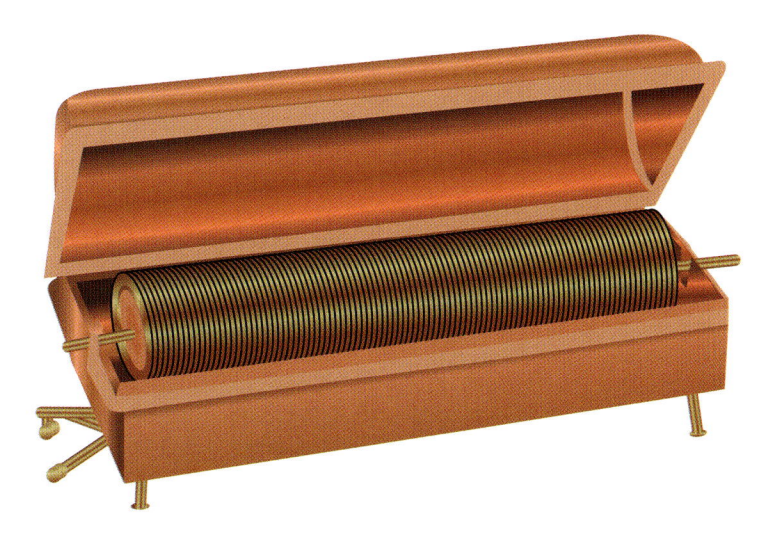

Figure 2-10. Disc oxygenator with a 3-day turn around.

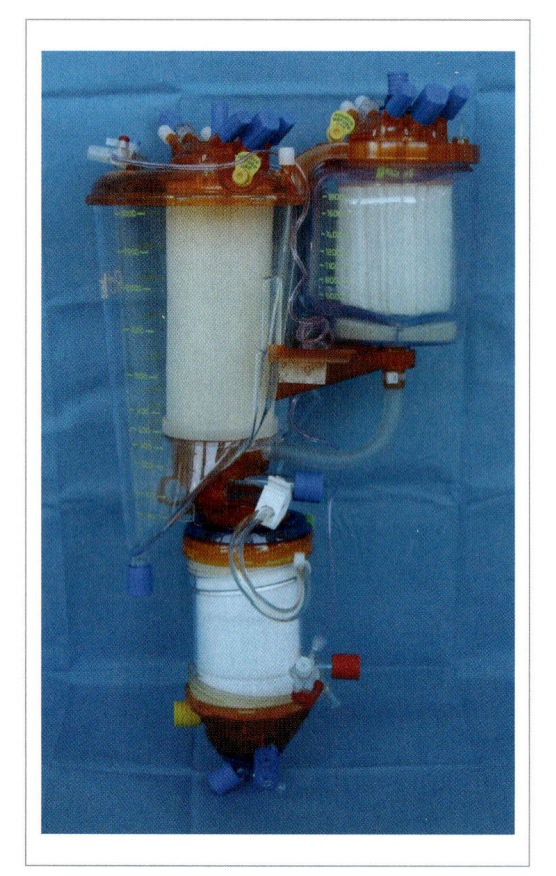

Figure 2-11. Microporous membrane oxygenator (positioned under venous reservoir system).

surface inhibiting plasma loss and third the surface tension of the blood counters seepage.

True Membranes

A pure membrane consists of silicone rubber sheets coiled in a cylindrical fashion. The silicone is non-porous making for a complete barrier between gas and blood. There is a greatly reduced risk of fluid seeping to the gas side or conversely gas being entrained into the blood. Though a pure membrane benefits from non-plasma leakage it also stops large molecules from diffusing through the membrane. This can stop the anesthetic gas isoflourane from entering the blood supply. The membranes are expensive to manufacture and high volume of prime is required. However, its longevity makes it an ideal membrane for long-term support,

known as extracorporeal membrane oxygenation, discussed later.

Heat Exchangers

Like the oxygenator, the increase in surface area increases efficiency. For this reason most heat exchangers are concentinated. Common materials are stainless steel, aluminum (both of which can be plastic coated), or polypropolene. Water is pumped at a controlled temperature around 10 L/min on one side of this heat exchanger membrane and this dictates the temperature of the blood on the other side of the membrane and therefore patient temperature. As mentioned earlier many patients are cooled at the start of CPB (sometimes as low as 12°C for major aortic work) and then rewarmed to normothermia (37–37.5°C). Arterial blood temperature should never exceed 37.5°C and the gradient between the water and the blood temperature should not exceed 10°C. This reduces the risk of cerebral injury, enzyme, and protein breakdown from this source.

Arterial Line Filters

The arterial line filter is the last filtration point on the CPB circuit before the blood is returned to the patient. It is designed to remove any microemboli above 40 μm (the most common ALF size). While this level of filtration has already occurred in the filters of the venous reservoir, the ALF will catch any microemboli (gaseous or particulate) generated from that point onward. This filtration is important because the diameters of the vessels in the patient's arterial network progressively decrease in size distally to the heart. As large bubble travel down this network, it will break into smaller bubbles that possess a greater surface tension. There is a critical point when the bubble size has decreased to a point where the surface tension becomes greater than the force that can be applied on it by the pressure of blood. It now acts as a plug and is treated as a foreign body, instigating an inflammatory response. Consequently the tissue downstream of the blockage becomes ischemic and eventually cell death occurs. If this occurs in the brain neurological, impairment is the result (see complications). Filter size should not venture much smaller than 40 µm due to concerns of filtering out and becoming blocked with blood components.[3]

Protecting the Myocardium

The ideal cardiac operating field is a blood free, stationary heart. This is achieved by positioning a large cross-clamp on the aorta above the coronary arteries and before the aortic cannula from the CPB circuit. This stops blood flow in the coronary arteries and therefore the myocardium must be protected. The two principle forms of myocardial protection are cross-clamp fibrillation and cardioplegia.

Cross-Clamp Fibrillation

Cross-clamp fibrillation involves passing a current into the heart to induce controlled ventricular fibrillation. The fibrillating or 'nearly still' heart can then be operated on. Additional myocardial protection is provided by the systemic cooling of the patient to 32°C, reducing the metabolic demands of the myocardium. This technique only allows the blood supply to the heart to be stopped for up to 15 min and is therefore only suitable for CABG operations. While gradual revascularization and ischemic preconditioning are advantageous, the drawbacks are multiple, potentailly damaging applications of the cross-clamp to the aorta.

Cardioplegia

Cardioplegia involves infusing a hyperkalemic solution into the isolated coronary system causing diastolic arrest. The 'completely still' heart has therefore a very small metabolic requirement. Cardioplegia is given as one large initial dose and subsequent maintenance doses. This can prolong the cross-clamp or ischemic time for longer than 1 hour if required. The hyperkalemic solution can be given mixed with the patient's own blood or as a crystalloid solution and either warm or cold.

Whole Body Hypothermia

This technique is actually whole body protection (all organs) rather than just myocardial protection. It is mainly used for major aortic work and involves the patient being cooled as low as 12°C. At this temperature, the patient's metabolic rate is extremely low and the patient can be drained of all their circulating blood to give the ideal blood free-operating field. Surgery can then be performed on the head and neck vessels and around the arch of the aorta. It is widely accepted that at this temperature circulatory arrest is possible for 20 min without having to use any isolated organ perfusion (e.g., cerebral, visceral).[4]

Monitoring During CPB

Venous Reservoir Level

The volume of blood in the venous reservoir is influenced by two variables: the inlet flowrate of blood from the right atrium via the venous line and the outlet flowrate of the CPB pump (roller or centrifugal). The later is relatively constant and controlled by the perfusionist, while the inlet flowrate is dictated by the patient's systemic vascular resistance, the position of the heart, surgical, and anesthetic intervention. To maintain a level in the venous reservoir the two variables must be the same, the responsibility of the perfusionist. If this does not happen the reservoir level will either increase (not immediately dangerous) or drop, a situation resulting in air entrainment into the CPB circuit. For an average patient, a reservoir level of 400 ml could disappear in just over 4 s with gross air entering the patient 12 s later. The issue surrounding gross air embolism cannot be overstated.

Activated Clotting Time

The importance of ensuring anticoagulation cannot be understated. There are many emergency situations that arise during CPB that the cardiac team can overcome. A patient's blood clotting during CPB is not a recoverable situation. Full anticoagulation is required to prevent clotted blood blocking the CPB circuit. Heparin is an anticoagulant that is ideal for this purpose: it has an affect that is easily measurable by activated clotted time (ACT), well tolerated, is relatively cheap and is easily reversible with protamine. Heparin binds to anti-thrombin III;

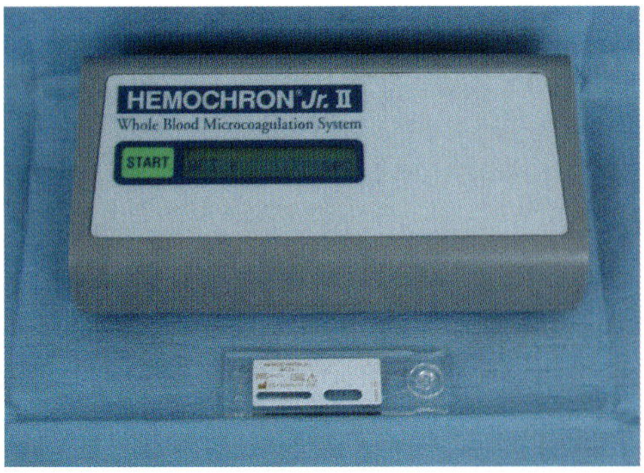

Figure 2-12. Modern ACT monitoring.

300-units/kg body weight is given at the anesthetic end as well as some in the CPB circuit prime. The level of anticoagulation is measured using an activated clotting time. This measures the time to clot formation of a known quantity of blood accelerated by a known amount of activator (kaolin and/or celite). The ACT-monitoring equipment shown in Figure 2-12 uses a cuvette system (which reduces user variability) to provide an accelerated real-time activated clotting result. Having an early real-time result is especially important to confirm adequate anticoagulation in an emergency situation. The threshold level for satisfactory anticoagulation varies from unit to unit but three times the patient's baseline ACT is an accepted minimum. The ACT is monitoring prior to heparin, post-heparin (pre-bypass), at least every 30 min during CPB and finally following. As well as avoiding a lack of anticoagulation, ensuring good anticoagulation will help protect the patients clotting factors and reduce the risk of small cell aggregates forming which can potentially block smaller capillaries. Once the patient has been disconnected from the CPB circuit that heparin is reversed using protamine. Protamine should be administered slowly as it has a number of adverse effects, including anaphylaxis, vasodilatation, pulmonary hypotension, and complement activation.[5]

Arterial Pump Flow

Arterial pump flow or cardiac output during CPB must be maintained between a range that ensures the patients metabolic demands at met without increasing blood damage and microemboli delivery. Extracorporeal support facilitates a very acute control over the patients cardiac output. The patients cardiac output (and therefore blood pressure) can be reduced to almost zero for short periods of time. Prolonged underperfusion can result in organ damage, for example, the kidneys, the liver, the gut, and the brain. As a guide the patients target cardiac output is calculated using the body surface area multiplied by a cardiac index of 2.4 L/min/m^2. This cardiac index can be reduced as the patient's temperature and therefore metabolic demand is reduced. The monitoring and decisions with regards to pump flow are intrinsically linked to arterial pressure and circulating blood volume. Most pumps used in cardiac centers worldwide deliver continuous not pulsatile flow.

Gas Flows in Flowmeter

Like pump flow, gas exchange, principally the oxygen and carbon dioxide levels of the blood must be maintained between limits. These must ensure that patients metabolic demands are met without exceeding the oxygen content of the blood or removing to much carbon dioxide. The efficiency of the gas exchange devices makes high O_2 levels (risk of cell damage and gas coming out of solution) and low CO_2 levels (interference with cerebral auto regulation) a real threat. These parameters are checked at least every 15 min via a blood gas analyzer (see Figure 2-13 showing examples of good and poor blood chemistry). In addition, some cardiac units have in-line blood gas monitoring which monitors the blood chemistry every 5 s using spectrophotometry.

Arterial Pressure

Arterial pressure or perfusion pressure is influenced by both blood flow and SVR. The pump is controlled as previously described, while the SVR is controlled pharmacologically using vasoconstrictors and vasodilators. A mean pressure of 70 mmHg is widely accepted as a target arterial pressure as the research dictates that this pressure provides adequate perfusion for the major organs. There is room to move below this, specifically for the brain which

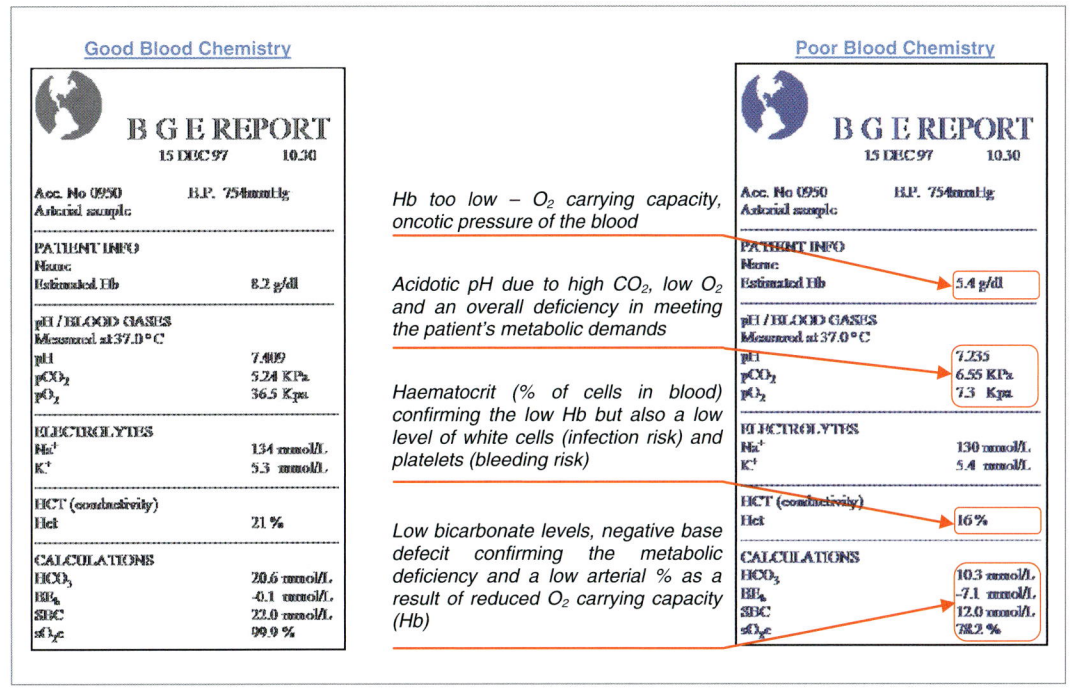

Figure 2-13. Labeled examples of good and poor blood chemistry during CPB.

autoregulates but not below 50 mmHg for any length of time. A pressure above a mean of 70 mmHg can make the surgery more difficult, especially with regards to the visualizing the operating field. There is still not a definitive answer with regards to the effect on the organs of non-pulsatile flow during CPB (see Figure 2-14). The main questions surround not only organ function but the ability to generate pulsatile flow in the patient's circulation and the blood damage it causes.

Venous Pressure

The central venous pressure (CVP) gives a direct indication of the amount of blood in the heart. This is important to ensure that we do not overfill the heart when we are gradually terminating CPB and asking the heart to do its own work again. It also provides advance warning when blood is not draining properly from the heart alerting the perfusionist to an impending reduction in venous reservoir level. For most cardiac operations, the CVP will be zero or negative due to the gravity drainage. The right atrium is not designed to deal with negative pressures and while this clearly upset the patient's oncotic balance, some of the other potential non-physiological effects are still not clearly defined.

Urine Output

Urine output is one of the key markers for kidney function but also plays a role in the patient's

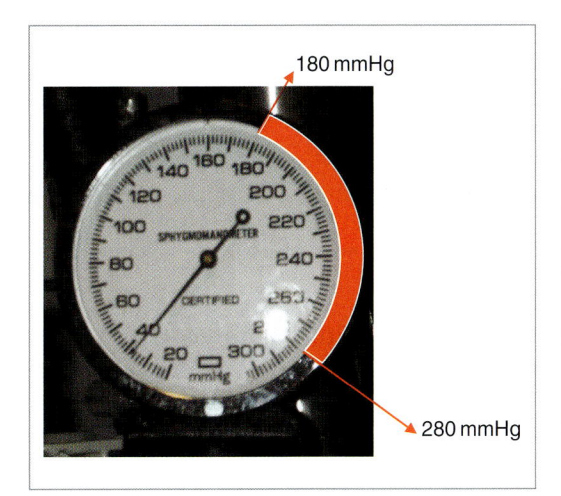

Figure 2-14. The arterial Tycos gauge showing operating thresholds.

total fluid balance as well as influencing many other CPB decisions. These include appropriate fluid use, whether the patient requires higher perfusion pressures or flows, whether pharmacological intervention is required, and the potential need for an artificial hemoconcentrator. Hemoconcentration provides a similar function to dialysis but fluid removal is based on the principle of convective solute transport across a semipermeable membrane compared to dialysis, where the driving force is solute osmotic pressure. With hemoconcentration access is more straightforward as the patient is on extracorporeal support and therefore has a faster filtration rate.

'Tycos' Pressure

The Tycos pressure is a direct measurement of the pressure at the tip of the aortic cannula. It provides information about the positioning of the cannula throughout the case as well as any obstructions (for example, aortic cross-clamp). This area of interaction between the CPB circuit and the patient's aorta is extremely non-physiological and has a knock on effect for the fluid dynamics throughout the circulation. The starting point during normal circulation is the aortic valve annulus (about 21 mm in diameter) with an axial exit flowrate of around 5 L/min (0.24 m/s). CPB changes this starting point to a tube (about 8 mm) angled off the aortas axis still with a flowrate of around 5 L/min but with a 7-fold increase blood velocity of 1.66 m/s. While the knock on effect with regards to the change in fluid dynamics in the organs is unclear, the positional aspect of the cannula must be considered. It is important to avoid blood jetting at 1.66 m/s against the wall of the aorta, especially a weak aorta or one heavily calcified due to athero-sclerosis.

ECG

With the heart isolated from the circulation by the cross-clamp the cardiac team have a very different aim than other medical teams in terms of target ECG, namely the maintenance of VF (cross-clamp fibrillation) or the maintenance of asystole. Once the cross-clamp is removed and blood supply to the myocardium is resumed, sinus rhythm is the goal. If sinus rhythm is not

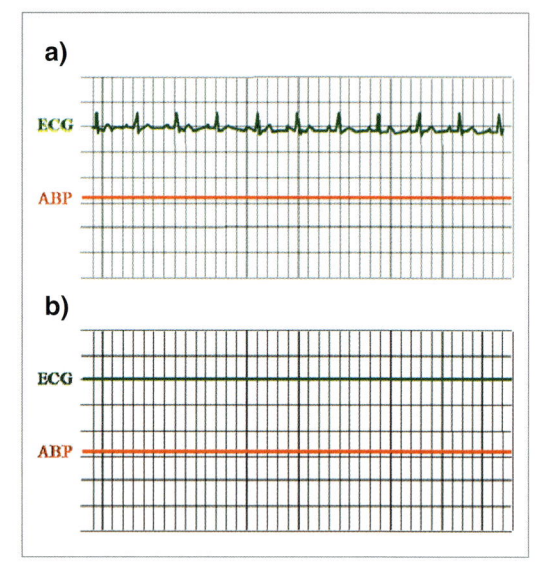

Figure 2-15. ECG and Arterial Blood Pressure on CPB: (**a**) x-clamp off and (**b**) x-clamp on.

forthcoming prior to the cessation of CPB, then epicardial pacing wires and temporary pacing will be used in the post-operative period. An example each of the ECG and arterial pressure traces during CPB is shown in Figure 2-15.

Arterial and Venous Saturations

These are monitored to ensure that the extracorporeal circuit is not only adding oxygen but meeting the patient's metabolic demands. Arterial saturations above 98% and venous saturations above 70% are the thresholds used.

Arterial and Venous Blood Temperature

These are monitored closely to ensure good global cooling and rewarming of the patient without exposing patients to the temperate risks discussed in the section on heat exchangers.

CPB Safety Features

All of the monitored parameters have either operator or mechanical safety devices. These safety features vary from an audible alarm to stopping the arterial pump. The mechanical alarm are detailed below:

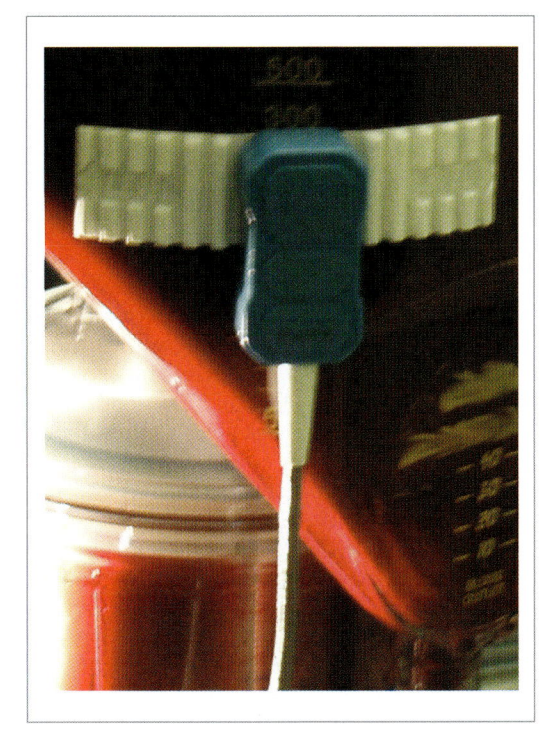

Figure 2-16. Level sensor that uses capacitance to detect level falling – will stop arterial pump.

- Venous reservoir level – level and/or bubble alarm stops arterial pump (see Figure 2-16)
- Arterial pump flow – audible alarm warns of high/low flows
- Gas flows – audible alarm
- Arterial (Tycos pressure) – pressure alarm stops arterial pump
- Arterial and venous saturation – audible alarm
- Arterial and venous temperature – audible alarm

The operator or clinical perfusionist is the overall safety device as well as ensuring the extracorporeal support is as physiological as possible. Clinical perfusionists are trained to have a unique blend of in-depth cardiac-specific medical knowledge and advanced technical skills. Accreditation varies across the world but always involves a balance between clinical and theoretical training.

Non-physiological Aspects of Cardiopulmonary Bypass

It is clear that extracorporeal support exposes both the patient and the patient's blood to forces and an environment not experienced in normal physiological. It is a testament to the bodies resilience that it can withstand such an insult. Acute non-physiology can result in mortality and moderate non-physiology can result in morbidity.

- Anticoagulation
- Exposure of the blood to air
- Exposure of the blood to shear stresses
- Exposure of the blood to non-physiological pressures
- Exposure of the aortic wall to non-physiological pressures and shear stresses
- Exposure of the organs to non-pulsatile perfusion
- Hemodilution
- Exposure of the right atrium to negative pressure
- Generation of gaseous and particulate microemboli

Complications of the Non-physiological Aspects of Cardiopulmonary Bypass

The in-hospital mortality varies depending on the operation, for example, CABG – 2–3%, isolated valve surgery – 4.3%, and combined CABG and valve surgery – 7.6%. Many of the non-physiological aspects of CPB contributed to the following post-operative problems.

Bleeding

The complex alterations of hemostasis lead to platelet dysfunction and increased fibrinolysis. These alterations can result in the requirement for donor blood products like red blood cells, platelets, and fresh plasma, all of which are associated with risk. About 1–3% of patients require re-exploration for persistent bleeding.

Neurological Events

As many as 75% of patients suffer subtle, reversible neurological deficits post-operatively. Stroke as a result of a macroembolism, intracerebral hemorrhage, or thrombotic occlusion is seen in <1% of patients below 70 years and 5% of patients above 70 years. Cerebral complications are associated with poor long-term outcome and increased mortality and morbidity.[6]

Kidney Dysfunction

Kidney or renal dysfunction is associated with hemodilution, hypothermia, and endocrine effects during CPB. About 1–5% of cardiac surgical patients require acute renal failure and require dialysis.[7]

Low Cardiac Output

This can present itself in several forms, namely low blood pressure, bradycardia or tachycardia, acidosis, and reduced urine output. CPB can contribute to many of the underlying reasons for low cardiac output, for example, inadequate circulating volume, myocardial injury, abnormal ECG, and electrolyte imbalance. It is important that the underlying reason is identified and the low cardiac output is avoided/reversed.[8]

Pulmonary Complications

Most patients suffer a mild reduction in lung function post-operatively. Many of the non-physiological aspects of CPB contribute to this. The main CPB contributor to major pulmonary dysfunction (about 2% of patients) is the inflammatory response caused by exposure to non-physiological surfaces and air. The inflammatory response created by the non-physiological surface still occurs even though there have been advances in surface biocompatibility over the last 5 years. Many of the modern circuits have a coating on all surfaces to increase biocompatibility. Some coatings attempt to mimic endothelium (phosphorylcholine), while others are coated with heparin (carmeda). Good anticoagulation with systemic heparin offers some protection against post-operative inflammatory response and associated morbidity but it acts near the end of the clotting cascade and therefore does not suppress the activation of the upstream protease cascades (bleeding issues).[9]

ECG Complications

The most common ECG irregularity is atrial fibrillation (reported in 25–30% of CABG patients on the second or third post-operative day). From the CPB point of view, this can be a result of poor myocardial protection, magnesium, and/or potassium imbalance. If AF persists the risk of microemboli generation (clot) should be reduced pharmacologically or via electrocardioversion.

Long-Term Circulatory Support

Patients in cardiogenic shock or who fail to wean from bypass may require post-CPB support as a bridge to recovery or transplant. Commonly used circulatory support strategies are intra-aortic balloon (IAB) counterpulsation and ventricular assist devices (VAD).

IAB counterpulsation involves a catheter with a 34 or 40 cc balloon at one end being inserted into the descending aorta via the femoral artery. The balloon sits just below the head and neck vessels and above the renal arteries. It uses the ECG as a trigger to inflate during diastole (the period of aortic valve closure during the cardiac cycle – dicrotic notch to the onset of the next cycle) and deflate during systole. This not only increases the diastolic pressure and therefore blood supply to the myocardium during inflation but also reduces the pressure the heart must work against by deflating. IAB counterpulsation can only provide up to 1.5 L/min of cardiac output support. IAB placement and the influence on the cardiac cycle are shown in Figure 2-17. Figure 2-17b shows three cardiac cycles and the influence of the IAB on both the second and the third cycles. The first cycle is shown for reference.

VAD technology can be applied to the left, right, or to both sides of the heart. It is more invasive than an IAB as relevant cannulation sites are required to remove and return blood. The extracorporeal circuit incorporates a centrifugal pump that can supply up to 6 L/min of cardiac output support (for a period of months), i.e., the heart does not need to contribute any of the work itself. They are used as a bridge to recovery or a bridge to transplant. Some of the longer-term VAD's use pneumatic or hydraulic chamber technology in an attempt to provide more physiological support. Finally extracorporeal membrane oxygenation (ECMO) or extracorporeal carbon dioxide removal (ECO_2R) incorporate a gas exchange device as well as a pump. The success rate of these techniques is considerably higher in pediatrics than adult surgery. The basic principles of these circuits are the same as the shorter-term circuits, only the materials differ

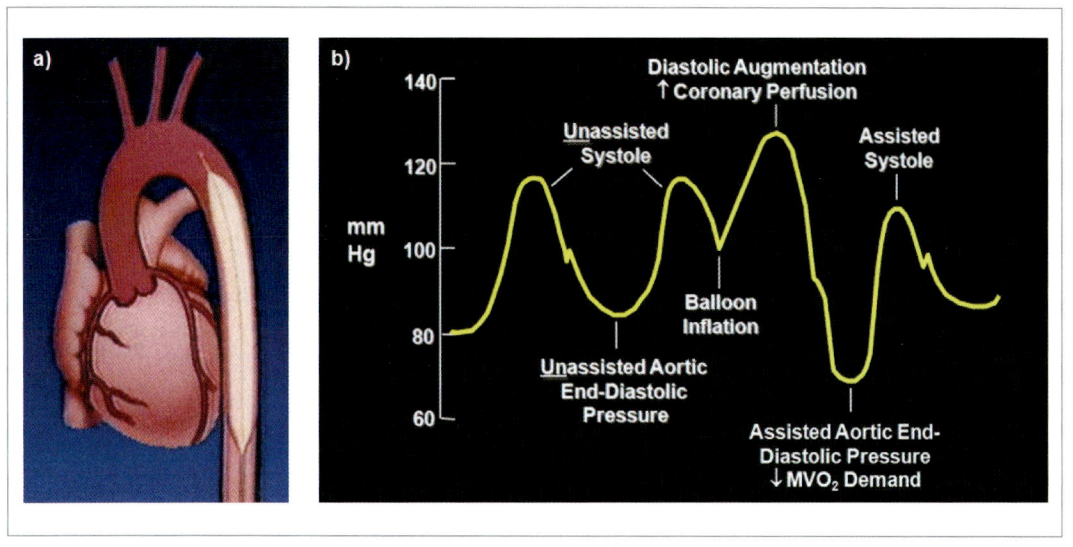

Figure 2-17. (a) IAB placement in the descending aorta and (b) influence of IAB on the cardiac cycle.

slightly. The key to success of long-term extracorporeal support is not found in the technology of the circuits, but the clinical/medical management of the patients.

References

1. Edmunds LH. *Adult Cardiac Surgery*. New York: McGraw-Hill Education; Jan 1997. ISBN-10: 0070189633, ISBN-13: 978-0070189638.
2. Ward J. *Oxygen delivery and demand. Surgery.* 2006;24(10):354–60.
3. Gravlee GP, Davis RF, Utley JR, Kurusz M. *Cardiopulmonary Bypass: Principles and Practice*, 2nd ed. Philadelphia: Lippincott/Williams & Wilkins; May 2000.
4. *Cardiopulmonary Bypass: Principles and practise, 2nd ed.* Gravlee, GP., Lippincot/Williams&Wilkins, Philadelphia; 2000.
5. Shannon M. Anticoagulation. *Surgery.* 2007;25(4): 150–4.
6. Kenneth G. Shann, Donald S. Likosky, John M. Murkin, et al. An evidence-based review of the practice of cardiopulmonary bypass in adults: A focus on neurologic injury, glycemic control, hemodilution, and the inflammatory response. *J Thorac Cardiovasc Surg.* 2006;132:283–90.
7. Delbridge MS, Raftery A. *Access for dialysis. Surgery.* 2004;22(11):277–83.
8. *Cardiovascular Physiology, 8th ed.* Berne, RM. CV Mosby, St. Louis; 2000.
9. Casthely PA, Bregman D. *Cardiopulmonary Bypass: Physiology, Related Complications, and Pharmacology.* Mount Kisco, NY: Blackwell/Futura; November 1991. ISBN-10: 0879933968, ISBN-13: 978-0879933968.

The Artificial Kidney

Christopher Kirwan and Andrew Frankel

Introduction

Approximately 100 individuals, per million population, per year, reach end-stage renal failure in the United Kingdom, with many more who have used hemodialysis for short-term treatment of acute renal failure or as a bridge to renal transplantation. An increase in prevalence of conditions such as diabetes means that in the future more and more people will be diagnosed with renal failure and will require renal replacement therapy.[1]

Most of the patients who receive hemodialysis would die without it and owe their lives to the artificial kidney. This chapter reviews the history of and the progression of the technology associated with the artificial kidney and ending with consideration of possible future technical advances.

The Kidney

The known functions of the kidney can be separated into four main categories: excretory, regulatory, endocrine, and metabolic (Table 3-1). The principle role is the elimination of waste material and the regulation of the volume and composition of body fluid.

The endocrine and metabolic functions of the kidney can be replaced with medications. Recombinant erythropoietin (r-epo) in combination with iron supplementation can help to control anemia. Calcium homeostasis is impaired because a diseased kidney cannot perform the second hydroxylation of vitamin D to its active component calcitriol or 1,25 di-hydroxycholecalciferol. Calcitriol can be replaced by tablets.

The challenge for physicians and engineers was to create a system that could replace the excretory and regulatory role of the failing kidney.

The kidney receives approximately 25% of cardiac output or 1300 ml of blood every minute. The functioning unit of the kidney is called a nephron. There are approximately one million nephrons in each kidney, and each nephron is made up of a filtering unit (the glomerulus) and its associated tubule, which regulates the filtrate produced from the glomerulus (Figure 3-1).[2]

Within the glomerulus, a hydrostatic pressure gradient of approximately 10 mmHg provides the driving force for the ultrafiltration of a virtually protein and fat-free fluid across the glomerular capillary wall into the renal tubule. The total ultrafiltration is more commonly known as the glomerular filtration rate (GFR) and in a healthy person this equates to the ultrafiltration of approximately 180 L of water a day.

The selective secretion and re-absorption of water, essential electrolytes, glucose, and amino acids occur as the filtrate moves along the renal tubule. Virtually all of the potassium, bicarbonate amino acids, and glucose are reabsorbed in the proximal renal tubule along with 60–80% of filtered water. Further water and sodium chloride are reabsorbed more distally with fine tuning of salt water balance occurring in the distal tubule and the collecting duct under the influence of aldosterone and antidiuretic hormone. This leaves approximately 2 L of urine a day. As renal failure progresses, the GFR falls and eventually dialysis is required to replace the excretory and regulatory functions.

N. Hakim (ed.), *Artificial Organs*, New Techniques in Surgery Series 4, DOI 10.1007/978-1-84882-283-2_3,
© Springer-Verlag London Limited 2009

Table 3-1. The Functions of the Kidney

Excretory	- excretion of waste products and drugs
Regulatory	- control of body fluid volume and its composition
Endocrine	- production of erythropoietin, renin and prostaglandins
Metabolic	- metabolism of vitamin D

The Artificial Kidney

In order to appreciate how the artificial kidney is developed, it is necessary to understand the basic components required (Table 3-2).

In this article, by concentrating on each component individually, we can build up a picture of how a successful artificial kidney has evolved over the years, allowing the expansion of hemodialysis into a recognized and readily available treatment.

The Semipermeable Membrane

An understanding of osmosis, diffusion, and semipermeable membranes began to emerge in the mid-1800s. There are two ways solutes can be moved through a membrane: diffusion and convection (Figure 3-2). Diffusion of solutes from a high concentration to a low concentration eventually leaves an equal concentration on both sides of the membrane. Convection pulls solution and solutes across a membrane. Thomas Graham, a professor of chemistry in Glasgow, first coined the phrase dialysis in 1854 when he described the movement of various types of solutes through a membrane forced by osmotic pressures.[3] Graham used ox bladders for his first membranes but later used vegetable parchment coated with albumin. A year later Adolf Fick described two equations which quantified that the flow of mass by diffusion (i.e., the flux) across a plane was proportional to the concentration gradient of the diffusant across that plane.[4] The membrane, or plane, he used in his studies was colloidin.[4] Colloidin is syrup-like liquid made from cellulose, nitric acid, alcohol, and ether and when it dries it forms a porous film.

In 1913, John Abel, a renowned pharmacologist at Johns Hopkins University USA, published an article describing hemodialysis in animals using a semipermeable membrane made of colloidin.[5] This was the first "Artificial Kidney".

Soon the first reports of dialysis in humans appeared. George Haas a German physician, dialyzed six patients over a colloidin membrane between 1924 and 1925, but none of them survived.[6–8] Two further patients were dialyzed over colloidin in 1928 when Haas experimented with heparin as an anticoagulant, but he described the results as disappointing, citing technical difficulties and opposition from colleagues.[9]

In 1923, Heinrich Necheles tried a prepared peritoneum (Gold-beater's skin), often from a sheep or an ox, as a membrane when dialyzing uremic dogs,[10] but this technique did not progress.

It became clear that a membrane had to be robust, easily sterilized without damage to the material or alterations in its properties and have a long shelf life. Colloidin performed badly in all of these areas but conveniently an alternative was already in use in the food and packaging industry.

In 1839, cellulose was the name given to the compound that "fills the cells that make up wood".[11] It was first purified from wood in 1885 and subsequently cellulose acetate was synthesized around 1895. It is thought that as early as 1910 it was available in sheet form under the name cellophane. Cellophane was used for laboratory studies of dialysis in sheet form by Freda Wilson of the University of British Columbia in 1927 and she showed how easy it was to sterilize.[12] This versatile and cheap product was already being made into tubing for the manufacture of sausages by the Visking Company of Chicago. It was tough, did not burst under moderate pressures and even in its commercial form was relatively free of microscopic holes. Andrus used the sausage skin in laboratory dialysis experiments and it proved to have excellent diffusion characteristics.[13] During the 1930s, many papers (reviewed by Fagette[14]) were published on the physical and dialysis characteristics of various forms of cellulose membranes.

In 1937, a New York hematologist, William Thalhimer, began to use cellophane tubing 2 cm wide and 30 cm long, in an artificial kidney similar to the one Abel constructed, to dialyze dogs. Along with his work into heparin, this provided the vital realization that commercially available cellophane could be used for in vivo hemodialysis.[15,16]

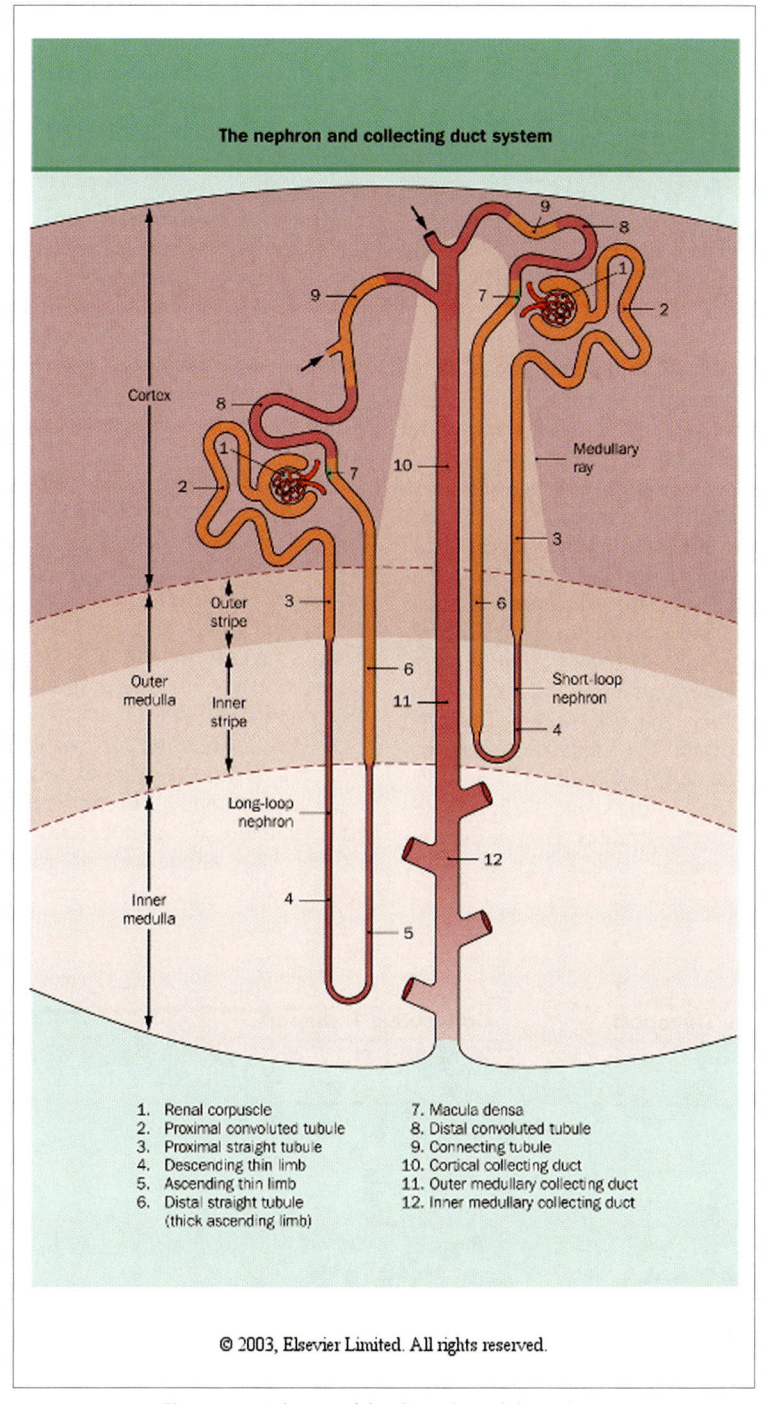

Figure 3-1. A diagram of the glomerulus and the nephron.

Cellulose acetate or cellophane was universally used as the membrane in dialysis machines up until around the 1960s. There were frequent leaks and a number of reports of ruptured cellophane membranes which constantly fuelled the search for other materials. Frederick Kiil was the first to use a new membrane called cuprophan. Cuprophan membranes had a greater

Table 3-2. Basic Components of an Artificial Kidney

- Semipermeable membrane separating blood and dialyzate
- Membrane support structure
- Blood compartment
  - Anticoagulation
  - Access to the blood stream
- Dialyzate compartment
  - Dialyzate composition
  - Water

porosity for solutes and water than other materials. Initially it was only available as flat sheets but by 1966 there was standardized industrial production of these dialysis membranes, and in 1969, the success had stimulated the production of the cuprophan tubular membrane.

Concurrently, 1964 saw the production of the next major step in the development of the artificial kidney, the hollow fiber dialyzers. Richard Stewart began to explore the medical applications of cellulose acetate hollow fibers.[17,18] These ultrathin fibers were approximately 200 μm in diameter and 5 μm thick. The fiber wall represented the dialysis membrane. The artificial kidney that he designed contained 11000 fibers[18] and the version that was used in the clinical trial in 1967 is very similar to current designs. He also demonstrated that substances could be selectively removed from the blood as well as excess water. The capillary sized fibers allowed the production of a dialyzer with a much larger surface area for blood to membrane contact while using relatively small amounts of extra corporeal blood (Figure 3-3). This resulted in increased efficiency of dialysis.

Hollow fiber dialyzers began a revolution in the way dialysis was considered and offered. The change in membrane type and size runs parallel with the reduction in size of the support structure for the artificial kidney, development of new polymers for the fibers, and a clearer understanding of the physiological effects and consequences of dialysis at a microscale level.

The human glomerular basement membrane has a higher permeability and larger ultrafiltration coefficient than the classical cellulose membranes. In the late 1970s, the polymer polysulfone was introduced as the next generation membrane and its benefits of large sieving coefficients for inulin and ß2 microglobulin were reported a few years later along with improved biocompatibility.[19]

Acetate, diacetate, Hemophan®, and Helixone®, as well as the original polysulfone, are just a few of the many different polymers that are now available for membranes in the artificial kidney. They all work in roughly the same way

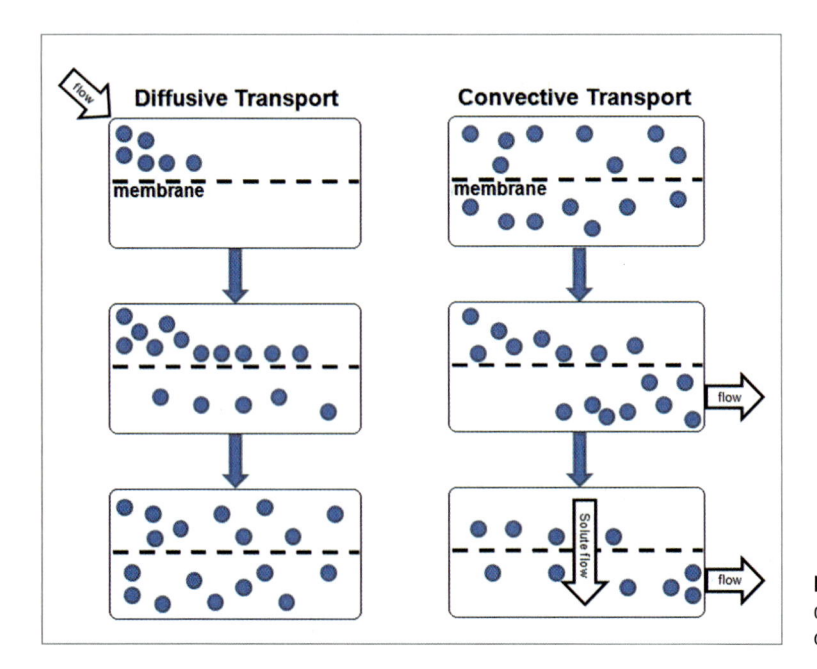

Figure 3-2. A diagram illustrating the difference between diffusion and convection.

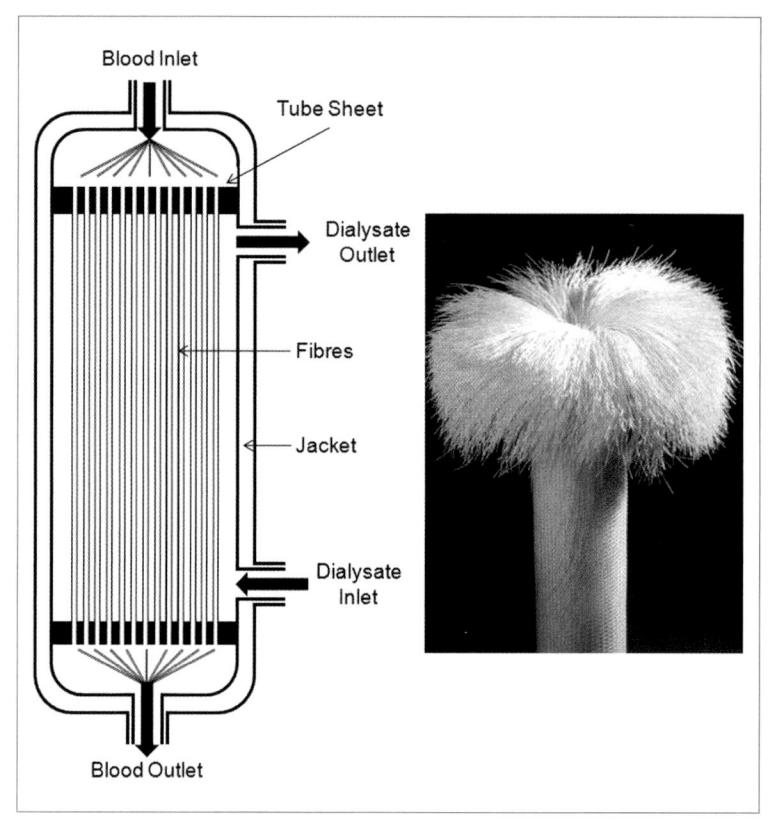

Figure 3-3. A diagram of a capillary fiber membrane with its support structure and a photo of a membrane that has been cross sectioned.

with varying degrees of efficiency. The modern Helixone® membrane (Fresenius Medical Care), for example, is a polysulfone-based high flux membrane in which the porosity of the inner layer is finely controlled at the nanoscale by nanotechnology. Nanotechnology is an atomically precise, functional machine system that is developed on the scale of the nanometer (1 nm = 1/1,000,000,000 m). In more general terms it is any technology related to features of nanometer scale such as thin films, fine particles, chemical synthesis, and advanced microlithography.[20] The Helixone® membrane is produced using a nano-controlled spinning procedure, which produces a significant effect on the structure of the skin layer of the membrane at the nanoscale level.[20] The result is an increased number of membrane pores where the spectrum of pore diameters is narrowed and concentrated around the desired values.[21] This enables the increased removal of medium sized molecules such as ß2-microglobulin, with virtually no albumin leak at all.[22] The membranes also span a range of surface areas from 0.7 to 1.8 m². They can be labeled low flux or high flux depending on whether they are specific for the removal of ß2-microglobulin (high flux).

Therefore the history of the artificial kidney, from an experiment to a widely used therapy, closely follows the development of the dialysis membranes and the ability to manufacture them in reproducible conditions on an industrial scale.

Membrane Support Structure

The support structure allows the membranes to perform the functional role of dialysis between the patients' blood and the dialyzate. In order to make dialysis a reality, the technology relating to the support structure for the membranes had to progress at the same rate as the membranes. In 1913, Able constructed the first dialysis machine it was extremely basic and was the basis for the machine that Haas used on humans in 1928 (Figure 3-4).

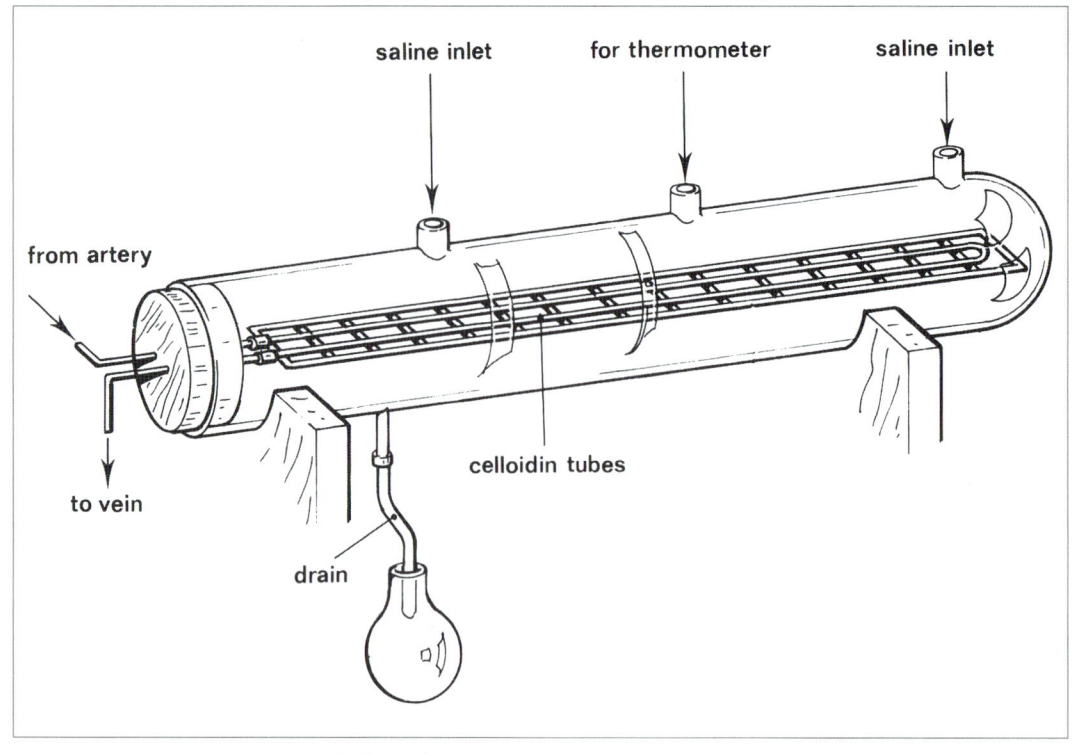

Figure 3-4. The first artificial kidney used on humans developed by Haas in 1928.

In 1943, William Kolff, a Dutch physician constructed the rotating drum dialyzer which was the first artificial kidney to be successfully used regularly on humans.[23] This device resembled a drum barrel made of slats with open spaces between the slats. Approximately 30–40 m of cellulose acetate tubing was wrapped around a small drum which was then partially immersed into a 100 L bath of dialyzate (Figure 3-5).

The patient's heart and own blood pressure forced blood into the cellulose acetate tubing. As the drum turned, it propelled the blood from one end of the tubing to the other. This allowed the diffusion of molecules from blood to dialyzate and vice versa. The blood was then collected in a glass cylinder with an open nipple at the lower end which was connected by rubber tubing to the patient's venous access. By alternating lowering and raising the cylinder, blood was collected and drained back into the patient's vein.

The procedure required a large volume of blood circulation outside the body during dialysis and required priming with at least 2 units of transfused blood.

Kolff gave away several of the rotating drum kidneys to promote the concept of dialysis. Some of the first published reports of patients treated with this artificial kidney came from the Royal Postgraduate Medical School at Hammersmith Hospital, London.[24]

The innovative Canadian surgeon Gordon Murray (1894–1976) is often forgotten when

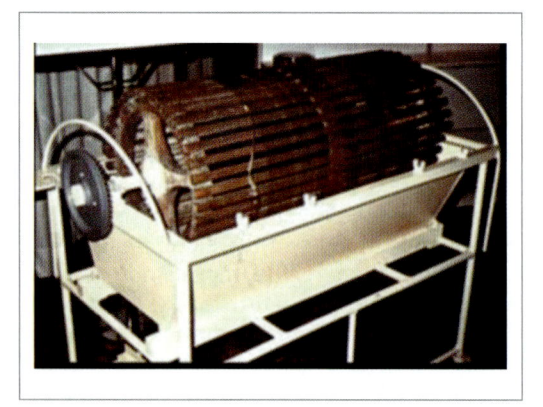

Figure 3-5. A picture of the rotating drum dialyzer invented by Kolff. (Cannot find copyright owner.)

discussing the history of dialysis. He is credited with having performed the first successful hemodialysis in humans in North America but neither he nor Kolff were aware of each other's work during the mid-1940s when wartime hampered communication. Murray's extensive investigations and experience in the use of heparin in vascular surgery laid the groundwork for the use of this anticoagulant with the artificial kidney. In 1945, he first designed a coil dialyzer in which cellophane tubing was wound about a steel frame. This machine, however, was confined to a basement after only a few treatments due to general lack of enthusiasm. In 1952, with resurgence in interest, he developed his second-generation apparatus. This was a plate dialyzer constructed with the help of Walter Roschlau and independent of Leonard Skeggs and Jack Leonards who are mentioned later. In all, he performed dialysis on only 11 patients with presumed acute renal failure, 5 of whom survived. He felt this was a relative failure and his treatments were dismissed by his colleagues. Murray finally lost interest in the artificial kidney when he discovered his idea had been marketed independently by a German researcher, Erwin Halstrup, who had worked with him for a while. The two machines were locked away and only resurfaced after his death.[25,26]

Until Nils Alwall produced his dialyzer in 1946 there was no controlled way to remove fluid from the patients' blood. This process, known as ultrafiltration, was achieved by using pressure to squeeze water from the plasma through the dialyzer membrane. In previous machines pressure from the cardiovascular system alone was not high enough to instigate ultrafiltration but had it been, the membranes would not have been strong enough to withstand it. The Alwall Dialyzer was similar to the rotating drum. Approximately 11 m of cellulose acetate tubing was wrapped around a stationary, vertical drum made of a metal screen. The membranes, in this situation, could withstand higher pressures because of their positioning between the metal plates of the screen. The membranes were enclosed in a tightly closed cylinder so that pressure adjustments to the dialyzate, in addition to the pressure coming from the cardiovascular system, could be tailored to control ultrafiltration.

In parallel to the increased availability of dialysis membranes two design variations began to emerge during the 1950s: (1) modifications of the original rotating drum dialyzer and (2) the twin coil dialyzer and the new flat plate dialyzers.

Rather than passing blood through membranous tubes, plate dialyzers directed the flow of dialysis solution and blood through alternating layers of membranous material.

In 1948, Skeggs and Leonards developed the first parallel flow artificial kidney.[27] The artificial kidney was designed to have a low resistance to blood flow and to have an adjustable surface area. Two sheets of membrane are sandwiched between two rubber pads in order to reduce the blood volume and to ensure uniform distribution of blood across the membrane. Using multiple layers added to its efficiency. The device had a very low resistance to blood flow and it could be used without a blood pump.

A siphon on the effluent of the dialyzing fluid allowed water to be removed from the blood in the artificial kidney. This is the first reference to negative pressure dialysis. This is different to ultrafiltration because negative pressure from the dialyzate is used to draw fluid off the human plasma rather than positive pressure in the blood stream to push fluid out of the plasma.

Meanwhile, Kolff sent his blueprints to George Thorn at the Peter Brigham Hospital in Boston, USA. During the Korean War in the 1950s, the Kolff–Brigham dialyzer, a modification of the original rotating drum dialyzer, was used to treat injured American soldiers (Figure 3-6). The membrane surface area could be adjusted by increasing or decreasing the number of wraps of tubing and a hood was added to better control the blood temperature.[28]

Von Garrelts had constructed a dialyzer in 1948 by wrapping a cellulose acetate membrane around a core. The layers of membrane were separated by rods. It was very bulky and weighed over 100 pounds and thus not used.

In 1952, Inouye and Engelberg took this concept and miniaturized it by wrapping the cellulose acetate tubing around a beaker and separating the layers with fiberglass mesh. He placed this "coil" in a pressure cooker in order to enclose it and control the temperature. There were openings in the pot for the dialyzing fluid. With the use of a vacuum on the dialyzate leaving the pot, he was able to draw the excess water out of the patient's blood. A blood pump, assisting the patients' blood pressure, was required to overcome resistance within the device.[29] Blood pumps are now an integral part of modern dialyzers.

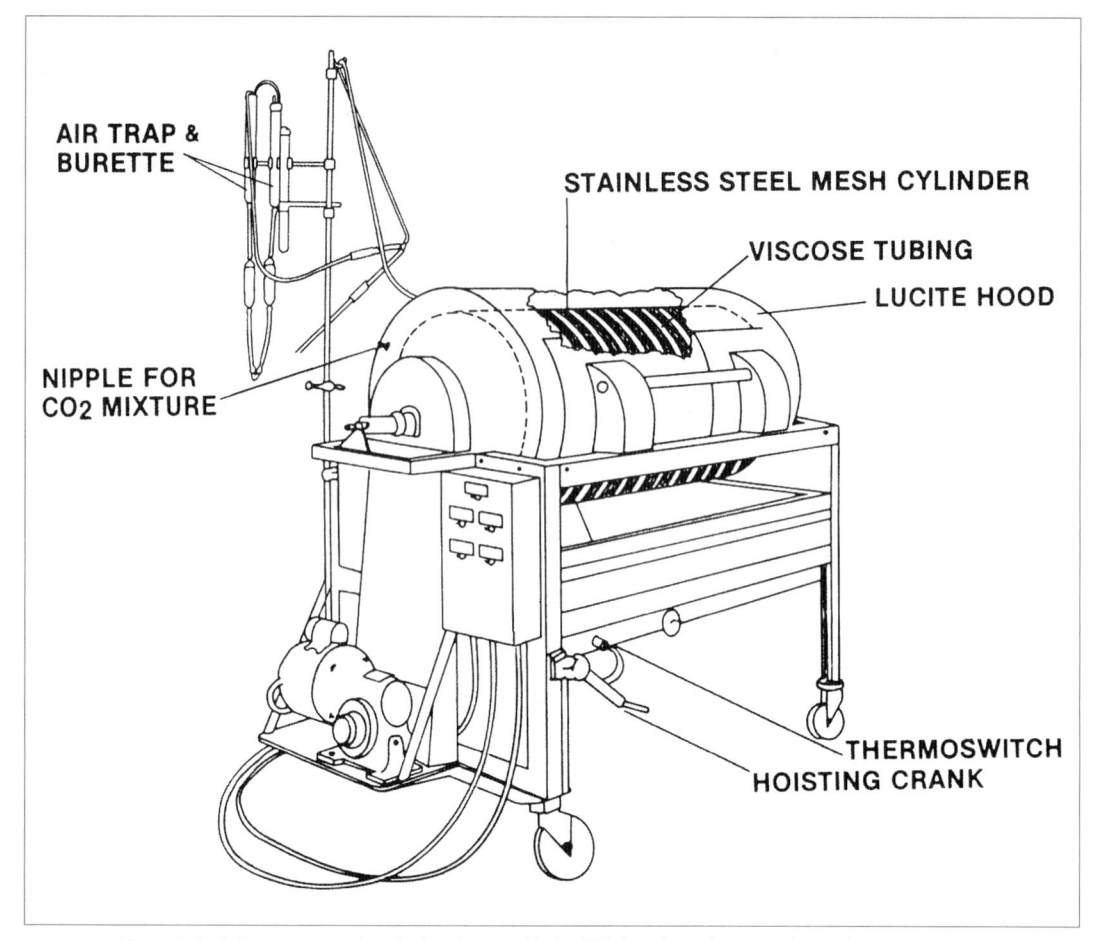

Figure 3-6. A diagram representing the Bringham-modified Kolff kidney, better known as the Kolff Brigham dialyzer.

This machine had to be abandoned, but using some of the concepts of the pressure cooker kidney and the principles of the Alwall machine, the Kolff–Travenol disposable twin coil dialyzer emerged in 1952. This device consisted of a twin coil seated in a big cylindrical steel tank that could hold about 100 L of water. The twin coil was pre-assembled and sterilized, but it required a liter of blood to prime it and had a high compliance to pressure changes. Hot water and cold water were mixed together, when making the dialyzate, to get the correct temperature as the block heater was only able to maintain a given temperature. It also necessitated a blood perfusion pump and a significant arteriovenous pressure differential across the membranes developed, which resulted in an uncontrolled ultrafiltration. There were no alarms, temperature or pressure monitors, full function checks, blood leak detectors, or air embolism detectors, all of which are standard on today's machines. It was, however, robust and kept in use in Edinburgh until the late 1980s![30]

Concurrently, in 1952, Guarino and Guarino developed an artificial kidney which would reduce the amount of blood outside of the body and to eliminate the need for pumping the blood through the device. In reverse to previous designs the dialyzing fluid was directed inside the cellulose acetate tubing and the blood cascaded down over the membrane having entered the device from the top. The metal tubing inside the membrane gave structural support. The artificial kidney had a very low blood volume but it had limited use because there was concern regarding the possibility of the dialyzing fluid leaking into the blood.

In 1960, Fredrik Kiil provided the definitive plate dialyzer[31] which was still used in some clinics until the 1990s. Three or more "Kiil" boards were used with two sheets of, the newly available, cuprophan membrane sandwiched between each pair of boards. The grooves in the boards directed the blood between the layers of membrane and the dialyzate outside the membrane envelope in opposite directions from one end of the boards to the other. The priming volume was less than 300 ml, but often the patients would have to construct the device themselves. This was complex and time consuming confining the patient for an extra 4 hours for any individual 10 hour dialysis session (Figure 3-7). As improvements in access to the patients' blood stream improved no blood pump was needed to drive this device. Excess fluid was removed by the use of negative pressure on the dialyzate effluent line.

As the dialysis program expanded this type of device was used for overnight, unattended hemodialysis that was pioneered by Belding Scribner[32] and his group in Seattle, USA. A totally monitored dialyzate system was required to automatically mix the dialyzate and to control temperature and conductivity. This delivery system was developed by Albert Babb, while at the University of Washington.

Following on from the knowledge gained with the Kiil dialyzer, Babb designed and developed the Milton-Roy Model A, built by the Milton Roy Company in St. Petersburg, Florida in 1964. It was also designed to perform nocturnal home hemodialysis. It was made in a wooden veneer to have a furniture appearance for the home. It featured automatic hot water disinfection (up to 90°c), automatic alarm checks, solid-state (diode) logic, and acoustic tile inside to reduce noise.

This instrument became the first of a series of negative pressure single patient systems, which was modified to use hollow fiber membranes, culminating in the hemodialysis machines seen today.

The introduction of hollow fiber dialyzers, during the 1960s, marked a change in dialysis machines from their initial development by dedicated artisans, who were engineers and physicians, to highly sophisticated machines and components that rely on large production series and standardized manufacturing processes. The

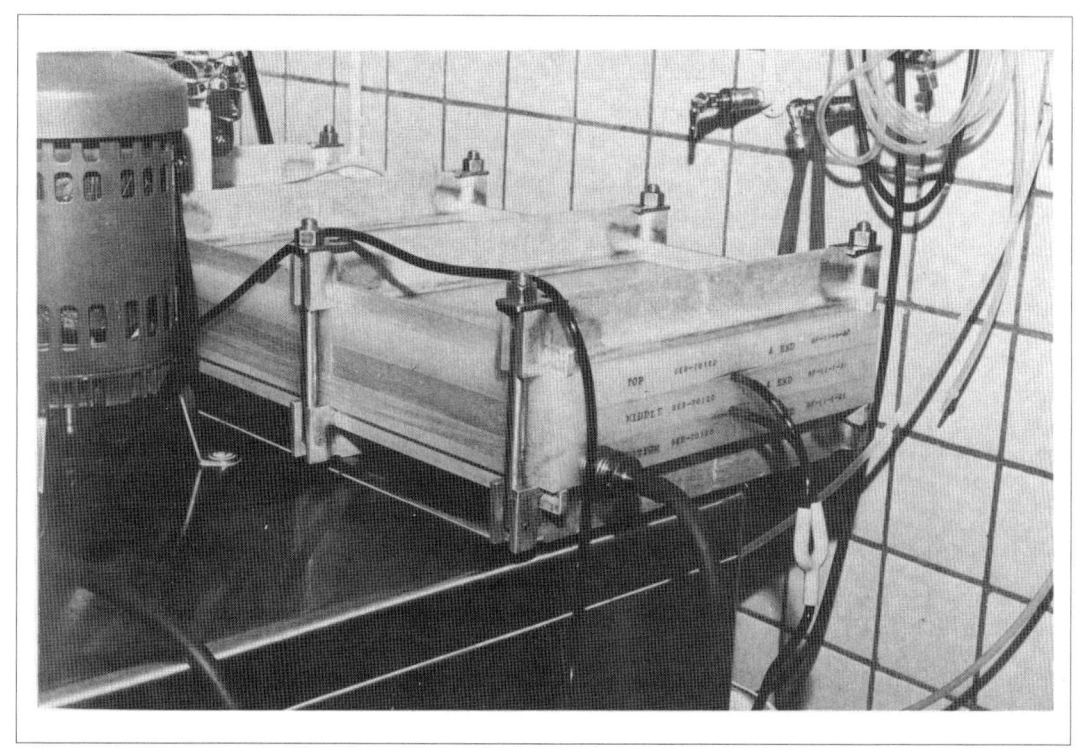

Figure 3-7. Modified two layer Kiil dialyzer during hemodialysis (1964).

artificial kidney is now not just the component that "filters the blood" but also includes blood access system, smooth and biocompatible blood pathways and circuit design, standardized thickness and porosity of membranes with accurate pump, alarm, and failure systems. A myriad of machines are now produced by a number of different companies (Figure 3-8).

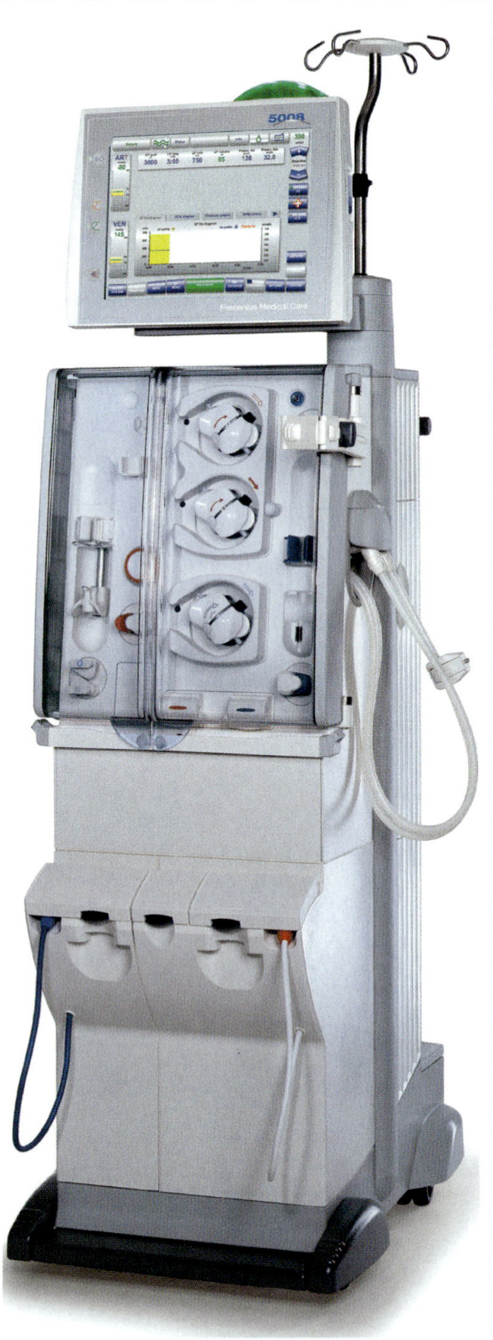

Blood Component

Anticoagulation

Preventing the blood from clotting once it had entered the extracorporeal circuit of a dialysis machine was one of the first major barriers in the development of the artificial kidney. George Haas initially used hiruidin, which is found in the saliva of leeches, as an anticoagulant for blood. Hiruidin was not practical for human use as it caused allergic reactions and was difficult to purify.

Jay Maclean was a medical student who discovered heparin in 1915 while studying pro-thrombotic agents.[33] He isolated a substance from the liver that seemed to prevent coagulation but his pharmacology professor James Howell controversially omitted his name from the two papers that first used the term heparin.[34,35] Howell eventually realized that heparin was more readily available from other tissues such as lung or intestine and not a phospholipid as originally thought, by this time, however, the name had already stuck! After purification and standardization, heparin became readily available in 1937. William Thalhimer, as mentioned above, was the first person to use heparin in exchange transfusion for the alleviation of uremia[16] and then for hemodialysis[15] in nephrectomized dogs. With this much more effective and less toxic anticoagulant, Kolff could now develop hemodialysis as a realistic treatment modality.

Access to the Blood Stream

Intermittent chronic hemodialysis also requires regular, reusable access to the patients' blood in order for it to pass through the artificial kidney. Modern hemodialysis processes 70–110 L of blood in a 4–5-hour period, which requires easy and reusable access to the blood stream. When Kolff first designed his machine the methods for extracting blood and returning it to the body rapidly exhausted the patients' arteries and veins. This meant that initially

Figure 3-8. A 'state of the art' Fresenius 5008, one of the most advanced dialysis machines available today.

dialysis was only suitable for acute renal failure and the chronic health of the patient relied on the recovery of renal function. A move toward chronic renal replacement therapy could only occur with safe, reliable, and reusable access to the patients' blood supply.

Developments began in 1960 with the Scribner shunt[36] (Figure 3-9).[37] Permanent cannulae were placed in the vein and an artery of the forearm of a patient. When they were not being used for dialysis, they were linked together with a Teflon tube to allow blood to flow across.

In 1966, Brescia and colleagues created the arteriovenous fistula (AVF) by joining an artery in the arm with a nearby vein[38] (Figure 3-10).[39] The vein, which is normally part of a low-pressure system, becomes arterialized, swells, and develops a thickened wall. Needles can easily be placed into the fistula, which is just under the surface of the skin, to allow repeated access. The AVF remains the gold standard of permanent dialysis access today.

Semipermanent access such as the PermCath® catheter and the Tesio® catheter are venous cannulae which are tunneled under the skin from their point of entry to a large central vein. These are often placed under fluoroscopy by physicians or radiologists and provide access to the blood stream in patients' who cannot have an AVF or when their AVF has failed. The main advantage of these forms of access is they can be used immediately. The main disadvantages include repeated infections and limited life span.

As another alternative, the LifeSite® Haemodialysis Access System combines unique valve technology with a cannulae connection system to the blood stream. The LifeSite® system consists of an implantable valve and cannulae. The valve is implanted subcutaneously and is attached to a patient's blood vessel via the venous cannulae and can be used immediately. The valve is made of medical grade materials that include titanium alloy, stainless steel, and silicone elastomers. The cannulae material used in the LifeSite® System is similar to other venous catheters. The valve has a dimpled entrance in the center of its domed top to accept a standard 14-gauge fistula needle (Figure 3-11).[40] Insertion of the fistula needle opens the valve and allows blood flow. When the fistula needle is withdrawn, the valve closes and blood flow stops. The dialysis needle is inserted into the same site each treatment resulting in the formation of a fibrous tract or "buttonhole". This access system is designed to eliminate the disfigurement associated with AV fistulae and grafts, as well as, the lifestyle impairments associated with protruding permanent catheters.

Dialyzate

Composition

The dialyzate is the chemical bath that is used to draw waste products out of the blood. Diffusion moves waste products in the blood across the membrane into the dialyzate compartment, where they are carried out of the body. At the same time, electrolytes and other chemicals in the dialyzate solution cross the membrane into the blood compartment. The purified, chemically balanced blood is then returned to the body.

Since the inception of a chronic dialysis programme, there has been a realization that the composition of the dialyzate is as important as all the other components of the artificial kidney. In 1913, when Abel and Rowntree first tried dialysis using animal blood the dialyzate was a

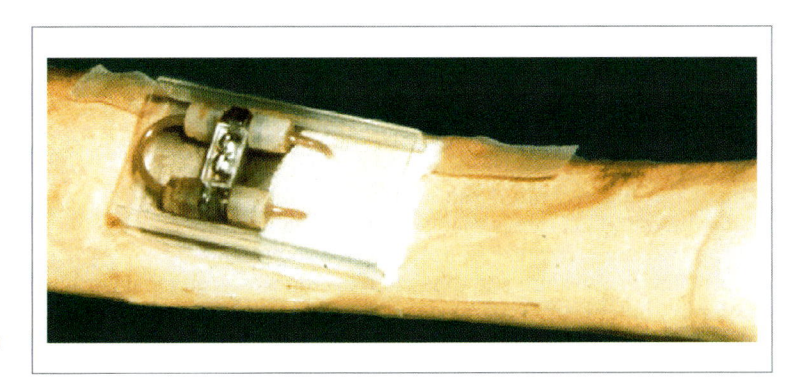

Figure 3-9. A Scribner shunt in patients forearm.

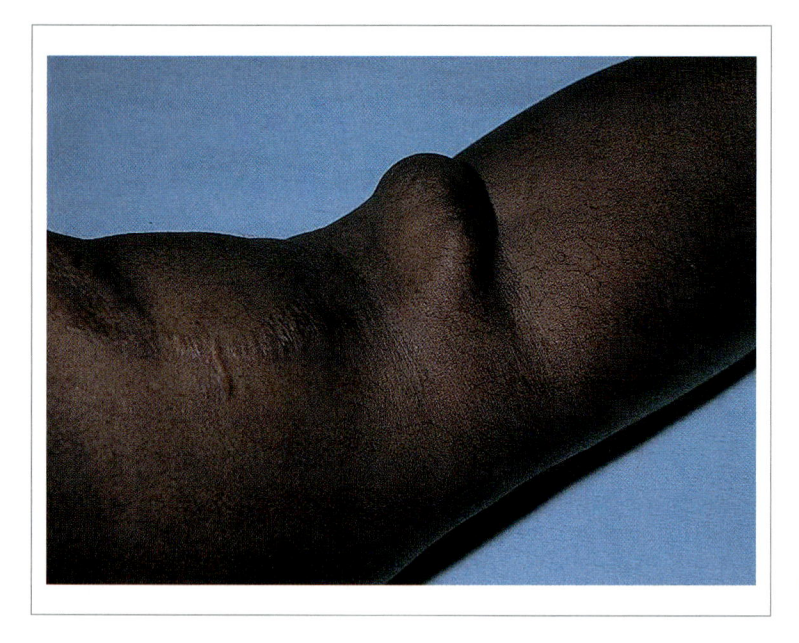

Figure 3-10. A left brachial arteriovenous fistula (AVF).

solution of normal saline and potassium. Gordon Murray, in his few attempts at dialysis realized that he had to use a dialyzate that contained physiological similarities to plasma and settled for Ringers solution.[26] For many years, dialyzate was mixed by hand in large vats that the various membranes passed through. As the membranes and their support structures improved, it could be mixed in a large communal vat and actively passed across a number of membranes at once.

Now dialyzate solutions are mixed to various prescriptions by the dialysis machines and the buffer added after mixing with a sterile water supply. The concentrations of sodium, potassium, and calcium are carefully chosen in the dialyzate to match the patients need. Along with the buffer these make up the most important features of the dialyzate. We know that the correct prescription of dialyzate can improve the cardiovascular stability of patients receiving hemodialysis treatment.[41]

Another important role of the dialyzate is to correct the patients' metabolic acidosis. This is done by the diffusive influx of the buffer supply, mainly bicarbonate, rather than through hydrogen ion clearance. Because of precipitation with calcium and magnesium and the risk of bacterial contamination, bicarbonate was abandoned and replaced by acetate during the first two decades of dialysis therapy. The key advantages were its equimolar conversion to bicarbonate, a bacteriostatic effect, and low cost. However, acetate-induced side-effects have been reported in a large number of studies during the 1980s due to the limitations in hepatic acetate metabolism in some patients.[42] In the last two decades, technical improvements, avoiding carbonate salt precipitation, and the development of high flux/high efficiency dialysis with worsened acetate-induced side-effects have gradually led to the reintroduction and generalization of bicarbonate as the preferred dialyzate buffer.

Direction of dialyzate flow as well as its composition is important. The Skeggs Leonards Plate Dialyzer was the first to push blood through the blood compartment in one direction and suction or vacuum pressure pulls the dialyzate through the dialyzate compartment in the opposite direction.[27] This countercurrent system is the most efficient mechanism of ultrafiltration and works to drain excess fluid out of the bloodstream and into the dialyzate and is now standard practice.

Water

Water has an enormous role in the delivery of safe, good dialysis. In modern machines, the dialyzate is pumped over the membrane at approximately 800 ml per minute.

For a unit that dialyses 90 patients a day, spread over three separate shifts, approximately 17,000 L of water will pass across the dialysis membranes and patients' blood in that period. It is therefore imperative that the water is free of infection and as pure as possible. This is a main focus within dialysis units, who have their own purification systems with national standards and strict quality control systems that have to be adhered to. In the 1970s, as dialysis became an established form of therapy, nephrologists realized the importance of water through a series of clinical incidents.

Sporadic outbreaks of encephalopathy in several dialysis units around the country were associated with aluminium toxicity.[43] Aluminium hydroxide, along with filtration, is used to improve the taste of "peaty" water and subsequently throughout the country, the drinking water aluminium concentration varied. This water was then used to mix the buffer solution of the dialyzate. To overcome this problem mains water is now treated using softeners, reverse osmosis, or ion exchange to remove the aluminium.[44] Water and plasma aluminium content is monitored routinely as part of the quality control systems and "dialysis dementia" in the United Kinhdom is a thing of the past.

Similarly hemolytic anemia was identified as a problem in hemodialysis patients in the 1970s.[45,46] Chloramine is formed when ammonia is added to water that contains free chlorine. This process is used by water companies to disinfect drinking water. Chloramine lasts a long time in water to more effectively remove pathogens such as bacteria and virus'. Water that contains chloramine is safe for people to drink, bathe, and cook in because the digestive process neutralizes it. Chloramine can, however, easily harm patients if it enters the blood stream during the dialysis process causing hemolytic anemia. Recently, recombinant erythropoetin resistance has been recognized as an insidious presentation of chloramine toxicity.[47]

Chloramine continues to cause problems in dialysis centers[48–50] and often it is because its concentration in the water tends to vary throughout the year. Levels are increased by water companies when bacterial contamination increases and the carbon filters, which easily remove chloramine, subsequently become insufficient.

The Future

Renal transplantation is the preferred treatment for many people with chronic renal failure; however, due to lack of donor organs and the unsuitability of a significant proportion of patients, hemodialysis will continue to be a common therapy. In the United Kingdom, hemodialysis commonly occurs in 4-hour sessions, three times a week and despite the progress that has been made in the last 50 years, hemodialysis is widely recognized as unphysiologic[51] and continues to be associated with high morbidity and mortality.

Since the invention of hollow fiber dialyzers the major areas of development have been new materials with enhancement of the delivery in dialysis using better machines cumulating in improved efficiency. We now provide safer and better tolerated dialysis but without the decrease in mortality we would desire.[52,53]

An ideal device for renal replacement therapy would mimic the function of the natural kidney (Table 3-3). It would be continuously operating, it would remove solute with a molecular weight spectrum, it would be flexible and remove water and solutes on an individual patient need, it would be wearable or implantable, and it must be biocompatible.

Nissenson and collegues[54] recently published an article about their vision for the future of the artificial kidney. In order to achieve the ambitious specifications they have pursued nanotechnology in the development of their artificial kidney, the Human Nephron Filter (HNF). As mentioned above, the hollow fiber membranes are already introducing aspects of this technology in artificial kidneys.

Table 3-3. Criteria for the Ideal Artificial Kidney

- Continuous
- Remove solutes with a wide range of molecular weights
- Function relative to individual patient needs
- Portable/wearable/implantable
- Biocompatible
- Light weight
- Low cost
- Safe
- Reliable

The HNF consists of two membranes operating in series within one device. The G membrane mimics the function of the glomerulus, using convection to generate plasma ultra filtrate containing all solutes approaching the molecular weight of albumin. The T membrane mimics the functions of the renal tubule, selectively reclaiming designated solutes to maintain body homeostasis, again by convection (Figure 3-12)[54]

Although only in developmental stages the authors have an animal prototype and many of the breakthrough aspects such as the chemistry, the pores, and the membranes are almost in place.

Progress continues to be made with living membranes. The ultimate goal of this approach is to replace the metabolic activity of the kidney to improve biological homeostasis, including immunologic, cardiovascular, and mineral metabolism. This all depends on the ability to isolate and expand in culture tubule cells from adult kidneys[55] and then incorporate them onto a standard hemofiltration cartridge.[56] In vitro and ex vivo animal experiments[56-58] have allowed an initial trial of the "renal tubule cell assist device" (RAD) in critically ill humans receiving continuous veno-venous hemofiltration in the ICU with encouraging results[59] leading to a phase II trial.

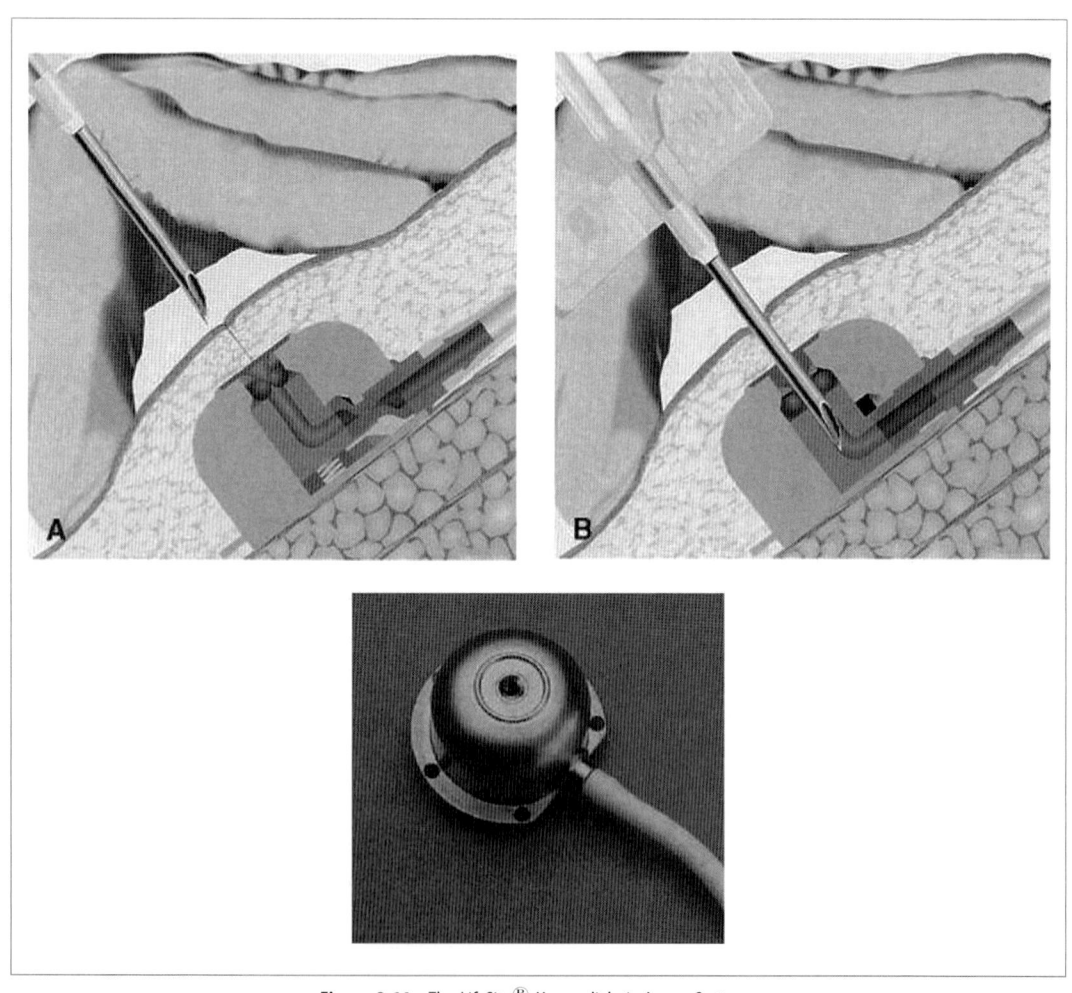

Figure 3-11. The LifeSite® Haemodialysis Access System.

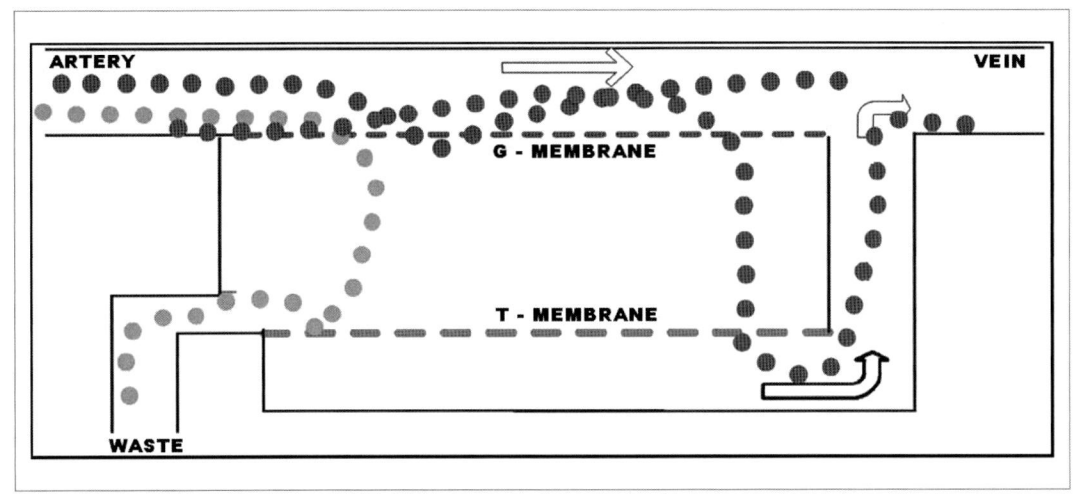

Figure 3-12. A diagram showing how the human nephron filter utilizes two membranes to mimic the renal tubule.

Conclusions

The development artificial kidney has progressed rapidly since its application to humans while the need for hemodialysis has continued to grow. The availability and variety are such that the nephrologist can tailor dialysis to the physiological need of the patient by using different combinations of membranes, dialyzate solutions, and pump speeds. There is, however, still progress to be made in morbidity, mortality, and quality of life for hemodialysis patients but the future of the artificial kidney looks exciting as new technologies emerge.

References

1. Ansell D, Feest T, Tomson C, Will E, Williams AJ. UK Renal Registry Report 2005.
2. Johnson R, Feehally J. Comprehensive Clinical Nephrology. London: Elsevier; 2003.
3. Graham T. The Balkerian Lecture: On Osmotic Force. *Phil Trans R Soc Lond.* 1854;144:177–228.
4. Fick A. Ueber Diffusion. *Annalen derPhysik un Chemie.* 1855;170:59–86.
5. Abel J, Rowntree L, Turner B. On the removal of diffusible substances from the circulating blood of living animals by means of dialysis. *J Pharmacol Exp Ther.* 1912;5:275–283.
6. Haas G. Dialysieren des strömendes Blutes am Lebenden. *Klin Wochenschr.* 1925;2:1888.
7. Haas G. Versuche der Blutauswaschung am Lebenden mit Hilfe der Dialyse. *Klin Wochenschr.* 1925;4:13–14.
8. Haas G. Ueber Versuche der Blutauswaschung am Lebenden mit Hilfe der Dialyse. *Archiv Exp Path Pharmakol.* 1926;106:158–172.
9. Haas G. Die Methoden der Blutauswaschung. *Aberhalden's Handb Biol Arbeitsmethoden Abt V teil.* 1935;8:717–754.
10. George C.R.P. Hirudin, heparin and Heinrich Neceles. *Nephrology.* 1998;4:225–228.
11. 'En effet, il y a dans les bois le tissu primitif, isomère avec amidon, que nous appelerons cellulose, et de plus une matière qui en remplit les cellules, et qui constitue la matière ligneuse véritable'. [The committee was formed of Brogniart, Pelouze and Dumas, and reported to the Académie on 14th January 1839: C R Acad Sci Paris1839; VIII: 51. It appears that the author of the word glucose, and presumably also cellulose, was Dumas, the rapporteur of the committee.]. In: eds. Book 'En effet, il y a dans les bois le tissu primitif, isomère avec amidon, que nous appelerons cellulose, et de plus une matière qui en remplit les cellules, et qui constitue la matière ligneuse véritable'. [The committee was formed of Brogniart, Pelouze and Dumas, and reported to the Académie on 14th January 1839: C R Acad Sci Paris1839; VIII: 51. It appears that the author of the word glucose, and presumably also cellulose, was Dumas, the rapporteur of the committee.].
12. Wilson F.L. Experiments with cellophane as a sterilisable dialysable membrane. *Arch Pathol Lab Med.* 1927;127:239.
13. Andrus F.C. Use of Visking sausage casing for ultrafiltration. *Proc Soc Exp Biol Med.* 1929;27:127–128.
14. Fagette P. Hemodialysis 1912–1945: no medical technology: before its time: part I. *ASAIO J.* 1999;45:238–249.
15. Thalhimer W, Solandt DY, Best CH. Experimental exchange transfusion using purified heparin. *Lancet.* 1938;2:554–557.
16. Thalhimer W. Experimental exchange transfusions for reducing azotemia: Use of artificial kidney for this purpose. *Proc Soc Exp Biol Med.* 1938;37:641–643.
17. Stewart RD, Cerny JC, Mahon HI. The Capillary "Kidney": Preliminary Report. *Med Bull (Ann Arbor).* 1964;30:116–118.

18. Stewart R, Cerny J, Mahon H. An artificial kidney made from capillary fibres. *Invest Urol.* 1966;5:614–624.
19. Streicher E, Schneider H. Polysulphone membrane mimicking human glomerular basement membrane. *Lancet.* 1983;2:1136.
20. Drexler KE. Nanosystems molecular machinery, manufacturing and computation. Chichester: Wiley; 1992.
21. Bowry SK. Nano-controlled membrane spinning technology: regulation of pore size, distribution and morphology of a new polysulfone dialysis membrane. *Contrib Nephrol.* 2002;137:85–94.
22. Bowry SK. Dialysis membranes today. *Int J Artif Organs.* 2002;25:447–460.
23. Kloff WJ, Berk HTJ, ter Welle M, van der Ley AJW, van Dijk EC, van Noordwijk J. The artificial Kidney: a dialyser with a great area. *Acta Med Scand.* 1944;117:121–134.
24. Bywaters EGL, Joekes AM. Artificial kidney: its application to treatment of traumatic anuria. *Proc Roy Soc Med.* 1948;41:420–426.
25. Clarke W. A Canadian giant: Dr. Gordon Murray and the artificial kidney. *CMAJ.* 1987;137:246–248.
26. McKeller S. Gordon Murray and the artificial kidney in Canada. *Nephrol Dial Transplant.* 1999;14:2766–2770.
27. Skeggs LT, Jr., Leonards JR. Studies on an Artificial Kidney: I. Preliminary Results With a New Type of Continuous Dialyzer. *Science.* 1948;108:212–213.
28. Murphy WP, Jr., Swan RC, Jr., Walter CW, Weller JM, Merrill JP. Use of an artificial kidney. III. Current procedures in clinical hemodialysis. *J Lab Clin Med.* 1952;40:436–444.
29. Inouye WY, Engelberg J. A simplified artificial dialyzer and ultrafilter. *Surg Forum.* 1953;4:438–442.
30. Wong D, Lambie AT, Winney RJ, Turner AN. Haemodialysis in Edinburgh 1957-1987. *J R Coll Physicians Edinb.* 2002;32:114–121.
31. Kiil F. Development of a parallel-flow artificial kidney in plastics. *Acta Chir Scand Suppl Suppl.* 1960;253:142–150.
32. Scribner BH, Buri R, Caner JE, Hegstrom R, Burnell JM. The treatment of chronic uremia by means of intermittent hemodialysis: a preliminary report. *Trans Am Soc Artif Intern Organs.* 1960;6:114–122.
33. Maclean J. The discovery of heparin. *Circulation.* 1959;19:75–78.
34. Howell WH. Heparin, an anticoagulant. *Am J Physiol.* 1923;63:434–435.
35. Howell WH, Holt E. Two new factors in blood coagulation: Heparin and pro-antithrombin. *Am J Physiol.* 1918;47:328–341.
36. Quinton W, Dillard D, Scribner BH. Cannulation of blood vessels for prolonged hemodialysis. *Trans Am Soc Artif Intern Organs.* 1960;6:104–113.
37. Scribner BH. Lasker Clinical Medicine Research Award. Medical dilemmas: the old is new. *Nat Med.* 2002;8:1066–1067.
38. Brescia MJ, Cimino JE, Appel K, Hurwich BJ. Chronic hemodialysis using venipuncture and a surgically created arteriovenous fistula. *N Engl J Med.* 1966;275:1089–1092.
39. Johnson R, Feehally J. Comprehensive Clinical Nephrology. London: Elsevier; 2003.
40. Schwab SJ, Weiss MA, Rushton F, Ross JP, Jackson J, Kapoian T, Yegge J, Rosenblatt M, Reese WJ, Soundararajan R, Work J, Ross J, Stainken B, Pedan A, Moran JA. Multicenter clinical trial results with the LifeSite hemodialysis access system. *Kidney Int.* 2002;62:1026–1033.
41. Locatelli F, Covic A, Chazot C, Leunissen K, Luno J, Yaqoob M. Optimal composition of the dialysate, with emphasis on its influence on blood pressure. *Nephrol Dial Transplant.* 2004;19:785–796.
42. Vinay P, Cardoso M, Tejedor A, Prud'homme M, Levelillee M, Vinet B, Courteau M, Gougoux A, Rengel M, Lapierre L, et al. Acetate metabolism during hemodialysis: metabolic considerations. *Am J Nephrol.* 1987;7:337–354.
43. Alfrey AC, LeGendre GR, Kaehny WD. The dialysis encephalopathy syndrome. Possible aluminum intoxication. *N Engl J Med.* 1976;294:184–188.
44. Petrie JJ, Fleming R, McKinnon P, Winney RJ, Cowie J. The use of ion exchange to remove aluminum from water used in hemodialysis. *Am J Kidney Dis.* 1984;4:69–74.
45. Botella J, Traver JA, Sanz-Guajardo D, Torres MT, Sanjuan I, Zabala P. Chloramines, an aggravating factor in the anemia of patients on regular dialysis treatment. *Proc Eur Dial Transplant Assoc.* 1977;14:192–199.
46. Eaton JW, Kolpin CF, Swofford HS, Kjellstrand CM, Jacob HS. Chlorinated urban water: a cause of dialysis-induced hemolytic anemia. *Science.* 1973;181:463–464.
47. Fluck S, McKane W, Cairns T, Fairchild V, Lawrence A, Lee J, Murray D, Polpitiye M, Palmer A, Taube D. Chloramine-induced haemolysis presenting as erythropoietin resistance. *Nephrol Dial Transplant.* 1999;14:1687–1691.
48. Calderaro RV, Heller L. [Outbreak of hemolytic reactions associated with chlorine and chloramine residuals in hemodialysis water]. *Rev Saude Publica.* 2001;35:481–486.
49. Pyo HJ, Kwon YJ, Wee KS, Kwon SY, Lee CH, Kim S, Lee JS, Cho SH, Cha CW. An outbreak of Heinz body positive hemolytic anemia in chronic hemodialysis patients. *Korean J Intern Med.* 1993;8:93–98.
50. Tipple MA, Shusterman N, Bland LA, McCarthy MA, Favero MS, Arduino MJ, Reid MH, Jarvis WR. Illness in hemodialysis patients after exposure to chloramine contaminated dialysate. *ASAIO Trans.* 1991;37:588–591.
51. Kjellstrand CM, Evans RL, Petersen RJ, Shideman JR, von Hartitzsch B, Buselmeier TJ. The "unphysiology" of dialysis: a major cause of dialysis side effects? *Kidney Int.* 1975;Suppl:30–34.
52. Ronco C, Ghezzi PM, La Greca G. The role of technology in hemodialysis. *J Nephrol.* 1999;12(Suppl 2):S68–81.
53. Woffindin C, Hoenich NA. Hemodialyzer performance: a review of the trends over the past two decades. *Artif Organs.* 1995;19:1113–1119.
54. Nissenson AR, Ronco C, Pergamit G, Edelstein M, Watts R. Continuously functioning artificial nephron system: the promise of nanotechnology. *Hemodial Int.* 2005;9:210–217.
55. Humes HD, Krauss JC, Cieslinski DA, Funke AJ. Tubulogenesis from isolated single cells of adult mammalian kidney: clonal analysis with a recombinant retrovirus. *Am J Physiol.* 1996;271:F42–49.
56. Humes HD. Tissue engineering of a bioartificial kidney: a universal donor organ. *Transplant Proc.* 1996;28:2032–2035.
57. Humes HD, Buffington DA, MacKay SM, Funke AJ, Weitzel WF. Replacement of renal function in uremic animals with a tissue-engineered kidney. *Nat Biotechnol.* 1999;17:451–455.

58. Humes HD, Fissell WH, Weitzel WF, Buffington DA, Westover AJ, MacKay SM, Gutierrez JM Metabolic replacement of kidney function in uremic animals with a bioartificial kidney containing human cells. *Am J Kidney Dis.* 2002;39:1078–1087.

59. Humes HD, Weitzel WF, Bartlett RH, Swaniker FC, Paganini EP, Luderer JR, Sobota J. Initial clinical results of the bioartificial kidney containing human cells in ICU patients with acute renal failure. *Kidney Int.* 2004;66:1578–1588.

4

Liver Substitution

Sambit Sen and Roger Williams

Introduction

Liver failure, whether occurring de novo without pre-existing liver disease (acute liver failure, ALF) or as an acute episode of decompensation superimposed on a chronic liver disorder (acute-on-chronic liver failure, ACLF), carries a high mortality. The lack of the detoxification, metabolic, and regulatory functions of the liver leads to life-threatening complications, including kidney failure, hepatic encephalopathy (HE), cerebral edema, severe hypotension, and susceptibility to infections culminating in multi-organ failure.[1,2] The only established therapy for patients of ALF who fail to improve with supportive management is liver transplantation (LTx), but currently one-third of these patients die while waiting for a transplant and the organ shortage is increasing.[3] Living-related donor transplantation has proved encouraging,[4] yet a suitable donor is found in time in only 30% of cases (of living-related donor transplantation).[5] Many patients of ACLF are not eligible for LTx, and current management focuses on treatment of the individual organ dysfunction. However, liver failure, whether of the acute or acute-on-chronic variety, is to some extent reversible. A supportive therapy which can tide over the acute period of crisis (and act as a bridge to liver transplantation in cases of ALF) can possibly be life-saving,[6] and the search for an effective liver support system continues. Essentially, two types are under development: artificial devices, based on the removal of albumin-bound toxins, and bioartificial devices, using hepatocytes to perform the functions of the failing liver.

However, one has to first consider whether liver support can be expected to work and provide worthwhile clinical benefit in the setting of liver failure in man. A recent review looks at the history of the development of liver support, elegantly tracing the quest for the elusive ideal liver support system.[7] Early studies demonstrated that cross-circulation of the patient with baboons or healthy human subjects led to recovery from coma.[8,9] Similarly, extracorporeal animal liver perfusion was found to be of help in supporting ALF patients,[10,11] as was single plasma exchange therapy.[12] Amongst the many other therapies tried, hemoperfusion over charcoal and, more recently, high-volume plasmapheresis[13] (which showed reduction of plasma bilirubin and arterial ammonia,[14] with improvement of peripheral hemodynamics[15] and cerebral blood flow[16]) have all been the subject of encouraging results, although with charcoal hemoperfusion this could not be confirmed in a controlled trial. Most substances are non-selectively removed by these various techniques, including some which are important physiologically (growth factors, clotting factors),[17,18] and with charcoal hemoperfusion, the filters causing activation of leucocytes with consequent cytokine release may have predisposed to bleeding and disseminated intravascular coagulation.[19]

There also exists a vast amount of published literature relating to the testing of bioartificial liver (BAL) devices in in vitro and animal models.[19–23] Thus studies with rat models of liver failure have shown improvement of parameters like serum bilirubin, albumin, and clotting factor production. A carefully controlled study with the Academic Medical Center-BAL (Amsterdam) in pigs with hepatic ischemia-induced ALF showed improvement of blood ammonia and bilirubin levels, with prolongation of survival (longest surviving animal kept alive up to 63 h).[24] A subsequent controlled study performed in anhepatic pigs with the same device[25] showed that those treated with BAL containing autologous hepatocytes survived longer (mean 65 h) compared to animals not treated with BAL (46 h) or treated with the BAL device without incorporating hepatocytes (43 h). The treatment was also associated with a significant decrease of arterial ammonia. What is perhaps surprising and certainly worth commenting upon is that in the long history of developing devices for liver support, despite beneficial effects in various animal models (large and small) of ALF, most of the devices have remained unproven when used subsequently in patients with ALF.

Functions Required of a Liver Support System

Liver failure leads to impairment of all aspects of hepatic function, including detoxifying and synthetic functions, as well as bile excretion. Altered hepatic metabolism is probably central to this.[26] For example, impaired gluconeogenesis and glycogenolysis predisposes to hypoglycemia. Albumin synthesis is hampered, as is the production of clotting factors. The impaired urea cycle leads to accumulation of ammonia in the body, and the metabolism of protein breakdown products is also impaired. This leads to the accumulation of a whole variety of toxins in the body, most of which, apart from a few like ammonia and lactate, are albumin-bound in the plasma (Table 4-1). This means that they cannot be adequately removed by conventional techniques of hemofiltration/hemodialysis. The importance of these toxins may be related to their role in the development of associated end-organ failures, especially affecting the brain, the circulation, and the kidneys, which considerably worsen the outcome in both ALF and ACLF.

The observation that these end-organ dysfunctions can be reversed following LTx has led to the hypothesis that the hepatic dysfunction is central to their pathogenesis, with the accumulation of toxins as the immediately responsible mechanism.[1] A liver support system which can remove these toxins could potentially prevent or reverse end-organ failure, and significantly improve outcome in liver failure, particularly if these toxins also cause further damage to the liver.[27] Clearance of these toxins from the body could potentially interrupt this vicious cycle leading to further hepatic function deterioration as well as end-organ failure. A system favorably modulating humoral and molecular mechanisms of liver regeneration (with reduction of plasma levels of regeneration-inhibitory substances like transforming growth factor (TGF) β) is ideally desirable,[28] as would one which could reasonably duplicate the role of the liver in the biotransformation and metabolism of various drugs and intermediate metabolites. While replacing lost biosynthetic functions would also be important, most substances produced by the liver can be given exogenously by intravenous infusion, and this particular aspect of liver synthetic function may not be of primary concern.[29]

Assessment of Current Liver Support Systems

The several liver support systems that are currently under investigation are considered under the two main categories of artificial and bioartificial. Despite natural concerns to try every possible therapy in an individual patient suddenly struck down by liver failure, especially ALF, the value of such devices can only be properly assessed in the setting of a controlled clinical trial. Such trials need to be adequately powered in the number of cases, with strict criteria for entry and with survival as the primary end point. However, the critical clinical condition of liver failure patients as well as the rarity of ALF generally makes performing such a study difficult.

Table 4-1. Some of the Endogenous Albumin-Bound Toxins, Which Accumulate in Liver Failure, Which Can Be Potentially Removed by Albumin Dialysis or Fractionated Plasma Separation and Adsorption

Aromatic amino acids
Bile acids
Bilirubin
Digoxin-like substances
Endogenous benzodiazepines
Indols
Mercaptans
Middle- and short-chain fatty acids
Nitric oxide
Phenols
Prostacyclins
Tryptophan

Patients with different degrees of severity of the syndrome are often grouped together within trials, and intensive care regimes are difficult to standardize. Furthermore LTx, when indicated, is likely to be performed at different times in the clinical course of patients and will hugely influence survival. Thus surrogate markers, rather than survival, are often used in assessing the efficacy of therapy. All these need to be kept in mind when interpreting the results of clinical trials of liver support systems. The reason why ALF figured prominently in previous studies was because it was considered that the chances of survival were so low that any possible therapy could be justified. The recent trials on artificial systems have been in the much more common condition of ACLF, which is the major cause for liver failure and is responsible for increasing numbers of hospital admissions worldwide. Therefore, one would expect ACLF to be the main clinical indication where liver support would be required.

Bioartificial Systems

Design of Devices

By utilizing viable hepatocytes these systems should reproduce the synthetic, detoxifying as well as excretory functions of the liver. Unfortunately human liver cells, which would be the best to use, are difficult to obtain and are difficult to grow in culture, becoming phenotypically unstable and rapidly losing liver-specific gene expression. The minimum quantity of cells required is not known, but based on the experience of hepatic resection in humans,[30] around 150–450 g of cells (or 10^{10} hepatocytes), providing the function of 10–30% of the normal liver mass, is required to support the failing liver[19,29] (though some experimental data in animal models have suggested that smaller quantities of cells may be enough to enhance spontaneous recovery, possibly by reducing plasma levels of regeneration-inhibitory substances like TGF-β[31]). Most of the current devices are based on the use of hepatocytes from other species, particularly pigs (as in the Demetriou BAL device HepatAssist (Circe Biomedical, Lexington, MA), using 6–10 $\times$ 10^9 cells, or 30–50 g).[23] A great advantage of porcine hepatocytes, unlike human liver cells, is that they can be satisfactorily cryopreserved, with cell isolation at a convenient time followed by storage at a clinical site prior to use, thereby avoiding the costs and contamination risks of long-term hepatocyte culture.[32] Cryopreservation is associated with caspase activation and apoptosis, which can be prevented by adding caspase inhibitors (ZVAD-fmk).[33] Another approach has been with genetically engineered human hepatocytes to produce cells with the desired functional and survival capabilities. Thus, the C3A hepatocyte line, a sub-clone of the ubiquitous HepG2 hepatoblastoma cell line, has been used in one system (4 $\times$ 10^{10}, or 200 g in each bioreactor cartridge of the Sussman device (extracorporeal liver assist device (ELAD, Vitagen, La Jolla, CA)).[22] Another immortalized human hepatocyte cell line under investigation is HHY41, which retains many liver-specific functions, protein synthesis, gluconeogenesis, and cytochrome P450 activity and is particularly resistant to acetaminophen.[34–36]

At the heart of the design for a BAL is the bioreactor (Figure 4-1). The simplest type, and one used most commonly, consists of a column containing hollow fiber capillaries through which flows the patient's plasma. In the extracapillary space lie the hepatocytes, either alone[22] or attached to microcarrier beads.[23] Plasma can be separated, warmed, and oxygenated in the secondary circuit before being perfused through the bioreactor capillaries. Free exchange of molecules can occur between plasma/blood and hepatocytes in the bioreactor across a membrane with a cut-off selected to allow the movement of most toxins as well as transport proteins like albumin (66 kDa molecular weight), while preventing passage of immunoglobulins (100–900 kDa), complements (>200 kDa), or viruses and cells. Most groups have used cut-offs between 50 and 150 kDa.[2,19] The hepatocytes extract oxygen and nutrients and detoxify toxins from the plasma, and their metabolites are simultaneously passed back into the plasma. The Demetriou system also incorporates two charcoal columns in the circuit prior to the bioreactor for removal of toxins which could damage or impair the function of the pig hepatocytes.

The more sophisticated system developed by Gerlach et al.[37] (Modular Extracorporeal Liver Support (MELS, Hybrid Organ, Berlin, Germany)) uses three sets of capillary tubes – one to provide oxygenation, and two to carry inflowing and outflowing plasma. The hepatocytes (400–600 g of primary human hepatocytes from explanted livers found unsuitable for LTx) remain in the extracapillary space. A detoxification module allows

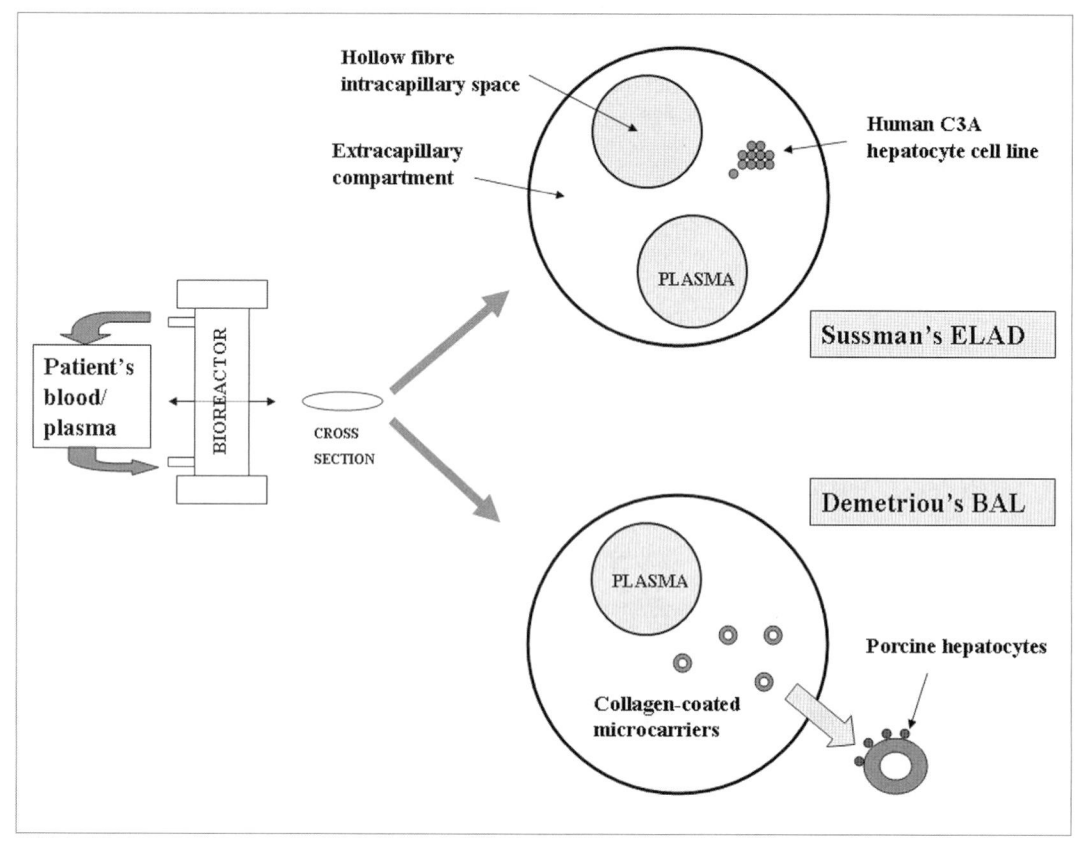

Figure 4-1. Schematic showing the structure of bioreactors in Sussman's extracorporeal liver assist device (ELAD) (*top*) and Demetriou's HepatAssist bioartificial liver (BAL) (*bottom*).

single-pass albumin dialysis to be performed, and continuous veno-venous hemodiafiltration can be included. The Academic Medical Center-BAL (AMC-BAL, Hep-Art, Amsterdam, The Netherlands) developed by Chamuleau et al.[38] incorporates a spirally wound polyester matrix sheet that includes an integral hollow fiber compartment for oxygenation and uses 220×10^6 porcine hepatocytes (Figure 4-2). In addition to these hollow fiber-based bioreactors, some others have tried designs based on "flat plates and monolayers," "perfused beds/scaffolds," and "encapsulation and suspension."[19] A porcine hepatocyte-based BAL using a "radial-flow" bioreactor (RFB) has been developed in Italy[39] and has undergone phase I clinical trials.

Clinical Trials

The first clinical use of a BAL device, comprising a kidney dialysis unit loaded with cryopreserved rabbit hepatocytes, was in 1987 to treat a single patient with ALF. The serum bilirubin decreased, neurological status improved, and the patient was ultimately discharged from hospital.[40] Of the many clinical studies of the different devices since then, only those relevant to currently available devices are included in the following assessment. The numerous difficulties associated with performing such trials in this extremely sick group of patients have already been referred to.

Porcine Hepatocyte-Based BAL

One of the first trials using this system (1996), which was developed by Demetriou and colleagues at the Cedars-Sinai Medical Center, USA, described 12 ALF patients, all of whom could be bridged over to LTx.[41] Following treatment lasting for 21–96 h, reversal of decerebration was observed in all 11 patients who were in grade 4 encephalopathy, with significantly improved

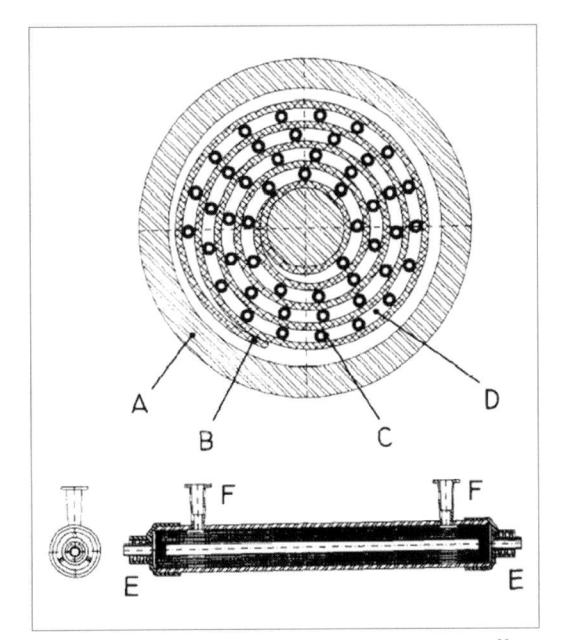

Figure 4-2. Schematic of Chamuleau's AMC-bioartificial liver.[38] (**A**) polysulfon dialysis housing; (**B**) three-dimensional non-woven polyester matrix for high-density hepatocyte culture; (**C**) polypropylene hollow fiber membranes for oxygen supply and CO_2 removal; (**D**) hollow fibers act as spacers between layers of the 3D matrix, creating numerous channels for the uniform flow and distribution of medium; (**E**) endcaps via which bioreactor is perfused with culture gas; (**F**) side-ports via which medium is perfused through the extra-fiber bioreactor space and is in direct contact with hepatocytes.

intracranial pressure (from a mean of 18.2 to 8.5 mmHg) and cerebral perfusion pressure. While improvement of the neurological state was most prominent, some important biochemical changes were noted as well. Serum ammonia (155.6–121.6 μmol/l) and bilirubin (21.6–18.2 mg/dl) improved, although the prothrombin time did not. Interestingly, two patients who underwent total hepatectomy to reduce the necrotic tissue mass were successfully maintained on BAL until they were transplanted. The results were less promising in eight ACLF patients, six of whom died within 14 days of the last BAL treatment. In another report by the same group (1997)[42] data were given on 18 ALF patients treated with BAL, of whom 16 could be successfully bridged over to transplantation, while 1 patient recovered sufficiently not to need it.

A more recent French study with BAL (using 5×10^9 porcine hepatocytes in each bioreactor) in 10 ALF patients[43] again reported changes predominantly in the neurological state, with improvement of Glasgow Coma Score in 6 (mean of 6.5–9.6). Serum bilirubin level was reduced (486.6–347 μmol/l), without any other changes in liver function tests. Arterial ammonia did not improve significantly, and there was no evidence of improved protein synthesis. On the contrary, serum albumin worsened significantly (27.8–22.7 g/l) after the first session of BAL treatment. Five patients had bleeding complications, probably explained by the significant reduction of both platelets (194.7–140 × 10^9/l) and fibrinogen (0.96–0.47 g/l) after the first session. Six patients had transient episodes of hemodynamic instability, although ultimately all patients could be bridged over to transplantation, and eight were alive and well at 18 months.

The device was further developed to make use of cryopreserved cells and include a larger number of hepatocytes (HepatAssist, Circe Biomedical), and has been evaluated in a large multi-center randomized controlled trial in 171 patients (fulminant hepatic failure – 147, primary graft non-function – 24), conducted in the United States and Europe.[44] While some improvements in intracranial pressure and consciousness level were seen, there was little evidence of improved synthetic function. Most disappointingly, a survival advantage was evident only in the sub-group with acetaminophen etiology (n=39) (BAL – 70% vs controls – 37%). Thirty-day survival in the entire study population was 62% for controls vs 71% for BAL-treated patients, while among fulminant liver failure patients alone, it was 59% vs 73%, respectively (p=0.1). However, this primary end point was confounded by the major impact of LTx; 54% of the entire study population was transplanted. Thirty-day survival with LTx (n=90) was 84% (BAL – 89% vs controls – 80%), while that without LTx (n=81) was 46% (BAL – 51% vs controls – 40%). A covariate time-dependent proportional hazard model with time-to-death as end point was therefore employed to account for the impact of LTx and other factors predictive of survival (including etiology, stage of encephalopathy) and showed a 47% reduction in mortality favoring BAL treatment (p=0.03) in the fulminant hepatic failure group (n=147).

Hepatoblastoma-Based Extracorporeal Liver Assist Device (ELAD)

The ELAD device developed by Sussman and colleagues was tried in one early randomized controlled study in London[45]; 24 ALF patients were enrolled, comprising 17 patients not fulfilling criteria for transplantation (predicted survival 50%) – group-I, and 7 patients fulfilling criteria (predicted survival <10%) – group-II. The device proved safe, without causing coagulopathy or hemodynamic instability to any significant extent. Arterial ammonia fell marginally in the ELAD group after 6 h treatment, and the rise in serum bilirubin over the period of the trial was more pronounced in the controls, but not significantly so. Worsening of encephalopathy was less in the ELAD-treated patients (3/12, 25%) compared to controls (7/12, 58%). However, a clear survival advantage was not shown. Survival in group-I was 7/9 (78%) with ELAD and 6/8 (75%) for controls, the much higher figure than anticipated making it difficult to show a survival advantage. There were only a small number of patients in group-II, and one each of three treated and four control patients survived. Interestingly, a significant improvement in galactose elimination capacity was demonstrated during the 6 h of ELAD treatment (compared to a decrease in controls), along with a fourfold increase of growth hormone levels (which decreased in the controls). Transforming growth factor levels did not change.

Since then, the device has undergone modifications, with plasma, rather than whole blood, being used for perfusion of the bioreactor hollow fibers, increase of the hepatocyte volume to 600–800 g, and introduction of an oxygenation system (VitaGen Inc). The results of a randomized controlled phase I trial in patients with fulminant hepatic failure were reported (still in abstract form[46]). Patients were stratified into those listed for LTx (n=19) and those not listed (n=5). Of the 19 patients listed for LTx, 12 received ELAD therapy; 11/12 (92%) ELAD patients went on to receive LTx, while only 3/7 (43%) controls were transplanted (p<0.05); 10/12 (83%) ELAD patients also achieved the primary end point of 30-day survival, compared to 3/7 (43%) controls (p=0.12). The device appeared to be safe and, though the study was not powered to look at outcome, showed a significant advantage for patients receiving a LTx in the ELAD group and a trend toward improved survival for those patients listed for LTx. On this basis, a phase II randomized controlled trial has been started in the United States.

Other Devices

Based on the encouraging results of carefully controlled studies of the AMC-BAL (Amsterdam) in large animal models, a phase I clinical trial with the device was carried out in Italy.[47] Seven ALF patients with grade 3–4 encephalopathy, listed for LTx, were treated for 8–35 h. Neurological improvement was observed in all patients. Serum bilirubin decreased by a mean of 31% (range 3–62%), as did arterial ammonia (44%, range 9–66%). The only adverse effect observed was transient hypotension in two patients immediately after starting the device. One of the patients improved sufficiently not to require LTx, while the remaining six were transplanted.

Early experience with the Modular Extracorporeal Liver Support (MELS) (Berlin) in eight patients has been reported.[48] Two patients each with ALF and ACLF were successfully bridged over to LTx, and one of two others with ACLF who were not eligible for transplant survived. Two patients with primary non-function of their liver grafts were bridged over to re-transplant. Overall treatment time varied between 7 and 144 h. No adverse events were noted. Neurological improvement, as well as some improvement of renal function and coagulation status, was observed. The Berlin group has also been working on a hybrid liver support system with extracorporeal plasma separation and perfusion through a bioreactor using 500 g of primary porcine hepatocytes from specific pathogen-free pigs. Results in a group of seven ALF patients (with grade 2–4 encephalopathy) who were listed for LTx have recently been published.[49] After treatment for 8–46 h, all seven could be successfully bridged to LTx. Interestingly, ammonia uptake and urea synthesis by the bioreactor were observed, along with some influence on glucose metabolism. Glucose uptake by the bioreactor increased when the plasma glucose rose, while it was released when the plasma levels dropped. These fascinating results have led to a phase I trial being carried out, where eight patients with ALF were bridged to LTx using this system.[50] The treatment was found to be safe and well-tolerated. Thrombocytopenia was the only significant side effect noted. Screening of patients' sera for antibodies specific for porcine endogenous retroviruses (PERVs) showed no reactivity.

Some of the other bioartificial systems which have undergone phase I clinical trials are the "radial-flow" bioreactor (RFB, Italy)[39] device, the TECA-HALSS (China), the HBAL (China), and the BLSS (Excorp Medical, Minneapolis, MN) systems.[51]

Safety Concerns

Any extracorporeal blood purification system has potential complications associated with its use. These include problems related to catheterization and anti-coagulation, thrombocytopenia and coagulopathies, susceptibility to infections and cardiac dysrhythmias, as well as hemodynamic, metabolic, and hypothermia-related consequences of the volume of blood circulating through the extracorporeal circuit.[2,19,52]

In addition, there are specific safety concerns regarding the use of the hepatocyte component, namely immune reactions to foreign antigens, xenozoonosis, and escape of tumorigenic cells into the patient. Antibodies directed against porcine antigens are detectable in the sera of patients treated with pig hepatocyte-containing BAL.[53] However, high titers are not generated for 1 (IgM) to 3 (IgG) weeks, indicating that this would become a problem clinically only with repetitive treatments. A similar response has been observed following ex vivo cross-species liver perfusion, with, in one case, an anaphylactic reaction being seen after 16 such perfusions over 2.5 months.[54] Where the aim is to provide long-term liver support, a human hepatocyte-based BAL (or an artificial device) will need to be used.

The issue regarding xenozoonosis is more complicated. PERV is ubiquitous among bred pigs, and transmission to humans via BAL has been a persistent fear. So strong have been the objections raised that trials using these systems, while permitted in the United States, remain on hold in the United Kingdom and most parts of Europe. PERV DNA and RNA have been detected in the supernatant of pig hepatocyte culture systems.[55] In vitro studies have found that these viruses can infect human cell lines.[55–60] However, PERV transmission to humans was not demonstrable in in vivo studies.[61–63] A recent study also could not find any evidence of PERV infection, using reverse transcriptase polymerase chain reaction, 6 months after BAL treatment.[43] The low membrane cut-off probably filters off any viable virus particles which might be present. Nyberg et al. have shown that a pore size of 5 nm (corresponding to a cut-off of 50–100 kDa) prevents PERV infection in human cells for 7 days[59] (while treatments are meant to last for not more than 1 day). Although the threat of PERV will probably not translate into reality, there might, quite conceivably, be other unknown viruses posing a greater threat.

The escape of tumorigenic cells from the human hepatoblastoma cell line is a potential hazard in the ELAD system. However, the addition of downstream cell filters to remove immortalized cells from the circulating fluid is generally regarded as being an adequate safety measure against seeding.

Artificial Extracorporeal Systems

The safety concerns and the high costs associated with hepatocyte-containing devices have led to a renewed interest in artificial liver support devices. The main difference in the newer systems is an increased selectivity of the detoxifying capacity, based on the removal of albumin-bound toxins.

The Importance of Albumin

The mechanisms underlying the development of the multi-organ dysfunction of liver failure are, as yet, poorly understood. The toxin hypothesis" implicates a variety of toxins which accumulate as a result of impaired hepatic metabolism/detoxification. Ammonia, protein breakdown products (aromatic amino acids, tryptophan, indole, mercaptan, phenol), and endogenous benzodiazepines, among others, are implicated in the development of hepatic encephalopathy. Nitric oxide (NO) and prostanoids are believed to be important in the pathogenesis of circulatory and renal dysfunction. Pro-inflammatory cytokines probably have wide-ranging influences, and oxidative stress has effects ranging from increased capillary permeability to modulating cell death.[6] However, the vast majority of these toxins (except possibly ammonia) are water-insoluble and albumin-bound (Table 4-1), and conventional renal replacement therapy cannot effectively remove them.

Intravenous albumin administration is of benefit in the treatment of patients with cirrhosis,[64–66] and improves survival in those with spontaneous bacterial peritonitis[67] or with hepatorenal syndrome,[68], [69] but the benefits exceed what could have been expected if it was acting simply as a volume expander. Indeed, it has been suggested that albumin is an important molecule involved in detoxification and binds various substances[70] and is perhaps more important in liver diseases than was previously thought.[71] This is the basis for the use of albumin as a binding and scavenging molecule in devices based on albumin dialysis or fractionated plasma separation and adsorption (FPSA), and therefore the trial of such devices in patients with liver failure.

Design of Devices

Molecular Adsorbents Recirculating System (MARS)

The first of the newer artificial liver support devices was based on the use of albumin dialysis with a membrane having a sufficiently small pore size. This makes the system specific for albumin-bound substances, which form the majority of the toxins accumulating in liver failure[72] (Table 4-1). At the same time, larger molecules (immunoglobulins, growth factors) which might be physiologically important are prevented from crossing over, thus eliminating one of the main problems with the earlier devices.[17,18]

MARS (Gambro AB, Lund, Sweden),[73,74] which has been developed over the last decade, is currently under extensive investigation and clinical trial. This uses a hollow fiber dialysis module where the patient's blood is dialyzed across an albumin-impregnated polysulfone membrane (with a cut-off of 50 kDa), while maintaining a constant flow of 20% albumin as dialysate in the extracapillary compartment (Figure 4-3). The premise is that toxins bound to albumin in the patient's blood will detach and bind to the binding sites on the membrane, as albumin, when attached to polymers, have a higher affinity for albumin-bound toxins.[75] These then pass on to the albumin in the dialysate (where albumin is present at a concentration (200 g/l) five to seven times that in the plasma). The dialysate, carrying a quantity of toxins, is then cleansed by perfusing over activated charcoal and anion-exchange resin. These take up most of the albumin-bound substances. Water-soluble toxins are removed by passage through a hemodialysis/hemofiltration module, which is run in conjunction with the albumin dialysis module. The dialysate is thus regenerated and once more capable of taking up more toxins from the blood. This recirculation component of the MARS system, using a fixed volume (600 ml) of albumin, is considerably more cost-effective than a single-pass albumin dialysis system would be.

Early in vitro studies showed that this method resulted in effective removal of unconjugated bilirubin, drugs with a high protein-binding ratio (sulfobromophthalein, theophylline), and a protein-bound toxin (phenol).[73] Further studies demonstrated that the system effectively removed strongly albumin-bound toxins like unconjugated bilirubin or free fatty acids from plasma and blood in vivo as well.[76] A subsequent study[74] looked at the in vivo effect of MARS on

(a) the amino acid profile,
(b) (i) physiologically important high molecular weight proteins (albumin, α-1-glycoprotein, α-1-antitrypsine, α-2-macroglobulin, transferrin), (ii) hormone-binding proteins (thyroxine-binding globulin [TBG]), and (iii) hormone systems (thyroxine and thyroid-stimulating hormone [TSH]) (to evaluate the relative selectivity of the albumin-mediated detoxification), and
(c) albumin-bound toxic substances (bilirubin, bile acids, free fatty acids, tryptophan).

The results showed that there was an improvement of the amino acid profile, with relative clearance of the aromatic amino acids (which accumulate in hepatic insufficiency) and an improved ratio of branched chain amino acids to aromatic amino acids. There was no significant removal of the physiologically important proteins or TBG, nor was there a significant change of the thyroid hormone profile. There was, however, a significant removal of all the albumin-bound toxins, which was most effective for fatty acids, followed by bile acids, tryptophan, and bilirubin.

Single-Pass Albumin Dialysis (SPAD)

The newly developed SPAD system (Fresenius Medical Care AG, Bad Homburg, Germany) (Figure 4-4) dialyses blood/plasma against a 4.4% solution of albumin, which is disposed of after a single pass. A standard renal replacement therapy machine is used without any additional

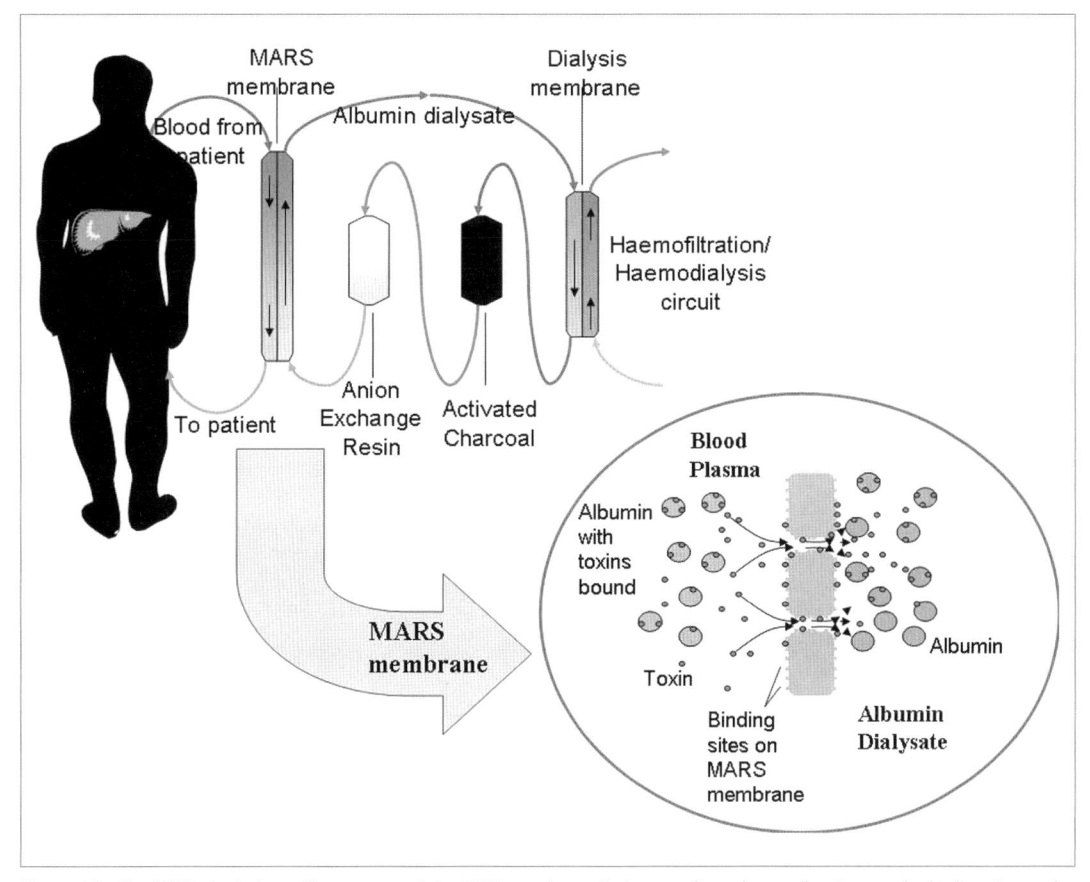

Figure 4-3. The MARS circuit. Inset: The structure of the MARS membrane. Toxins pass from plasma albumin onto the binding site on the membrane, and then to the albumin in the dialysate.

perfusion pump system, making the equipment required simpler. This fact, and the use of considerably more diluted albumin as the dialysate (4.4%, as opposed to 20% in case of MARS), offsets the cost of not recirculating the dialysate. Continuous veno-venous hemodiafiltration can be undertaken in conjunction as well. A point to note is that in MARS dialysis, the albumin dialysate is precleansed by passing through the adsorbent columns for ~30 min prior to starting treatment, potentially freeing up more binding sites on the albumin molecule. This does not occur in SPAD, which, at least theoretically, is a disadvantage.

Prometheus

The fractionated plasma separation and adsorption (FPSA)[77] system, introduced in 1999, removes albumin-bound toxins by fractionation of the plasma with the subsequent detoxification of the native albumin by adsorption. It uses an albumin-permeable membrane with a cut-off of 250 kDa. Albumin and possibly other plasma proteins with their bound toxins cross the membrane and pass through special adsorbers (one or two columns in series in the secondary circuit, containing a neutral resin adsorber and an anion exchanger) that remove the toxins. The cleansed albumin is returned to the plasma. In the commercially produced Prometheus system (Fresenius Medical Care AG, Bad Homburg, Germany)[78] (Figure 4-5) the FPSA method is combined with high-flux hemodialysis (of the blood directly, as opposed to the MARS system, where hemodialysis/filtration of the albumin dialysate is performed).

It is worthwhile noting some salient differences between FPSA and albumin dialysis. No albumin solution is required as a dialysate in FPSA. This would probably result in lower running costs. The patient's own albumin is separated from the

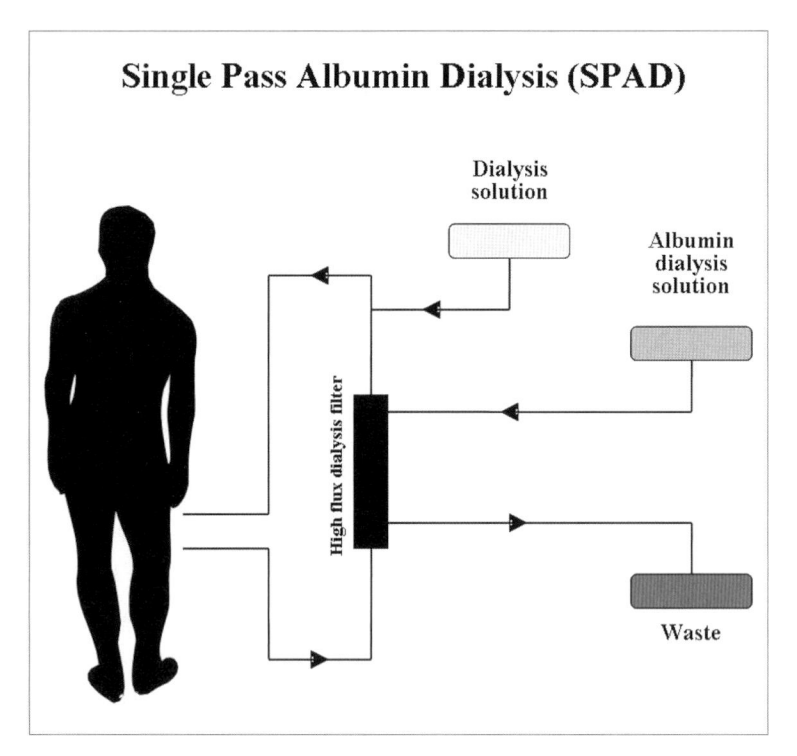

Figure 4-4. Schematic of the single-pass albumin dialysis (SPAD) system. Plasma from a reservoir is dialyzed against a 4.4% solution of albumin, which is disposed of after a single pass. A standard renal replacement therapy machine is used to run the circuit.

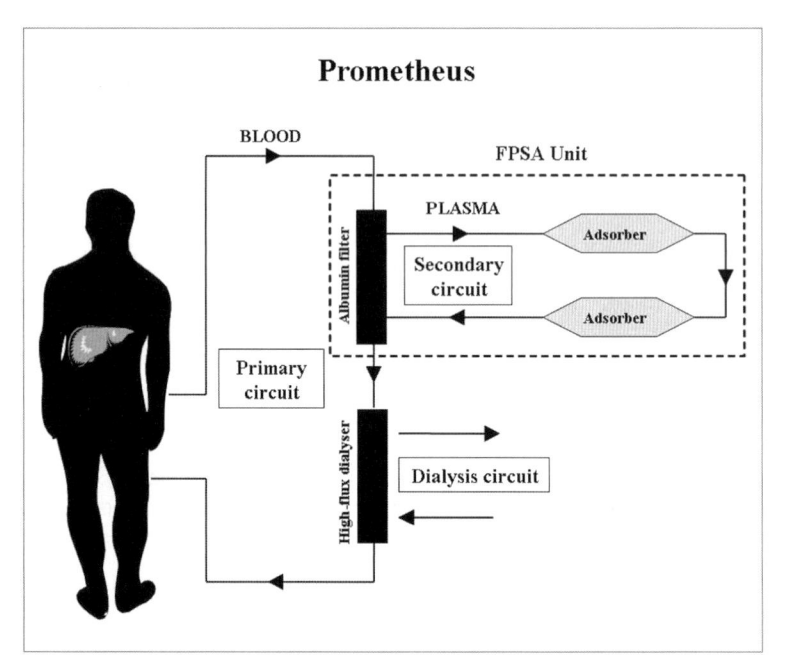

Figure 4-5. Schematic of the Prometheus circuit, utilizing the principle of fractionated plasma separation and adsorption (FPSA). The plasma is fractionated across an albumin-permeable membrane, with the subsequent detoxification of the native albumin by adsorption of bound toxins across one or two adsorber columns (containing a neutral resin adsorber and an anion exchanger) in the secondary circuit. The cleansed albumin is returned to the plasma. The reconstituted blood subsequently undergoes high-flux hemodialysis before being returned to the patient.

plasma and then detoxified in contact with adsorbent columns. This means that FPSA uses a far less selective membrane than albumin dialysis (MARS or SPAD). Loss of the patient's albumin into the circuit is a more real risk in the former compared to the latter. This also means that using potent though unselective adsorbers such as activated charcoal in FPSA (in contact with the patient's own plasma fraction, and therefore risking the possible removal of biologically useful molecules) would be far more hazardous than their use in albumin dialysis (where contact would be only with the albumin solution of the dialysate). This probably explains why charcoal, used in the earlier version of FPSA, was replaced by a neutral resin adsorber, while it continues to be used safely in MARS. Finally, while heparin continues to be used as the anti-coagulant of choice in MARS and SPAD, it seems to have resulted in clotting problems with FPSA,[78] where citrate is being looked at as an alternative.[79]

Clinical Trials

MARS

Acute-on-chronic Liver Failure (ACLF). In the initial clinical trials MARS has predominantly been evaluated in the context of ACLF, even though most studies were small and uncontrolled. Improvement of hyperbilirubinemia, HE, circulatory, and renal functions have been observed.[80–82] The improvement of HE has been associated with a reduction of serum ammonia levels, decrease of intracranial pressures, and increase of cerebral perfusion pressures.[80–83] Circulatory changes following MARS treatment have manifested in the form of increased mean arterial pressure and systemic vascular resistance and decreased cardiac output.[80,81,84,85] A recent study demonstrated clinically significant, acute reduction of portal pressure in severe alcoholic hepatitis.[86]

The largest series of patients with ACLF (n=26), with intrahepatic cholestasis (bilirubin level > 20 mg/dL), treated with MARS has been reported from Rostock.[87] The series included 10 patients with a United Network Organ Sharing (UNOS) status 2b, all of whom survived, and 16 patients with a UNOS status 2a, of whom 7 survived. Another study on patients with severe acute alcoholic hepatitis treated with MARS (n=8)[88] showed improvement of 3-month predicted mortality (pre-MARS: 76%, post-MARS: 27%), with 50% of patients (4/8) still surviving at 3 months.

The first randomized trial of MARS evaluated 13 ACLF patients with type-I hepatorenal syndrome who were treated with either MARS (n=8) or standard medical therapy including hemodiafiltration (n=5).[85] The mortality rate was 100% in the group receiving hemodiafiltration at day 7 compared with 62.5% in the MARS group at day 7 and 75% at day 30, respectively (p < 0.01). Mean survival was longer in the MARS group, which was accompanied by a significant decrease in serum bilirubin and creatinine, and increase in serum sodium and prothrombin activity. MAP at the end of treatment was significantly greater in the MARS group. Although urine output did not increase significantly in the MARS group, 4 of the 8 patients showed an increase compared with none of the control group.

A subsequent randomized controlled trial, performed in two centers (Rostock and Essen), included 24 patients with ACLF with marked hyperbilirubinemia (serum bilirubin>20 mg/dl [340 μmol/L]) who were randomized to receive standard medical therapy alone (n=12) or MARS in addition (n=12).[89] The primary end point of bilirubin <15 mg/dL for three consecutive days was reached in 5 of 12 MARS patients and in 2 of 12 control patients. Compared to controls, bilirubin, bile acids, and creatinine decreased and MAP and HE improved in the MARS group. Most importantly, albumin dialysis was associated with a significant improvement in 30-day survival (11/12 vs 6/11 in controls).

An FDA-controlled multi-center randomized trial (not yet published) on the role of MARS in advanced hepatic encephalopathy (grade III/IV) has recently been completed in 70 cirrhotic patients in the United States and Europe (reported only in abstract form).[90] MARS treatment (daily for 6 h over five consecutive days) significantly improved encephalopathy compared to standard medical therapy. The number of patients dying during the 180 days of follow-up and the number having LTx, however, were not significantly different in the two groups. Resolving coma within 5 days was shown to have a strong impact on the 2-week transplant-free survival: 81% compared with 34% in those remaining in coma (p<0.001).[91] A European multi-center randomized controlled trial evaluating the role of MARS in ACLF with mortality as the primary end point is awaiting completion.

Acute Liver Failure. In the context of ALF, no controlled studies have been performed as yet. Outcome data are available from three centers – Rome, Helsinki, and Gothenburg. Novelli et al.[92] from Rome have treated nine cases of fulminant hepatic failure. Three patients survived without requiring transplantation. The remaining six were transplanted, of whom four survived, while two died due to sepsis. The authors have extended the series to 24, in whom they report improvement of serum bilirubin, INR, and ammonia as well as neurological status (though outcome is not described).[93,94] Isoniemi[95] (Helsinki) has reported 45 cases of ALF managed with MARS; 80% of the patients survived, which is a strikingly high proportion. Native liver recovered in 23 cases, while 13 patients were transplanted successfully. Hemodynamic and neurological improvements were noted following MARS therapy in most cases. While these results are quite encouraging, especially in those with a toxic etiology, it is to be noted that at least in some of these cases MARS was started before the development of encephalopathy, and in the absence of matched controls such improvement is difficult to interpret. Felldin et al. (Gothenburg) describe 10 patients of ALF treated with MARS, of whom 7 survived. Beneficial effect was most evident in those who received 5 or more sessions of treatment (4/5 survivors).[96,97]

Among other studies, one has described improvement in encephalopathy, a reduction of cerebral edema and intracranial pressure, with increase of cerebral perfusion pressure in three ALF patients treated with MARS.[98] A recent small randomized controlled study in patients with hyperacute liver failure found that a single session of MARS treatment (n=8) improved systemic hemodynamics (mean arterial pressure, systemic vascular resistance, and cardiac output) compared to controls (n=5), who had only been mechanically cooled to match the MARS group.[99] A phase I trial from the United States evaluated a slightly modified system using continuous albumin dialysis with continuous hemodiafiltration in nine ALF patients (UNOS status 1: 5; status 2a: 4).[100] Of those with status 1, one recovered native hepatic function while three were bridged to transplantation.

Two recent studies have reported the use of MARS in ALF related to hepatitis B. A Chinese series describes ten such patients, of whom one was successfully bridged to LTx and three were alive at 3-month follow-up.[101] Hemodynamic, neurological, and biochemical improvements were noted. An Italian series describes MARS treatment in five patients of hepatitis B-related ALF in lymphoma patients undergoing chemotherapy.[102] Three were alive at 1-year follow-up, while MARS was thought to have been commenced too late in the two who died.

A recent report describes the interim analysis on the first 27 patients included in a randomized controlled single-center trial evaluating MARS in hypoxic liver failure due to cardiogenic shock following cardiac surgery.[103] Seven out of 14 patients (50%) in the MARS group survived, compared to 4 out of 13 (32%) in the non-MARS group. No significant difference in survival was found. A full report is awaited.

There are also individual case reports of the use of MARS (n=4)[104–106] or albumin dialysis (n=1)[107] to treat Wilson's disease with ALF (grade 3–4 encephalopathy, oligo-anuria, coagulopathy), all of whom were successfully bridged to transplantation after a period ranging from 9 to 59 days. MARS has also been used to treat ALF due to paracetamol overdose (n=3)[104,108,109] and mushroom intoxication (n=3),[104,110,111] where all survived without requiring transplantation, while a case of acute Budd–Chiari syndrome died in spite of MARS and transplantation.[104] A series of five MARS-treated paracetamol overdose patients report survival in four, with one patient dying of brain edema.[112]

Other Indications. Results with MARS in the treatment of primary graft dysfunction following liver transplantation are limited. One study[113] reported six such patients (primary non-function: n=4, delayed non-function: n=2), where MARS treatment led to a recovery in five cases, eliminating the need for re-transplantation. The sixth patient died. Another study[104] reported two patients of liver failure following transplantation, one due to primary non-function and the other due to severe graft dysfunction, both of whom were bridged to re-transplantation with MARS. The former died following sepsis, while the latter survived. Data available from four other centers describe eight cases of primary graft dysfunction treated with MARS, of whom three recovered and four were successfully bridged to re-transplantation.[114]

There have been reports of the use of MARS for the treatment of liver failure following hepatic resection (n=7),[104,115–117] but only one such patient survived.[104] There have also been anecdotal reports of the use of MARS in progressive intrahepatic cholestasis due to chronic graft-versus-host disease (n=1),[118] and in patients with heart failure, complicated by liver failure, awaiting heart transplantation.[119]

Newer Indications. Over the last 3 years, two new clinical indications for the use of MARS therapy appear to be emerging. Intrahepatic cholestasis with intractable pruritus can be an extremely debilitating condition, severely impairing the patient's quality of life. Therapeutic options are limited for cases which fail to respond to currently available medications. In this setting, MARS has given a rapid, significant, and reasonably well-sustained response.[120–122] Mullhaupt et al. described rapid resolution of pruritus following a single session of MARS in a patient with primary biliary cirrhosis, but with recurrence of symptoms within 5 days.[121] Macia et al. described a similar improvement with MARS in two patients with primary biliary cirrhosis and one patient with post-transplantation biliary stenosis, with the effect persisting for 3–8 weeks.[123] In one of these patients, out-patient follow-up with a MARS session every few months (after the initial therapy) was successful in achieving long-term improvement. Doria et al. reported three patients with hepatitis C-virus-related intractable pruritus, treated with seven sessions of MARS, where an improvement persisting for several months was noted.[122] Bellmann et al. recently described seven patients with post-transplantation intractable pruritus who were treated with three consecutive sessions of MARS.[124] Six patients responded, and the improvement was sustained for >3 months in three of them. The last two studies also demonstrated an associated reduction of serum bile acids, implicating this as a potential mechanism of the response. However, removal of plasma opioids such as met-enkephalins[125] may be responsible as well.

The other emerging indication for MARS therapy is in the setting of overdose/toxicity with protein-bound, especially albumin-bound, substances which are often non-dialyzable. We have reported the rapid clinical improvement following a single MARS session of a patient with phenytoin toxicity, associated with a linear rapid reduction of both total and free plasma phenytoin levels.[126] This observation was taken further in a subsequent study in an animal model of ALF, where we determined whether this detoxifying capacity was restricted to only albumin-bound substances or could be generalized to substances bound to other proteins as well.[127] The results demonstrated that fentanyl (85% bound to α-1-acid glycoprotein in the plasma) was removed as efficiently by MARS as midazolam (97% bound to albumin). These data provide the rationale to explore the role of MARS in the treatment of toxicities with a variety of protein-bound non-dialyzable substances.

Pathophysiological Basis. The pathophysiological basis of the development of the clinical manifestations of ACLF is only poorly understood. Similarly, very little is known about the mechanisms underlying the observed clinical improvements following MARS therapy. The improvement in HE may be due to the associated significant reduction of serum ammonia levels,[80–82] as a result of direct removal by the MARS system.[128] Another possible explanation might be a favorable alteration of the amino acids profile, with relative clearance of aromatic amino acids, as had been observed in the early in vivo studies.[74] A reduction of plasma nitrates and nitrites following MARS, probably due to direct removal by the system,[128] may contribute to the improvement of the circulatory status. Whether production of nitric oxide is altered as well following therapy is as yet not known. This systemic hemodynamic improvement may, at least in part, be responsible for the associated improvement of renal function. An alteration in the profile of inflammatory mediators and cytokines, either by removal by the MARS circuit or by altered production due to an "improved" internal environment following blood purification by MARS, might conceivably have a role to play. Preliminary data from one study failed to show any change of plasma levels of tumor necrosis factor (TNF)-α or its receptors following MARS treatment, in spite of their detection in the dialysate in fairly considerable amounts, indicating removal of these substances across the membrane.[128]

SPAD

In vitro studies suggest that its detoxifying capacity is similar to or even greater than (especially with regard to bilirubin and ammonia clearance) that of MARS.[129] However, would these results hold up in vivo too? As of now, there are only a few reports of its clinical use. One was a case of fulminant Wilson's disease, where it was found to efficiently clear bilirubin and copper, both protein-bound, from the plasma.[107] Subsequently, three cirrhotic patients were treated long term, resulting in two successful transplantations and one patient dying from sepsis after

140 days.[130] There is another case report of a successful short-term bridging to LTx from Berlin.[131]

Prometheus

Since Prometheus was first used successfully in a young patient with ALF and multi-organ failure due to ecstasy and cocaine intoxication (who was deemed ineligible for LTx),[132] more clinical data have emerged. The results of Prometheus treatment in 11 patients with ACLF and accompanying renal failure have been published.[78] Improvement of serum levels of conjugated bilirubin, bile acids, ammonia, cholinesterase, creatinine, urea, and blood pH occurred. A drop in blood pressure in two patients and uncontrolled bleeding in one patient were the adverse events noted. Another randomized cross-over study compared alternating treatments with MARS and Prometheus in eight patients with ACLF. Reduction ratios of both bilirubin and urea were more with Prometheus. Their safety profiles were found to be comparable.[133] In another study, the removal capacity and selectivity of the Prometheus system was evaluated in a clinical trial on nine patients of ACLF.[134] Levels of endogenous toxins (urea nitrogen, creatinine, total bilirubin, and bile acids) were found to decrease significantly. A subsequent report by the same group reported toxin removal in ACLF by Prometheus (n=9) to be more effective compared to that by MARS (n=9).[135] Prospective controlled trials are planned for the future.

Safety Profile

The safety of the MARS device has been evaluated through its use in over 3000 patients worldwide. The MARS Registry, which is maintained by the University of Rostock, contains data on about 500 patients treated with this device.[136,137] In general, the treatment is well tolerated and the only consistent adverse finding with the use of MARS is thrombocytopenia. Critical analysis of the data from the Registry in patients with ACLF suggests that its use should be contraindicated in those with established disseminated intravascular coagulation (DIC) or in those patients with "incipient" DIC characterized by progressive thrombocytopenia ($< 50 \times 10^9$/L) and/or coagulopathy (INR > 2.3). Another factor found in the interim analysis of the first multi-center European clinical trial in ACLF patients is the adverse influence on outcome of already established renal support.

The initial pilot trial looking at the safety of the Prometheus system found it to be generally safe and well tolerated.[78] A drop in blood pressure in two patients and uncontrolled bleeding in one patient were the adverse events noted. In general, a significant drop in mean arterial pressure was noted during Prometheus treatment, which returned to the pre-treatment levels by the following day. This might be related to the larger extracorporeal blood and plasma volume for Prometheus (because of the additional plasma volume in the secondary circuit) compared to either MARS or SPAD. A reversible increase of white cells (though no other signs of systemic inflammation), possible due to transient leukocyte activation by the membrane, was noted too. However, no case of thrombocytopenia (as has sometimes been seen with MARS therapy) was observed. Finally, heparin, which remains the anti-coagulant of choice in MARS and SPAD, seems to have resulted in clotting problems with Prometheus,[78] where citrate is being looked at as an alternative.[79]

Conclusion

Most of the benefits observed with liver support in the setting of ALF have been in the form of successful bridging to transplantation, rather than recovery of the native liver. The latter has been relatively more often achieved only in studies on patients with ACLF. While most studies with hybrid bioartificial systems have demonstrated their immediate safety, concerns persist, particularly regarding the acquisition of retroviral infections when porcine hepatocyte modules are used. The complexity of the circuits and the high costs involved inevitably will be a limiting factor to their use. Artificial systems are simpler, safer, and cheaper. The data supporting their use in ACLF are encouraging. However, only when a carefully conducted controlled clinical trial has shown proven benefit, including survival, can we be certain of its value, whatever the efficacy of toxin removal.

The difficulties in showing such a benefit with a controlled trial in ALF have already been referred to. LTx has a major influence on survival in the most severe group of cases, and the timing of it is inevitably going to differ from case to case and from center to center depending on the availability of organs. One group of patients that could be utilized for future trials in ALF would be patients who are early in the course of their disease, in whom subsequent improvement or deterioration can be correlated with the requirement for LTx as the primary end point. The main difficulty with such a trial is in setting the selection criteria for inclusion so that mortality is still sufficiently high in the control group for a benefit to be shown. Another category of ALF patients who could be studied are those who fulfill criteria for LTx, but who because of co-morbidity or other reasons are considered unsuitable for it. ALF from paracetamol hepatotoxicity has a different clinical course with lower requirement for LTx and higher incidence of spontaneous recovery than ALF due to other etiologies, and probably merits a separate and specifically designed trial, taking into account the percentage of cases that do go downhill rapidly. Whatever the inclusion criteria and design of the trial in ALF, the patients must be stratified for etiology, age, and rapidity of onset of encephalopathy.

As regards the setting of ACLF, well-designed controlled trials (especially with MARS) with survival as the primary end point have already been set up. The main point to note is that quite large numbers of patients (about 150–200) would need to be included for the trials to be adequately powered. This implies that these logistically complex studies need to be carried out in multiple centers while at the same time maintaining the basic homogeneity of the trial – which in practice can be more daunting than they would appear in theory.

As for the devices themselves, what of the future? While the search for an effective liver support system remains the Holy Grail for researchers in this area, the value of the present systems, whether hybrid bioartificial or entirely artificial, is still far from certain. What still remains a puzzle with the bioartificial devices is the lack of major discernible synthetic effect from the biological component. Further work on what underlies the improvement in consciousness levels with BAL, as well as of the various beneficial effects reported with MARS, is clearly essential. The shortage of human hepatocytes for use in BAL could be solved by the use of stem cells, especially hemopoietic stem cells, induced to differentiate into mature functional hepatocytes.[138] Reversible immortalization of tumorigenic human cell lines using the Cre-Lox genetic engineering system, with excision of the immortalizing gene, thus removing the threat of tumorigenesis,[139] is another approach which has already been tested experimentally. The viability and functional capacity of hepatocytes[138] has been shown to be improved by co-culture with non-hepatocytic/endothelial cells, and their presence would also help through the scavenging functions of the endothelial cells.[140] As to the improvement in the design of bioreactors, better provision for the functions of bile excretion could be of benefit. Interestingly, it has recently been reported that bile duct-like structures form in cultures of bile epithelial cells.[141,142] But all these possible developments will add even further to the complexity (and costs) of the hybrid bioartificial devices. As to improvements for the artificial devices like MARS, additional adsorption columns for removal of specific toxins, like copper for acute Wilson's disease, and modification to the membrane and its albumin impregnation so as to decrease quantities of albumin required and increase transport efficiency would be worthwhile. SPAD and FPSA are variations of these devices which are already being tested. Which of these systems will ultimately stand the test of time? Only the future will tell.

References

1. Sen S, Williams R, Jalan R. The pathophysiological basis of acute-on-chronic liver failure. *Liver*. 2002;22(Suppl 2):5–13.
2. Stockmann HB, IJzermans JN. Prospects for the temporary treatment of acute liver failure. *Eur J Gastroenterol Hepatol*. 2002;14:195–203.
3. www.optn.org.
4. Miwa S, Hashikura Y, Mita A, Kubota T, Chisuwa H, Nakazawa Y, Ikegami T, Terada M, Miyagawa S, Kawasaki S. Living-related liver transplantation for patients with fulminant and subfulminant hepatic failure. *Hepatology*. 1999;30:1521–6.
5. Baker A, Dhawan A, Devlin J, Mieli-Vergani G, O' Grady J, Williams R, Rela M, Heaton N. Assessment of potential donors for living related liver transplantation. *Br J Surg*. 1999;86:200–5.
6. Sen S, Williams R, Jalan R. The pathophysiological basis of acute-on-chronic liver failure. *Liver*. 2002;22(Suppl 2):5–13.
7. Williams R. The elusive goal of liver support–quest for the Holy Grail. *Clin Med*. 2006;6:482–7.

8. Abouna GM. Cross-circulation between man and baboon in hepatic coma. *Lancet.* 1968;2:729–30.
9. Motin J, Bouletreau P, Petit P, Latarjet J. [Hepatic assistance by means of inter-human cross circulation. Apropos of 6 cases]. *Minerva Chir.* 1974;29:989–93.
10. Abouna GM, Garry R, Hull C, Kirkley J, Walder DN. Pig-liver perfusion in hepatic coma. *Lancet.* 1968;2:509–10.
11. Ranek L, Hansen RI, Hilden M, Ramsoe K, Schmidt A, Winkler K, Tygstrup N. Pig liver perfusion in the treatment of acute hepatic failure. *Scand J Gastroenterol.* 1971;9:161–9.
12. Graw RG, Jr., Buckner CD, Eisel R. Plasma exchange transfusion for hepatic coma. *New technic Transfusion.* 1970;10:26–32.
13. Larsen FS, Hansen BA, Jorgensen LG, Secher NH, Kirkegaard P, Tygstrup N. High-volume plasmapheresis and acute liver transplantation in fulminant hepatic failure. *Transplant Proc.* 1994;26:1788.
14. Clemmesen JO, Kondrup J, Nielsen LB, Larsen FS, Ott P. Effects of high-volume plasmapheresis on ammonia, urea, and amino acids in patients with acute liver failure. *Am J Gastroenterol.* 2001;96:1217–23.
15. Clemmesen JO, Larsen FS, Ejlersen E, Schiodt FV, Ott P, Hansen BA. Haemodynamic changes after high-volume plasmapheresis in patients with chronic and acute liver failure. *Eur J Gastroenterol Hepatol.* 1997;9:55–60.
16. Larsen FS, Hansen BA, Ejlersen E, Secher NH, Clemmesen JO, Tygstrup N, Knudsen GM. Cerebral blood flow, oxygen metabolism and transcranial Doppler sonography during high-volume plasmapheresis in fulminant hepatic failure. *Eur J Gastroenterol Hepatol.* 1996;8:261–5.
17. O'Grady JG, Gimson AE, O'Brien CJ, Pucknell A, Hughes RD, Williams R. Controlled trials of charcoal hemoperfusion and prognostic factors in fulminant hepatic failure. *Gastroenterology.* 1988;94:1186–92.
18. McGuire BM, Sielaff TD, Nyberg SL, Hu MY, Cerra FB, Bloomer JR. Review of support systems used in the management of fulminant hepatic failure. *Dig Dis.* 1995;13:379–88.
19. Allen JW, Hassanein T, Bhatia SN. Advances in bioartificial liver devices. *Hepatology.* 2001;34:447–55.
20. Jauregui HO, Mullon CJ, Trenkler D, Naik S, Santangini H, Press P, Muller TE, Solomon BA. In vivo evaluation of a hollow fiber liver assist device. *Hepatology.* 1995;21:460–9.
21. Nyberg SL, Peshwa MV, Payne WD, Hu WS, Cerra FB. Evolution of the bioartificial liver: the need for randomized clinical trials. *Am J Surg.* 1993;166:512–21.
22. Sussman NL, Chong MG, Koussayer T, He DE, Shang TA, Whisennand HH, Kelly JH. Reversal of fulminant hepatic failure using an extracorporeal liver assist device. *Hepatology.* 1992;16:60–5.
23. Rozga J, Williams F, Ro MS, Neuzil DF, Giorgio TD, Backfisch G, Moscioni AD, Hakim R, Demetriou AA. Development of a bioartificial liver: properties and function of a hollow-fiber module inoculated with liver cells. *Hepatology.* 1993;17:258–65.
24. Flendrig LM, Calise F, Di Florio E, Mancini A, Ceriello A, Santaniello W, Mezza E, Sicoli F, Belleza G, Bracco A, Cozzolino S, Scala D, Mazzone M, Fattore M, Gonzales E, Chamuleau RA. Significantly improved survival time in pigs with complete liver ischemia treated with a novel bioartificial liver. *Int J Artif Organs.* 1999;22:701–9.
25. Sosef MN, Abrahamse LS, van de Kerkhove MP, Hartman R, Chamuleau RA, van Gulik TM. Assessment of the AMC-bioartificial liver in the anhepatic pig. *Transplantation.* 2002;73:204–9.
26. Arai K, Lee K, Berthiaume F, Tompkins RG, Yarmush ML. Intrahepatic amino acid and glucose metabolism in a D-galactosamine-induced rat liver failure model. *Hepatology.* 2001;34:360–71.
27. Hughes RD, Cochrane AM, Thomson AD, Murray-Lyon IM, Williams R. The cytotoxicity of plasma from patients with acute hepatic failure to isolated rabbit hepatocytes. *Br J Exp Pathol.* 1976;57:348–53.
28. Suh KS, Lilja H, Kamohara Y, Eguchi S, Arkadopoulos N, Neuman T, Demetriou AA, Rozga J. Bioartificial liver treatment in rats with fulminant hepatic failure: effect on DNA-binding activity of liver-enriched and growth-associated transcription factors. *J Surg Res.* 1999;85:243–50.
29. Strain AJ, Neuberger JM. A bioartificial liver–state of the art. *Science.* 2002;295:1005–9.
30. Nagasue N, Yukaya H, Ogawa Y, Kohno H, Nakamura T. Human liver regeneration after major hepatic resection. A study of normal liver and livers with chronic hepatitis and cirrhosis. *Ann Surg.* 1987;206:30–9.
31. Arkadopoulos N, Lilja H, Suh KS, Demetriou AA, Rozga J. Intrasplenic transplantation of allogeneic hepatocytes prolongs survival in anhepatic rats. *Hepatology.* 1998;328:1365–70.
32. Wu L, Sun J, Wang L, Wang C, Woodman K, Koutalistras N, Horvat M, Sheil AG. Cryopreservation of primary porcine hepatocytes for use in bioartificial liver support systems. *Transplant Proc.* 2000;32:2271–2.
33. Yagi T, Hardin JA, Valenzuela YM, Miyoshi H, Gores GJ, Nyberg SL. Caspase inhibition reduces apoptotic death of cryopreserved porcine hepatocytes. *Hepatology.* 2001;33:1432–40.
34. Kono Y, Yang S, Letarte M, Roberts EA. Establishment of a human hepatocyte line derived from primary culture in a collagen gel sandwich culture system. *Exp Cell Res.* 1995;221:478–85.
35. McCloskey P, Edwards RJ, Tootle R, Selden C, Roberts E, Hodgson HJ. Resistance of three immortalized human hepatocyte cell lines to acetaminophen and N-acetyl-p-benzoquinoneimine toxicity. *J Hepatol.* 1999;31:841–51.
36. McCloskey P, Tootle R, Selden C, Larsen F, Roberts E, Hodgson HJ. Modulation of hepatocyte function in an immortalized human hepatocyte cell line following exposure to liver-failure plasma. *Artif Organs.* 2002;26:340–8.
37. Gerlach JC, Schnoy N, Encke J, Smith MD, Muller C, Neuhaus P. Improved hepatocyte in vitro maintenance in a culture model with woven multicompartment capillary systems: electron microscopy studies. *Hepatology.* 1995;22:546–52.
38. Flendrig LM, la Soe JW, Jorning GG, Steenbeek A, Karlsen OT, Bovee WM, Ladiges NC, te Velde AA, Chamuleau RA. In vitro evaluation of a novel bioreactor based on an integral oxygenator and a spirally wound nonwoven polyester matrix for hepatocyte culture as small aggregates. *J Hepatol.* 1997;26:1379–92.
39. Morsiani E, Pazzi P, Puviani AC, Brogli M, Valieri L, Gorini P, Scoletta P, Marangoni E, Ragazzi R, Azzena G, Frazzoli E, Di Luca D, Cassai E, Lombardi G, Cavallari A, Faenza S, Pasetto A, Girardis M, Jovine E, Pinna AD. Early experiences with a porcine hepatocyte-based

40. Matsumura KN, Guevara GR, Huston H, Hamilton WL, Rikimaru M, Yamasaki G, Matsumura MS. Hybrid bioartificial liver in hepatic failure: preliminary clinical report. *Surgery*. 1987;101:99–103.
41. Chen SC, Hewitt WR, Watanabe FD, Eguchi S, Kahaku E, Middleton Y, Rozga J, Demetriou AA. Clinical experience with a porcine hepatocyte-based liver support system. *Int J Artif Organs*. 1996;19:664–9.
42. Watanabe FD, Mullon CJ, Hewitt WR, Arkadopoulos N, Kahaku E, Eguchi S, Khalili T, Arnaout W, Shackleton CR, Rozga J, Solomon B, Demetriou AA. Clinical experience with a bioartificial liver in the treatment of severe liver failure. A phase I clinical trial. *Ann Surg*. 1997;225:484–91; discussion 491–4.
43. Samuel D, Ichai P, Feray C, Saliba F, Azoulay D, Arulnaden JL, Debat P, Gigou M, Adam R, Bismuth A, Castaing D, Bismuth H. Neurological improvement during bioartificial liver sessions in patients with acute liver failure awaiting transplantation. *Transplantation*. 2002;73:257–64.
44. Demetriou AA, Brown RS, Jr., Busuttil RW, Fair J, McGuire BM, Rosenthal P, Am Esch JS, 2nd, Lerut J, Nyberg SL, Salizzoni M, Fagan EA, de Hemptinne B, Broelsch CE, Muraca M, Salmeron JM, Rabkin JM, Metselaar HJ, Pratt D, De La Mata M, McChesney LP, Everson GT, Lavin PT, Stevens AC, Pitkin Z, Solomon BA. Prospective, randomized, multicenter, controlled trial of a bioartificial liver in treating acute liver failure. *Ann Surg*. 2004;239:660–7; discussion 667–70.
45. Ellis AJ, Hughes RD, Wendon JA, Dunne J, Langley PG, Kelly JH, Gislason GT, Sussman NL, Williams R. Pilot-controlled trial of the extracorporeal liver assist device in acute liver failure. *Hepatology*. 1996;24:1446–51.
46. Millis JM, Kramer DJ, O'Grady J, Heffron T, Caldwell S, Hart ME, Maguire P. Results of phase I trial of the extracorporeal liver assist device for patients with fulminant hepatic failure. *Am J Transplantation*. 2001;1(suppl 1):391.
47. van de Kerkhove MP, Di Florio E, Scuderi V, Mancini A, Belli A, Bracco A, Dauri M, Tisone G, Di Nicuolo G, Amoroso P, Spadari A, Lombardi G, Hoekstra R, Calise F, Chamuleau RA. Phase I clinical trial with the AMC-bioartificial liver. Academic Medical Center. *Int J Artif Organs*. 2002;25:950–9.
48. Sauer IM, Zeilinger K, Obermayer N, Pless G, Grunwald A, Pascher A, Mieder T, Roth S, Goetz M, Kardassis D, Mas A, Neuhaus P, Gerlach JC. Primary human liver cells as source for modular extracorporeal liver support–a preliminary report. *Int J Artif Organs*. 2002;25:1001–5.
49. Mundt A, Puhl G, Muller A, Sauer I, Muller C, Richard R, Fotopoulou C, Doll R, Gabelein G, Hohn W, Hofbauer R, Neuhaus P, Gerlach J. A method to assess biochemical activity of liver cells during clinical application of extracorporeal hybrid liver support. *Int J Artif Organs*. 2002;25:542–8.
50. Sauer IM, Kardassis D, Zeilinger K, Pascher A, Gruenwald A, Pless G, Irgang M, Kraemer M, Puhl G, Frank J, Muller AR, Steinmuller T, Denner J, Neuhaus P, Gerlach JC. Clinical extracorporeal hybrid liver support–phase I study with primary porcine liver cells. *Xenotransplantation*. 2003;10:460–9.
51. Chamuleau RA, Poyck PP, van de Kerkhove MP. Bioartificial liver: its pros and cons. *Ther Apher Dial*. 2006;10:168–74.
52. Jalan R, Williams R. Bio-artificial liver support for acute liver failure: should we be using it to treat patients? *Transplantation*. 2002;73:165–6.
53. Baquerizo A, Mhoyan A, Shirwan H, Swensson J, Busuttil RW, Demetriou AA, Cramer DV. Xenoantibody response of patients with severe acute liver failure exposed to porcine antigens following treatment with a bioartificial liver. *Transplant Proc*. 1997;29:964–5.
54. Abouna GM, Boehmig HG, Serrou B, Amemiya H, Martineau G. Long-term hepatic support by intermittent multi-species liver perfusions. *Lancet*. 1970;2:391–6.
55. Nyberg SL, Hibbs JR, Hardin JA, Germer JJ, Platt JL, Paya CV, Wiesner RH. Influence of human fulminant hepatic failure sera on endogenous retroviral expression in pig hepatocytes. *Liver Transpl*. 2000;6:76–84.
56. Patience C, Takeuchi Y, Weiss RA. Infection of human cells by an endogenous retrovirus of pigs. *Nat Med*. 1997;3:282–6.
57. Martin U, Kiessig V, Blusch JH, Haverich A, von der Helm K, Herden T, Steinhoff G. Expression of pig endogenous retrovirus by primary porcine endothelial cells and infection of human cells. *Lancet*. 1998;352:692–4.
58. Wilson CA, Wong S, Muller J, Davidson CE, Rose TM, Burd P. Type C retrovirus released from porcine primary peripheral blood mononuclear cells infects human cells. *J Virol*. 1998;72:3082–7.
59. Nyberg SL, Hibbs JR, Hardin JA, Germer JJ, Persing DH. Transfer of porcine endogenous retrovirus across hollow fiber membranes: significance to a bioartificial liver. *Transplantation*. 1999;67:1251–5.
60. Martin U, Winkler ME, Id M, Radeke H, Arseniev L, Takeuchi Y, Simon AR, Patience C, Haverich A, Steinhoff G. Productive infection of primary human endothelial cells by pig endogenous retrovirus (PERV). *Xenotransplantation*. 2000;7:138–42.
61. Heneine W, Tibell A, Switzer WM, Sandstrom P, Rosales GV, Mathews A, Korsgren O, Chapman LE, Folks TM, Groth CG. No evidence of infection with porcine endogenous retrovirus in recipients of porcine islet-cell xenografts. *Lancet*. 1998;352:695–9.
62. Paradis K, Langford G, Long Z, Heneine W, Sandstrom P, Switzer WM, Chapman LE, Lockey C, Onions D, Otto E. Search for cross-species transmission of porcine endogenous retrovirus in patients treated with living pig tissue. The XEN 111 Study Group. *Science*. 1999;285:1236–41.
63. Patience C, Patton GS, Takeuchi Y, Weiss RA, McClure MO, Rydberg L, Breimer ME. No evidence of pig DNA or retroviral infection in patients with short-term extracorporeal connection to pig kidneys. *Lancet*. 1998;352:699–701.
64. Arroyo V. Review article: albumin in the treatment of liver diseases-new features of a classical treatment. *Aliment Pharmacol Ther*. 2002;16(Suppl 5):1–5.
65. Ruiz-del-Arbol L, Monescillo A, Jimenez W, Garcia-Plaza A, Arroyo V, Rodes J. Paracentesis-induced circulatory dysfunction: mechanism and effect on hepatic hemodynamics in cirrhosis. *Gastroenterology*. 1997;113:579–86.
66. Gines A, Fernandez-Esparrach G, Monescillo A, Vila C, Domenech E, Abecasis R, Angeli P, Ruiz-Del-Arbol L, Planas R, Sola R, Gines P, Terg R, Inglada L, Vaque P, Salerno F, Vargas V, Clemente G, Quer JC, Jimenez W, Arroyo V, Rodes J. Randomized trial comparing albumin, dextran 70, and polygeline in cirrhotic patients with

67. Sort P, Navasa M, Arroyo V, Aldeguer X, Planas R, Ruiz-del-Arbol L, Castells L, Vargas V, Soriano G, Guevara M, Gines P, Rodes J. Effect of intravenous albumin on renal impairment and mortality in patients with cirrhosis and spontaneous bacterial peritonitis. *N Engl J Med.* 1999;341:403–9.
68. Duvoux C, Zanditenas D, Hezode C, Chauvat A, Monin JL, Roudot-Thoraval F, Mallat A, Dhumeaux D. Effects of noradrenalin and albumin in patients with type I hepatorenal syndrome: a pilot study. *Hepatology.* 2002;36:374–80.
69. Ortega R, Gines P, Uriz J, Cardenas A, Calahorra B, De Las Heras D, Guevara M, Bataller R, Jimenez W, Arroyo V, Rodes J. Terlipressin therapy with and without albumin for patients with hepatorenal syndrome: results of a prospective, nonrandomized study. *Hepatology.* 2002;36:941–8.
70. Curry S, Mandelkow H, Brick P, Franks N. Crystal structure of human serum albumin complexed with fatty acid reveals an asymmetric distribution of binding sites. *Nat Struct Biol.* 1998;5:827–35.
71. Evans TW. Review article: albumin as a drug-biological effects of albumin unrelated to oncotic pressure. *Aliment Pharmacol Ther.* 2002;16(Suppl 5):6–11.
72. Mitzner SR, Stange J, Klammt S, Peszynski P, Schmidt R, Noldge-Schomburg G. Extracorporeal detoxification using the molecular adsorbent recirculating system for critically ill patients with liver failure. *J Am Soc Nephrol.* 2001;12 (Suppl 17):S75–82.
73. Stange J, Ramlow W, Mitzner S, Schmidt R, Klinkmann H. Dialysis against a recycled albumin solution enables the removal of albumin-bound toxins. *Artif Organs.* 1993;17:809–13.
74. Stange J, Mitzner S. A carrier-mediated transport of toxins in a hybrid membrane. Safety barrier between a patients blood and a bioartificial liver. *Int J Artif Organs.* 1996;19:677–91.
75. Hughes R, Ton HY, Langley P, Davies M, Hanid MA, Mellon P, Silk DB, Williams R. Albumin-coated Amberlite XAD-7 resin for hemoperfusion in acute liver failure. Part II: in vivo evaluation. *Artif Organs.* 1979;3:23–6.
76. Stange J, Mitzner S, Ramlow W, Gliesche T, Hickstein H, Schmidt R. A new procedure for the removal of protein bound drugs and toxins. *Asaio J.* 1993;39:M621–5.
77. Falkenhagen D, Strobl W, Vogt G, Schrefl A, Linsberger I, Gerner FJ, Schoenhofen M. Fractionated plasma separation and adsorption system: a novel system for blood purification to remove albumin bound substances. *Artif Organs.* 1999;23:81–6.
78. Rifai K, Ernst T, Kretschmer U, Bahr MJ, Schneider A, Hafer C, Haller H, Manns MP, Fliser D. Prometheus–a new extracorporeal system for the treatment of liver failure. *J Hepatol.* 2003;39:984–90.
79. Herget-Rosenthal S, Lison C, Treichel U, et al. Citrate anticoagulated modified fractionated plasma separation and adsorption: first clinical efficacy and safety data in liver failure (Abstract). *J Am Soc Nephrol.* 2003;14:729A.
80. Mitzner SR, Klammt S, Peszynski P, Hickstein H, Korten G, Stange J, Schmidt R. Improvement of multiple organ functions in hepatorenal syndrome during albumin dialysis with the molecular adsorbent recirculating system. *Ther Apher.* 2001;5:417–22.
81. Sorkine P, Ben Abraham R, Szold O, Biderman P, Kidron A, Merchav H, Brill S, Oren R. Role of the molecular adsorbent recycling system (MARS) in the treatment of patients with acute exacerbation of chronic liver failure. *Crit Care Med.* 2001;29:1332–6.
82. Stange J, Mitzner SR, Risler T, Erley CM, Lauchart W, Goehl H, Klammt S, Peszynski P, Freytag J, Hickstein H, Lohr M, Liebe S, Schareck W, Hopt UT, Schmidt R. Molecular adsorbent recycling system (MARS): clinical results of a new membrane-based blood purification system for bioartificial liver support. *Artif Organs.* 1999;23:319–30.
83. Schmidt LE, Svendsen LB, Sorensen VR, Hansen BA, Larsen FS. Cerebral blood flow velocity increases during a single treatment with the molecular adsorbents recirculating system in patients with acute on chronic liver failure. *Liver Transpl.* 2001;7:709–12.
84. Schmidt LE, Sorensen VR, Svendsen LB, Hansen BA, Larsen FS. Hemodynamic changes during a single treatment with the molecular adsorbents recirculating system in patients with acute-on-chronic liver failure. *Liver Transpl.* 2001;7:1034–9.
85. Mitzner SR, Stange J, Klammt S, Risler T, Erley CM, Bader BD, Berger ED, Lauchart W, Peszynski P, Freytag J, Hickstein H, Loock J, Lohr JM, Liebe S, Emmrich J, Korten G, Schmidt R. Improvement of hepatorenal syndrome with extracorporeal albumin dialysis MARS: results of a prospective, randomized, controlled clinical trial. *Liver Transpl.* 2000;6:277–86.
86. Sen S, Mookerjee RP, Cheshire LM, Davies NA, Williams R, Jalan R. Albumin dialysis reduces portal pressure acutely in patients with severe alcoholic hepatitis. *J Hepatol.* 2005;43:142–8.
87. Stange J, Mitzner SR, Klammt S, Freytag J, Peszynski P, Loock J, Hickstein H, Korten G, Schmidt R, Hentschel J, Schulz M, Lohr M, Liebe S, Schareck W, Hopt UT. Liver support by extracorporeal blood purification: a clinical observation. *Liver Transpl.* 2000;6:603–13.
88. Jalan R, Sen S, Steiner C, Kapoor D, Alisa A, Williams R. Extracorporeal liver support with molecular adsorbents recirculating system in patients with severe acute alcoholic hepatitis. *J Hepatol.* 2003;38:24–31.
89. Heemann U, Treichel U, Loock J, Philipp T, Gerken G, Malago M, Klammt S, Loehr M, Liebe S, Mitzner S, Schmidt R, Stange J. Albumin dialysis in cirrhosis with superimposed acute liver injury: a prospective, controlled study. *Hepatology.* 2002;36:949–58.
90. Hassanein T, Tofteng F, Brown RSJ, McGuire BM, Lynch P, Mehta R, et al. Efficacy of albumin dialysis (MARS) in patients with cirrhosis and advanced grades of hepatic encephalopathy: a prospective, controlled, randomized multicenter trial. *Hepatology.* 2004; 40:726A–727A.
91. Stange J, Hassanein TI, Mehta R, et al. Short-term survival of patients with severe intractable hepatic encephalopathy: The role of albumin dialysis. *Hepatology.* 2005;42:286A.
92. Novelli G, Rossi M, Pretagostini R, Poli L, Novelli L, Berloco P, Ferretti G, Iappelli M, Cortesini R. MARS (Molecular Adsorbent Recirculating System): experience in 34 cases of acute liver failure. *Liver.* 2002; 22(Suppl 2):43–7.
93. Novelli G, Rossi M, Pretagostini R, Novelli L, Poli L, Ferretti G, Iappelli M, Berloco P, Cortesini R. A 3-year experience with Molecular Adsorbent Recirculating System (MARS): our results on 63 patients with hepatic failure and color Doppler US evaluation of cerebral perfusion. *Liver Int.* 2003;23(Suppl 3):10–5.

94. Novelli G, Rossi M, Pretagostini M, Pugliese F, Ruberto F, Novelli L, Nudo F, Bussotti A, Corradini S, Martelli S, Berloco PB. One hundred sixteen cases of acute liver failure treated with MARS. *Transplant Proc.* 2005;37: 2557–9.
95. Lahdenpera A, Koivusalo AM, Vakkuri A, Hockerstedt K, Isoniemi H. Value of albumin dialysis therapy in severe liver insufficiency. *Transpl Int.* 2005;17:717–23.
96. Felldin M, Friman S, Backman L, Siewert-Delle A, Henriksson BA, Larsson B, Olausson M. Treatment with the molecular adsorbent recirculating system in patients with acute liver failure. *Transplant Proc.* 2003;35:822–3.
97. Felldin M, Friman S, Olausson M, Backman L, Castedal M, Larsson B, Henriksson BA, Siewert-Delle A. [Liver dialysis using MARS in acute hepatic failure. Promising results in a pilot setting]. *Lakartidningen.* 2003;100: 3836–8, 3841.
98. Abraham RB, Szold O, Merhav H, Biderman P, Kidron A, Nakache R, Oren R, Sorkine P. Rapid resolution of brain edema and improved cerebral perfusion pressure following the molecular adsorbent recycling system in acute liver failure patients. *Transplant Proc.* 2001;33: 2897–9.
99. Schmidt LE, Wang LP, Hansen BA, Larsen FS. Systemic hemodynamic effects of treatment with the molecular adsorbents recirculating system in patients with hyperacute liver failure: A prospective controlled trial. *Liver Transpl.* 2003;9:290–7.
100. Awad SS, Swaniker F, Magee J, Punch J, Bartlett RH. Results of a phase I trial evaluating a liver support device utilizing albumin dialysis. *Surgery.* 2001;130: 354–62.
101. Tsai MH, Chen YC, Wu CS, Ho YP, Fang JT, Lien JM, Yang C, Chu YY, Liu NJ, Lin CH, Chiu CT, Chen PC. Extracorporal liver support with molecular adsorbents recirculating system in patients with hepatitis B-associated fulminant hepatic failure. *Int J Clin Pract.* 2005;59:1289–94.
102. Novelli G, Rossi M, Ferretti G, Nudo F, Bussotti A, Mennini G, Novelli L, Ferretti S, Antonellis F, Martelli S, Berloco PB. Molecular adsorbent recirculating system treatment for acute hepatic failure in patients with hepatitis B undergoing chemotherapy for non-Hodgkin's lymphoma. *Transplant Proc.* 2005;37:2560–2.
103. El Banayosy A, Kizner L, Schueler V, Bergmeier S, Cobaugh D, Koerfer R. First use of the Molecular Adsorbent Recirculating System technique on patients with hypoxic liver failure after cardiogenic shock. *Asaio J.* 2004;50:332–7.
104. Lamesch P, Jost U, Schreiter D, Scheibner L, Beier O, Fangmann J, Hauss J. Molecular adsorbant recirculating system in patients with liver failure. *Transplant Proc.* 2001;33:3480–2.
105. Manz T, Ochs A, Bisse E, Strey C, Grotz W. Liver support – a task for nephrologists? Extracorporeal treatment of a patient with fulminant Wilson crisis. *Blood Purif.* 2003;21:232–6.
106. Sen S, Felldin M, Steiner C, Larsson B, Gillett GT, Olausson M, Williams R, Jalan R. Albumin dialysis and Molecular Adsorbents Recirculating System (MARS) for acute Wilson's disease. *Liver Transpl.* 2002;8:962–7.
107. Kreymann B, Seige M, Schweigart U, Kopp KF, Classen M. Albumin dialysis: effective removal of copper in a patient with fulminant Wilson disease and successful bridging to liver transplantation: a new possibility for the elimination of protein-bound toxins. *J Hepatol.* 1999;31:1080–5.
108. McIntyre CW, Fluck RJ, Freeman JG, Lambie SH. Use of albumin dialysis in the treatment of hepatic and renal dysfunction due to paracetamol intoxication. *Nephrol Dial Transplant.* 2002;17:316–7.
109. Siewert-Delle A, Henriksson BA, Baeckmann L. Albumin dialysis with the MARS for a patient with acute liver failure due to paracetamol intoxication: a case report. *Z Gastroenterol.* 2001;39(Suppl):48.
110. Shi Y, He J, Chen S, Zhang L, Yang X, Wang Z, Wang M. MARS: optimistic therapy method in fulminant hepatic failure secondary to cytotoxic mushroom poisoning–a case report. *Liver.* 2002;22(Suppl 2):78–80.
111. Catalina MV, Nunez O, Ponferrada A, Menchen L, Matilla A, Clemente G, Banares R. [Liver failure due to mushroom poisoning: clinical course and new treatment perspectives]. *Gastroenterol Hepatol.* 2003;26: 417–20.
112. Koivusalo AM, Yildirim Y, Vakkuri A, Lindgren L, Hockerstedt K, Isoniemi H. Experience with albumin dialysis in five patients with severe overdoses of paracetamol. *Acta Anaesthesiol Scand.* 2003;47:1145–50.
113. Novelli G, Rossi M, Pretagostini R, Poli L, Peritore D, Berloco P, Di Nicuolo A, Iappelli M, Cortesini R. Use of MARS in the treatment of acute liver failure: preliminary monocentric experience. *Transplant Proc.* 2001;33: 1942–4.
114. Stange J, Hassanein TI, Mehta R, Mitzner SR, Bartlett RH. The molecular adsorbents recycling system as a liver support system based on albumin dialysis: a summary of preclinical investigations, prospective, randomized, controlled clinical trial, and clinical experience from 19 centers. *Artif Organs.* 2002;26:103–10.
115. Kellersmann R, Gassel HJ, Buhler C, Thiede A, Timmermann W. Application of Molecular Adsorbent Recirculating System in patients with severe liver failure after hepatic resection or transplantation: initial single-centre experiences. *Liver.* 2002;22(Suppl 2):56–8.
116. Mullhaupt B, Kullak-Ublick GA, Ambuhl P, Maggiorini M, Stocker R, Kadry Z, Clavien PA, Renner EL. First clinical experience with Molecular Adsorbent Recirculating System (MARS) in six patients with severe acute on chronic liver failure. *Liver.* 2002;22(Suppl 2):59–62.
117. Delafosse B, Garnier E, Dumortier J, Boillot O. Edouard Herriot experience with the MARS in 5 patients experiencing hepatic failure. *Z Gastroenterol.* 2001;39:38.
118. Sen S, Jalan R, Morris EC, Steiner C, Mackinnon S, Williams R. Reversal of severe cholestasis caused by chronic graft-versus-host disease with the MARS liver-support device. *Transplantation.* 2003;75: 1766–7.
119. Notohamiprodjo M, Banayosy A, Kizner L, Schuller V, Korfer R. One year experience with MARS therapy in patients with multiorgan failure in Cardiac Center Bad Oyenhausen. *Z Gastroenterol.* 2001;39(Suppl):51.
120. Sturm E, Franssen CF, Gouw A, Staels B, Boverhof R, De Knegt RJ, Stellaard F, Bijleveld CM, Kuipers F. Extracorporal albumin dialysis (MARS) improves cholestasis and normalizes low apo A-I levels in a patient with benign recurrent intrahepatic cholestasis (BRIC). *Liver.* 2002;22(Suppl 2):72–5.
121. Mullhaupt B, Kullak-Ublick GA, Ambuhl PM, Stocker R, Renner EL. Successful use of the Molecular

Adsorbent Recirculating System (MARS) in a patient with primary biliary cirrhosis (PBC) and treatment refractory pruritus. *Hepatol Res.* 2003;25:442–446.
122. Doria C, Mandala L, Smith J, Vitale CH, Lauro A, Gruttadauria S, Marino IR, Foglieni CS, Magnone M, Scott VL. Effect of molecular adsorbent recirculating system in hepatitis C virus-related intractable pruritus. *Liver Transpl.* 2003;9:437–43.
123. Macia M, Aviles J, Navarro J, Morales S, Garcia J. Efficacy of molecular adsorbent recirculating system for the treatment of intractable pruritus in cholestasis. *Am J Med.* 2003;114:62–4.
124. Bellmann R, Graziadei IW, Feistritzer C, Schwaighofer H, Stellaard F, Sturm E, Wiedermann CJ, Joannidis M. Treatment of refractory cholestatic pruritus after liver transplantation with albumin dialysis. *Liver Transpl.* 2004;10:107–14.
125. Mela M, Mancuso A, Burroughs AK. Review article: pruritus in cholestatic and other liver diseases. *Aliment Pharmacol Ther.* 2003;17:857–70.
126. Sen S, Ratnaraj N, Davies NA, Mookerjee RP, Cooper CE, Patsalos PN, Williams R, Jalan R. Treatment of phenytoin toxicity by the molecular adsorbents recirculating system (MARS). *Epilepsia.* 2003;44:265–7.
127. Sen S, Ytrebo LM, Rose C, Fuskevaag OM, Davies NA, Nedredal GI, Williams R, Revhaug A, Jalan R. Albumin dialysis: a new therapeutic strategy for intoxication from protein-bound drugs. *Intensive Care Med.* 2004.
128. Sen S, Davies NA, Mookerjee RP, Cheshire LM, Hodges SJ, Williams R, Jalan R. Pathophysiological effects of albumin dialysis in acute-on-chronic liver failure: A randomized controlled study. *Liver Transpl.* 2004;10: 1109–19.
129. Sauer IM, Goetz M, Steffen I, Walter G, Kehr DC, Schwartlander R, Hwang YJ, Pascher A, Gerlach JC, Neuhaus P. In vitro comparison of the molecular adsorbent recirculation system (MARS) and single-pass albumin dialysis (SPAD). *Hepatology.* 2004;39:1408–14.
130. Seige M, Kreymann B, Jeschke B, Schweigart U, Kopp KF, Classen M. Long-term treatment of patients with acute exacerbation of chronic liver failure by albumin dialysis. *Transplant Proc.* 1999;31:1371–5.
131. Sauer IM, Zeilinger K, Pless G, Kardassis D, Theruvath T, Pascher A, Goetz M, Neuhaus P, Gerlach JC. Extracorporeal liver support based on primary human liver cells and albumin dialysis–treatment of a patient with primary graft non-function. *J Hepatol.* 2003;39:649–53.
132. Kramer L, Bauer E, Schenk P, Steininger R, Vigl M, Mallek R. Successful treatment of refractory cerebral oedema in ecstasy/cocaine-induced fulminant hepatic failure using a new high-efficacy liver detoxification device (FPSA-Prometheus). *Wien Klin Wochenschr.* 2003;115:599–603.
133. Krisper P, Haditsch B, Stauber R, Jung A, Stadlbauer V, Trauner M, Holzer H, Schneditz D. In vivo quantification of liver dialysis: comparison of albumin dialysis and fractionated plasma separation. *J Hepatol.* 2005;43:451–7.
134. Evenepoel P, Laleman W, Wilmer A, Claes K, Maes B, Kuypers D, Bammens B, Nevens F, Vanrenterghem Y. Detoxifying capacity and kinetics of prometheus–a new extracorporeal system for the treatment of liver failure. *Blood Purif.* 2005;23:349–58.
135. Evenepoel P, Laleman W, Wilmer A, Claes K, Kuypers D, Bammens B, Nevens F, Vanrenterghem Y. Prometheus versus molecular adsorbents recirculating system: comparison of efficiency in two different liver detoxification devices. *Artif Organs.* 2006;30:276–84.
136. Steiner C, Zinggrebe A, Viertler A. Experiences with MARS therapy in liver disease: analysis of 385 patients of the International MARS Registry. *Hepatology.* 2003; 38:239A.
137. Sen S, Steiner C, Williams R, Jalan R. Artificial liver support: Overview of Registry and controlled clinical trials. In: Arroyo V, Forns X, Garcia-Pagan JC, Rodes J, eds. Progress in the treatment of liver diseases. Barcelona: Ars Medica; 2003:429–35.
138. Mallet VO, Mitchell C, Mezey E, Fabre M, Guidotti JE, Renia L, Coulombel L, Kahn A, Gilgenkrantz H. Bone marrow transplantation in mice leads to a minor population of hepatocytes that can be selectively amplified in vivo. *Hepatology.* 2002;35:799–804.
139. Kobayashi N, Fujiwara T, Westerman KA, Inoue Y, Sakaguchi M, Noguchi H, Miyazaki M, Cai J, Tanaka N, Fox IJ, Leboulch P. Prevention of acute liver failure in rats with reversibly immortalized human hepatocytes. *Science.* 2000;287:1258–62.
140. Seternes T, Sorensen K, Smedsrod B. Scavenger endothelial cells of vertebrates: a nonperipheral leukocyte system for high-capacity elimination of waste macromolecules. *Proc Natl Acad Sci USA.* 2002;99: 7594–7.
141. Auth MK, Joplin RE, Okamoto M, Ishida Y, McMaster P, Neuberger JM, Blaheta RA, Voit T, Strain AJ. Morphogenesis of primary human biliary epithelial cells: induction in high-density culture or by coculture with autologous human hepatocytes. *Hepatology.* 2001;33: 519–29.
142. Sirica AE, Gainey TW. A new rat bile ductular epithelial cell culture model characterized by the appearance of polarized bile ducts in vitro. *Hepatology.* 1997;26: 537–49.

Glucose Sensors and Insulin Pumps: Prospects for an Artificial Pancreas

Martin Press

Introduction

Insulin is an extraordinary hormone. When we eat, as any medical student will tell you, insulin stimulates glucose uptake into insulin-sensitive tissues (muscle, fat, liver). What they often appreciate less is that this effect requires the high insulin levels which occur only transiently after meals. When we are not eating, there is a continued need for glucose homeostasis, and insulin then, at much lower concentrations, regulates glucose production, predominantly from glycogen stores in the liver. Patients are often baffled that they can wake up with higher glucose levels than those they went to bed with despite not having eaten anything, but hepatic glucose production, regulated by insulin, is the main determinant of fasting blood glucose levels. Insulin, in effect, does the work of two hormones.

It does so by having two quite different dose–response curves in different organs (Figure 5-1). The steep part of these respective curves is seen at concentrations which are some 10-fold apart. Thus, at fasting insulin concentrations, small changes in insulin, such as are constantly seen as the pancreatic β-cells respond to minute changes in glucose concentrations, have a negligible effect on glucose uptake. However, this same fluctuation in insulin levels modulates significant changes in hepatic glucose production and is thus able to rapidly correct any tendency for glucose levels to stray outside a very narrow physiological range. Following a meal, not only is glucose uptake stimulated, but hepatic glucose production is also almost completely suppressed.

It is not clear why it is that the liver has not evolved to be able to measure glucose levels itself and has to rely on the pancreatic β-cells to 'tell' it how much glucose to produce. So long as the pancreatic β-cells are working well it presents no problems. But if a diabetic patient gives himself too much insulin, the resultant high-circulating insulin levels are read by the liver as the signal that glucose levels are too high and hepatic glucose production promptly falls, resulting in hypoglycemia. Conversely, insulin deficiency as a result of pancreatic β-cell failure is the signal to the liver that glucose levels are low, with the result that hepatic glucose production increases inappropriately. In the extreme situation of diabetic ketoacidosis, when the pancreatic β-cells fail completely, the liver is pouring glucose into the circulation to try to correct a non-existent state of hypoglycemia.

Conventional Insulin Treatment

In vivo, insulin is secreted in pulses every 10–15 min. Given that the half life of insulin in the circulation is less than 5 min, this results in wide short-term variation in insulin concentrations which enables minute-to-minute regulation of blood glucose levels. While the replacement of other endocrine hormones with long half lives, such as thyroxine, does not present a great clinical problem, the idea of replacing a hormone such as insulin whose concentrations are constantly changing is another matter altogether and indeed it is amazing that in patients with Type 1 diabetes we manage as well as we do with just a few injections a day.

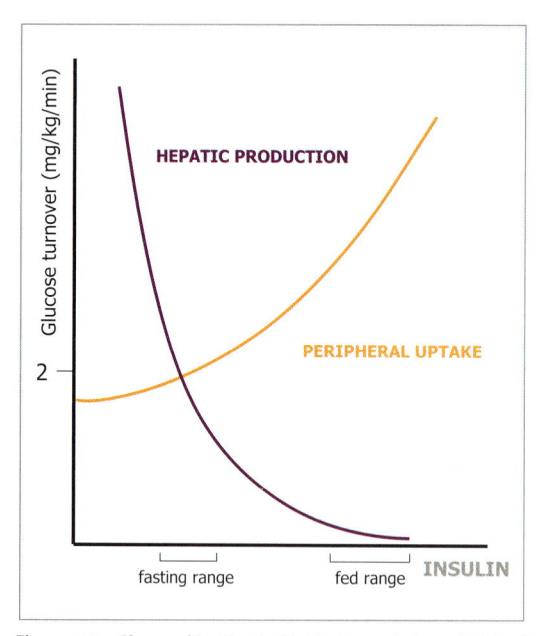

Figure 5-1. Glucose kinetics (with kind permission of Oxford University Press). Glucose uptake is stimulated by insulin, but only at the elevated concentrations seen after meals. At low insulin levels, glucose uptake is not zero because of insulin-independent uptake by tissues such as the brain, in particular. Glucose production, in contrast, is regulated at the low insulin levels typically seen in the fasting state, in which glucose production is the main determinant of fasting glucose levels.

Traditional insulin therapy has in the past involved relatively 'dirty' insulin preparations, purified from animal pancreases. When insulin was first introduced into clinical practice in the 1920s this did not matter as the impressive point was that one was preventing what would otherwise be inevitable death from diabetic ketoacidosis. However, the impure insulin preparations extracted from animal pancreases elicit an immunological response which involves insulin antibodies which tend to buffer sudden changes in insulin concentrations and may cause immunological reactions at the injection sites. With the appreciation that a more sophisticated approach was necessary in order to achieve adequate metabolic control to prevent diabetic complications and optimize quality of life, the shortcomings of the old insulin preparations became even more apparent.

In the 1970s, so-called mono-component insulins were introduced which contained very few impurities. These were extracted from pigs, whose insulin is only 1 amino acid different from man (compared to bovine insulin, which is 3 amino acids different). As a result, they elicited less in the way of an antibody response. Since then, there has been an almost complete move toward recombinant DNA technology to synthesize insulin de novo in the laboratory. The resultant insulin is 100% pure and is identical to naturally produced human insulin. Indeed, its original marketing bore a strong resemblance to that of Coca Cola in being 'the real thing'.

Because soluble, 'regular' insulin synthesized in this way elicits little or no significant antibody response, it tends to be shorter acting than extracted insulin. However, the recombinant DNA technology has been taken one step further and, by means of substitutions, deletions, or rearrangements within the molecule, manufacturers have been able to produce insulins with even shorter durations of action. There are currently three genetically modified ultra-short acting insulins on the British market, lispro, aspart, and glulisine, each the result of different molecular modifications, but all with essentially the same pharmacokinetics.

The physiological significance of this genetic engineering is that we now have insulins whose duration of action is sufficiently short as to mimic the narrow insulin peaks secreted physiologically with meals. Soluble (regular) insulin as injected exists as a hexamer and, since it takes some 30–40 min to dissociate into monomers and enter the circulation, the injection needs to be given 30–40 min before the patient wants to eat. This causes practical problems, especially with children. Even then, the biological effect of the insulin is still not fast enough to prevent a rapid rise in blood glucose levels, so that patients have to be encouraged to eat small meals and then a snack 3 or 4 h later, when the meal has gone but the insulin is still working, if they wish to avoid hypoglycemia before the next meal.

In contrast, with ultra-short acting analogues the dissociation is so rapid that there is an almost immediate rise in circulating insulin levels and the elevation in insulin levels lasts for only 3 or 4 h. When the meal effect is gone, so is the insulin. This means that the insulin can (indeed, must) be taken immediately before the patient eats, and mid-morning, mid-afternoon, and bedtime snacks are not necessary. The patient can eat (within reason) whatever they wish and adjust the insulin dose to the carbohydrate content of the meal so that the old idea of needing to restrict carbohydrate intake has been replaced with a philosophy of learning the carbohydrate content of foods and matching insulin doses to the carbohydrate intake.

As emphasized above, these high-insulin peaks are present for only a few hours after each meal. In between meals, low levels of insulin are still necessary to regulate hepatic glucose production and maintain normoglycemia. With conventional insulin regimens, this has always proved difficult due partly to the vagaries of absorption of depot insulin preparations with marked variation from one injection to the next and partly to the fact that insulin levels following an injection inevitably peak and then wane. The latter is particularly a problem overnight when insulin requirements are typically low in the first part of the night but rise in the second part (the so-called 'dawn phenomenon'), just when the effect of an intermediate acting insulin is waning.

What is ideally required therefore, is a system of administering insulin which provides a relatively constant 'basal' infusion of insulin around the clock, with 'boluses' of insulin which are given just before the patient eats. This is what the insulin pumps currently available seek to provide. They give a constant trickle of insulin as a basal rate with extra as boluses whenever told to do so. They can be programmed to give a different basal rate at different times of the day (a higher rate from 5 am until 8 am, for example) while at the same time giving complete flexibility with respect to the number of times the patient eats and the dose of insulin needed to balance the amount of carbohydrate the meals or snacks contain. A recent study showed that metabolic control was a direct function of the number of insulin boluses given[1].

Open Loop Insulin Pumps: History

The concept of a portable pump, permanently attached to the patient and under the patient's control, was first developed in the late 1970s. The first publication on 'continuous subcutaneous insulin infusion' (CSII), by Dr John Pickup of Guy's Hospital, was published in the British Medical Journal in 1978[2] and the pump that he used is now in the Science Museum in London.

At that time, small pumps were used to give in-patients morphine or other drugs for relatively short periods of time. They were designed to be left on the bedside table. Some of the first attempts to give insulin from a portable pump involved simply strapping these same pumps to the patient's belt but they were desperately heavy and crude. Smaller, lighter pumps were rapidly developed. The first studies in England were done predominantly with the Mill Hill infuser, while those in the USA used a purpose built pump made by Auto-Syringe in New Hampshire (Figure 5-2). Dean Kamen, who dropped out of college to start Auto-Syringe in 1979, has become better known recently for inventing the Segway personal transporter, from which George Bush famously fell off. He is in the great tradition of eccentric inventors.[3] He sold Auto-Syringe after a few years to Baxter International for $30 million and, with the money, bought an island off the coast of Connecticut, declared independence from the United States and appointed the founders of Ben and Jerry's as joint Ministers of Ice Cream!

MiniMed, the company which has dominated the development of diabetes technology since their first pump was launched in 1983, was also very much associated with one particular man. Mr. Al Mann personally funded the development of insulin pumps and glucose sensors by MiniMed for 20 years and without his personal commitment it is very doubtful that an artificial pancreas would even be on the horizon at this point.

While it was the technology that grabbed the headlines, equally important was the change in mindset whereby it was left to the patient to take responsibility for their diabetes, following changes in their blood glucose levels with self-administered finger pricks and a portable glucose meter. This in turn arose from Dr Clara Lowy's study, also published in 1978,[4] on women who monitored their diabetic control during pregnancy and who, to the doctors' astonishment, chose to continue to monitor their blood glucose levels afterwards because it put them in control.

All pumps currently available commercially use broadly the same principles. Inside a case the size of a small mobile phone is a battery and a small electric motor which drives a syringe pump. This delivers a near-continuous infusion of insulin through a long tube to a plastic cannula which is inserted through the skin into subcutaneous adipose tissue. The cannula is typically changed twice a week while the insulin reservoir has to be topped up at intervals which depend on the insulin requirements of the patient.

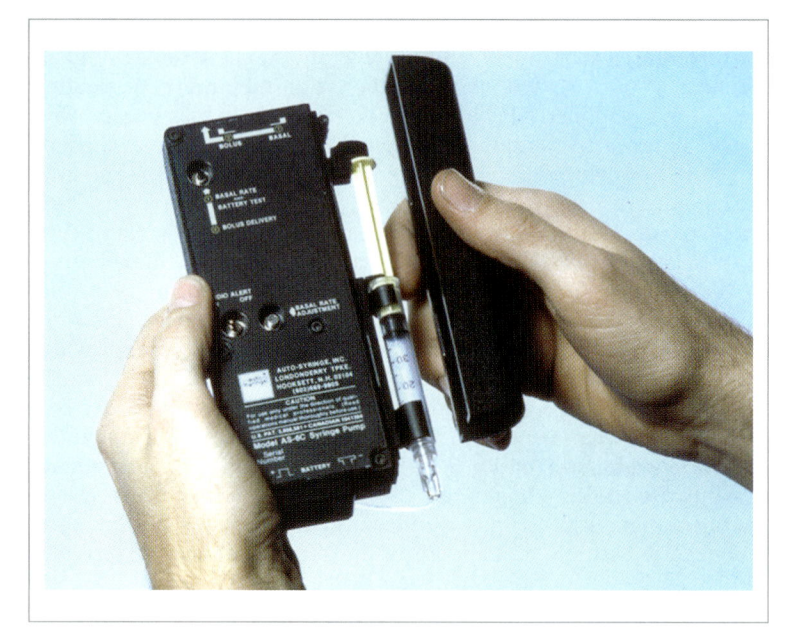

Figure 5-2. Original Auto-Syringe insulin pump, circa 1981. A small syringe filled with insulin was connected to a catheter inserted into subcutaneous fat via a fine tube. The syringe was driven by an electric motor the speed of which was dependent on the 'basal' and 'bolus' settings of the pump.

Several companies have brought insulin pumps to market over the years, and at present in Britain, there are at least four available. The original Auto-Syringe pump had only two buttons, labeled 'basal' and 'bolus' (Figure 5-2). The basal rate could be adjusted in steps of 1 unit per 24 h and it was a long time before other manufacturers offered such fine adjustment, which is necessary because the slope of the dose–response curve of glucose production versus insulin is so steep (Figure 5-1). Other aspects of pump development consisted largely of improved safety features and more sophisticated programmes for varying the shape and duration of bolus delivery. Roche offers the improved convenience of prefilled insulin syringes. Most centers now use ultra-short acting insulin analogues rather than insulin itself to take advantage of the narrowness of the post-meal insulin peak and the speed with which it is possible to change effective circulating insulin levels.

Open Loop Insulin Pumps: Pros and Cons

Compared to what is now regarded as a conventional regimen of multiple daily injections (MDI), pumps have both advantages and disadvantages. Thus, there is no need with the pump to inject yourself, but on the other hand you have to replace the giving set and cannula twice a week. There is no peaking or waning of insulin effect as seen overnight and in the inter-prandial periods with conventional regimens. On the other hand, if there is an interruption in insulin supply for more than an hour or two, there is rapid metabolic decompensation leading to hyperglycemia and ketosis since there is no subcutaneous insulin reserve.

Most studies comparing CSII and MDI have described either a reduction in glycated hemoglobin without a corresponding increase in the incidence of hypoglycemia or a reduction in hypoglycemia without a concomitant rise in HbA_{1c}.[5] However, to most patients on an insulin pump, the major advantage relates to flexibility and issues of lifestyle and quality of life rather than directly to the diabetic control itself.

Although CSII offers the convenience of being able to programme the pump to allow for reproducible fluctuations in insulin sensitivity, most centers start with a single daily basal rate, which is typically some 20–30% less than the patient has previously been receiving from their long-acting insulin because of better absorption. The pump makes it possible to allow for diurnal variation in insulin sensitivity (we are most insulin resistant in the early hours of the morning as the result of growth hormone secretion during deep sleep in the early part of the night). Disetronic (since taken over by Roche) took this concept to extremes with their philosophy of programming frequent changes in basal rate around the clock to match changes in average diurnal insulin sensitivity. This approach failed to take into account the fact that everyone is different and no one exactly follows the average. In practice, a single 24 h constant basal rate usually works surprisingly well and in order to do better, there is no alternative but to work out an individualized programme of basal rates for each patient. Even then, the necessary diurnal changes in basal rates vary from one day to another in a given patient, which is why perfect control is not attainable with an open loop system.

Overnight basal rates are adjusted to give satisfactory mean fasting glucose levels. So long as there is no mid-morning snack, morning basal levels are adjusted according to pre-lunch glucose levels and so on. Some centers omit the previous meal and meal bolus to adjust the basal rate but this may change insulin sensitivity and gives the whole procedure a spurious accuracy. Patients are not machines and do not give exactly the same results if tested more than once.

Meal boluses are calculated on the basis of meal carbohydrate content and we are not the only unit to have obtained excellent results by giving patients an intensive educational course, modeled on the principles of DAFNE (Dosage Adjustment For Normal Eating) and BERTIE (Bournemouth's Education Resources for Training in Insulin and Eating), to teach them to estimate the doses they are likely to need for a particular meal.

Just as with the basal rates, it is necessary to modify and adapt the formula used to calculate meal boluses in a particular patient. Thus, for example, the patient may start with, say, 1 unit per 10 g carbohydrate ingested and increase or decrease this as necessary according to their response. Sometimes it may be necessary to vary the ratio to allow for fluctuations in diurnal insulin sensitivity. Thus, for example, if they eat 60 g of carbohydrate for both breakfast and lunch, many patients find that while 6 units of insulin will be sufficient at lunchtime, they may need 7 or 8 units to cover breakfast. This may also reflect some 'carry-over' of insulin from the breakfast dose. Supper usually needs more insulin in any case because for most patients it is the biggest meal of the day.

The real beauty of the pump, however, is that it gives such great flexibility with respect to the timing and amount of meals. With a conventional insulin regimen, once the insulin injection has been given, one has to eat to match the insulin or risk hypoglycemia. Conversely, if one eats more than one had intended when the injection was given, one has to either accept that glucose levels will run high or give oneself an extra injection. With the pump, it is perfectly possible to give a bolus to cover one's main course and only when dessert comes to decide whether to give extra insulin to cover it. Extra small boluses of insulin to cover between-meal snacks can be given without any problem.

When we exercise, circulating insulin levels typically fall by some 30% and this, together with an increase in glucagon, adrenaline, and growth hormone, modulates the mobilization of the necessary metabolic fuels. In patients with Type 1 diabetes, there is no way of reducing insulin levels, which are determined by the previous injection of insulin, except with the pump. As alluded to above, the lack of a subcutaneous insulin reservoir is a drawback if the insulin supply from the pump is interrupted, with one exception. This is exactly what is wanted during exercise.

Patients taking injections have little choice but to take extra sugar to prevent hypoglycemia when they exercise. However, giving sets on modern pumps have a quick release connector which allows patients to simply disconnect the pump and take it off when they exercise. If they are going to exercise for more than half an hour, they should keep the pump on but can turn the basal rate down to mimic what normal β-cells would do.

Modern 'open-loop' insulin pumps are in no sense automatic. Just as a car does not go round a corner unless you turn the steering wheel, so a pump has to be told how much insulin to give. This in turn means that the patient has to do regular finger-prick glucose estimations. Unsurprisingly, the more finger-pricks the patient does, the better the control. One of the fashionable 'tools' available to patients on pumps who are prepared to do more than the minimum number of finger-pricks is to give correction doses to bring down a high glucose level. The disadvantage of this is first that it is difficult, when giving insulin without food, not to give too much, and overshoot into hypoglycemia, and second that it tends to make patients err on the cautious side with their meal doses. One might add that it encourages patients to do 8 or 10 finger-pricks a day, which some of us might think would be spending too much time and energy on their diabetes and too little on the rest of their lives!

The latest version of Medtronic's pump incorporates a 'Bolus Wizard' to help the patient to work out how much insulin they need (Roche market a similar bolus calculator and other manufacturers are also developing 'smart pumps'). It takes into account not only what your blood sugar level is and how much carbohydrate you are planning to eat but also calculates and allows for the amount of insulin still acting in your circulation from your previous meal bolus. Many patients find this ingenious piece of software invaluable although they have to realize that the Wizard's suggested doses are no more than a recommendation and they need to have the confidence to override the suggestions when necessary. Furthermore, high postprandial glucose levels as a result of not taking enough insulin with the previous meal come down anyway, and the idea of chasing them down faster carries the danger of making the patient more neurotic about the risk to their health of a brief post-prandial peak than is appropriate. I am personally much more concerned about a high fasting glucose value because it will probably have been high all night.

There are two other drawbacks which are unique to the pump. The first is cost. Most manufacturers charge roughly £2,500 for the pump itself but on top of this is the cost of giving sets and cannulas, which comfortably add another £1,000 per year, not to mention the strips for the glucose meter for the extra finger-pricks which are necessary if one is to take full advantage of what the pump has to offer. Both the pump manufacturers and the glucose meter manufacturers, like mobile phone manufacturers, tend to give the basic equipment away quite cheaply for what it is and then make their money on the supplies, sticks, or phone calls, respectively. In Britain, recommended targets for diabetes control which made the patient eligible for reimbursement for pumps and pump supplies were published in 2003. Patients who could not achieve levels of glycated hemoglobin below 7.5% (or 6.5% if they had other cardiovascular risk factors) 'without disabling hypoglycemia' were deemed eligible. The levels chosen meant that a far higher percentage of patients with Type 1 diabetes were eligible than the 2 or 3% currently on insulin pumps in the United Kingdom. Clearly there would be very substantial implications for the health-care budget if all such patients were started on CSII.

Finally, there is the issue of visibility and body image: the concept that one is wearing a badge of illness. Even if the pump is invisible to an outsider (and there is no reason why it should not be), it is a constant reminder to the patient himself of the fact that they have a medical problem. When pumps first became available on a large scale in the United States in the early 80s, the first people to want them were, unsurprisingly, those for whom this was not a big issue and who were keen to be part of the new technological revolution. Twenty-five years later, pumps are old hat (at least the open loop pumps available commercially) and it is much more a question of the attitude of the professional group managing the patient and whether the money will be reimbursed which decides whether a given patient goes onto an insulin pump.

Some groups start patients with newly diagnosed Type 1 diabetes on pumps from the beginning, even though such patients are usually relatively easy to manage for the first year or two because they have significant residual β-cell function. The logic for this is first that this is what they are going to need in due course and the sooner they get used to the idea the better, and second, that there is evidence that diabetic control in the first years of diabetes has a disproportionate influence on the risk of complications in later years.

Open-loop pumps have advantages over multiple injections,[5] particularly in patients whose life style varies considerably from one day to the next. When we put people on pumps, we always stress that this is an experiment and that, if they do not like it, they can go back to injections without having lost anything. Very few people do. Clearly the patients who go onto pumps have been selected because we think they will suit them but in practice, once a patient has got used to being attached to a gadget 24 h a day there is rarely any looking back.

Unfortunately, even with the most highly motivated patient, it is still not possible to achieve perfect control. Blood glucose is influenced by things of which we still have little understanding so that even a patient who eats exactly the same amount of exactly the same food, and who takes exactly the same amount of exercise at the same time each day, will have different glycemic profiles from one day to the next. Instability and unpredictability are the hallmarks of Type 1 diabetes. This high variance means that attempts to achieve completely normal average glucose levels are inevitably limited by the resultant increase in the frequency of hypoglycemic episodes.

This is quite simply the nature of Type 1 diabetes and does not imply failure on the part of either the patient or the medical team. Thus, the landmark Diabetes Control and Complications Trial (DCCT), which attempted to achieve the best possible control with either pumps or multiple injections, managed only an average HbA_{1c}, reflecting the average blood glucose for the past 2 months or so, of 7%, compared to an upper limit of normal for subjects without diabetes of 6.1.[6] This was because the incidence of severe hypoglycemia (defined as requiring the intervention of others) was 62 per 100 patient years (compared to 19 in the conventionally treated control group). Thus, the markedly increased incidence of hypoglycemia prevented normalization of HbA_{1c}, and it is hardly surprising that intensive treatment, while it reduced the incidence of complications, failed to prevent them altogether.

Intraportal Insulin Delivery

In the 1990s, three manufacturers (Siemens, Infusaid, and Minimed) explored whether there were advantages to infusing the insulin into the peritoneal cavity rather than into fat. The thinking was first that this would mimic physiological delivery of insulin into the portal vein so that the liver would see much higher concentrations than other organs, and second that an artificial pancreas would probably involve a fully implanted system, so that this would be the next logical step. Both Siemens and Infusaid dropped out in the 1990s because of prohibitive development costs while MiniMed went on to do a clinical trial of a closed loop system which used an intravenous sensor and intraperitoneal insulin delivery which was abandoned after a few years because of sensor problems.

Intraperitoneal insulin delivery has one major clinical advantage, which is a much reduced risk of hypoglycemia. At the same time, it has several major disadvantages. It requires a small operation to implant the pump. The insulin reservoir has to be refilled every few months in the hospital and further surgery is needed every few years to replace the batteries. There were major problems with insulin aggregation and blockage of the catheter tube with the specially manufactured 400 U/ml insulin which was necessary, necessitating a redesign of the pump with a side-port which could be used to flush the catheter. Intraperitoneal insulin delivery is arguably the best route by which to give insulin but at present it is out of fashion because of these drawbacks and current development work on artificial pancreases is focusing on subcutaneous insulin delivery with ultra-short-acting insulin analogues.

Need for Closed Loop System

Although subcutaneous insulin infusion pumps have been available since the early 1980s, there were major issues with the development of continuous glucose sensors and they did not become commercially available until 1999. They showed vividly just how bad glucose control is in patients with Type 1 diabetes. In an unselected group of patients, Bode showed that patients with Type 1 diabetes spend only 14.5 h per day in the euglycemic range (70–180 mg/dl, 3.9–10.0 mmol/l), with 2.3 h below and 7.2 h above these limits.[7] Apart from the increased risk of complications from the hyperglycemic values, patients will feel less well as the result of the fluctuation of their glucose levels while episodes of hypoglycemia may compromise their quality of life still further.

In order to achieve near-normal glucose control, and in particular to achieve it without hypoglycemia, one needs a closed loop system whereby blood glucose levels are monitored on a minute-to-minute basis and the amount of insulin infused into the circulation is also varied on a minute-to-minute basis to keep glucose levels normal. In the fasting state, insulin levels need to change very rapidly to counter changes in glucose levels. Furthermore, immediately after meals, when large amounts of glucose enter the blood stream from the digestion of starch, the magnitude of the necessary increase in insulin levels needs to be considerable. Conversely, an immediate fall in insulin levels is necessary in response to exercise to facilitate the mobilization of metabolic fuels. All of these are of course exactly what healthy pancreatic β-cells do very effectively.

Transplants

Replacement of the β-cells is perfectly possible either by transplanting a whole pancreas or, because the patient with Type 1 diabetes needs only the β-cell containing islets, by isolating and transplanting the islets alone. Whole pancreas transplantation carries a high chance of long-term insulin independence. The operation is reserved almost exclusively for patients needing a kidney transplant for end-stage diabetic nephropathy who will require a kidney.

Pancreatic islet transplantation is less invasive since the islets comprise only some 2–3 ml and they can be transplanted without the need for surgery. However, it is not easy to isolate sufficiently large numbers of viable islets from a cadaver pancreas. To compensate for the fact that so many islets are lost during the procedure of isolation and transplantation, more than one transplant is usually necessary, making the procedure currently somewhat extravagant. Although diabetes is stabilized and serious hypoglycemia is abolished, long-term insulin independence is achieved in only a minority of patients.

Most importantly, however, the need for long-term immunosuppression, with the inevitable drug side effects and increased incidence of infections and malignancies, makes either procedure less than ideal. One is effectively exchanging one problem for another and unless the diabetes is causing major problems this exchange is not justified. Furthermore, the shortage of donor organs means that transplantation is not going to be the solution except for a small minority of patients for the foreseeable future until a source of β-cells in quantity becomes available.

Closed Loop Insulin Pumps: History

The attraction of closed loop insulin pumps is that one will in theory have the advantages of a transplant without the drawbacks. The credit for the first closed-loop insulin pumps goes to Michael Albisser in Canada[8] and Ernst-Friedrich Pfeiffer in Germany in 1974. These initial experiments led to the development of the Biostator,[9] a large and cumbersome machine suitable only for bedside use (Figure 5-3). Heparin was infused very slowly through the central lumen of a double lumen catheter inserted into an antecubital vein, while blood was withdrawn, only slightly more quickly, through the other. One was thus able to withdraw heparinized blood without anticoagulating the patient. To avoid exsanguinating the patient, the flow rate had to be very slow, which in turn introduced a significant delay to the glucose measurements.

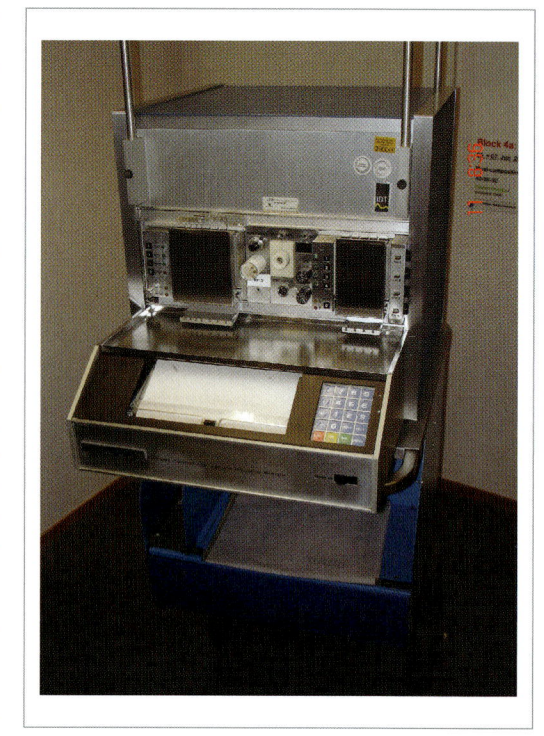

Figure 5-3. The **Biostator** dates from the mid-1970s and constituted one of the first attempts at a closed loop insulin pump. Glucose levels were measured on blood continuously withdrawn from an indwelling venous catheter. A computer with basic algorithms regulated the rate of delivery of insulin into a second catheter. Interestingly, it was the computer which was felt at the time to be the component which was unlikely ever to be miniaturized to the point at which a closed loop pump might become portable. (With kind permission of Prof Freckmann at the Institute of Diabetes Technology).

A glucose analyzer on one side of the machine contained the pump to withdraw the blood and measure glucose concentrations, while on the other side was a barely less cumbersome insulin infusion set-up. In the middle was a keyboard and what, by today's standards, was a very primitive computer. The apparatus could only be used for relatively brief acute procedures such as surgery or labor and the need to miniaturise the system was obvious. At the time, it was thought that it might be possible to miniaturise the glucose analyzer and insulin infuser, but it was felt that it would be the impossibility of miniaturizing a computer that would preclude the development of a portable artificial pancreas!

Nevertheless, when open-loop pumps came into widespread use in the early 1980s, it was widely believed that closed-loop pumps were only a matter of a few years away, and indeed the first description from Japan of a wearable closed-loop system in man in 1982[10] reinforced this belief. In that paper, the rate limiting step was perceived to be that of biocompatibility, meaning that the sensor had to be changed every few days. One felt at the time that the Japanese would soon solve the problem. They have not done so, however, and instead one now accepts that subcutaneous sensors have to be changed, just like insulin pump cannulae, up to twice a week.

The closed-loop comprises three components: the glucose sensor, the insulin pump, and the computer software telling the pump how much insulin to give. Unsurprisingly, each of these has its own problems. The fact that it has taken so long since 1982 vividly attests to these difficulties.

Glucose Sensors

Many attempts have been made to develop a non-invasive way to measure blood glucose. It would, in effect, allow patients to do finger-prick glucose measurements without having to prick their fingers. This would allow much more frequent checks on glucose levels which in turn would make it possible to monitor not only single levels but also trends. Unfortunately, despite attempts to use many different physical principles, including near-infrared spectroscopy, changes in tissue refractive errors (and hence in light scattering), fluorescence decay times, and many others, none of these methods has proved as accurate as the invasive methods. The methods simply have too little specificity and hence have to contend with too great a level of background noise. The reader is referred to the review in John Pickup's textbook if they wish to go into these methods in more detail[11].

The Glucowatch represented a way to measure glucose outside the body by a supposedly non-invasive method. In this technique, the gadget worn on the wrist applied a voltage between two electrodes which resulted in salt, water, and its contained glucose being sucked through the skin by a process of reverse iontophoresis. Unfortunately, it could only be used for a matter of hours at a time, tended to cause a mild burn and stopped working if the patient sweated. Given that sweating is a feature of hypoglycemia, exactly the situation in which one most needs an accurate glucose measurement, this represented a major drawback and Animas has now withdrawn the product.

The commonest implanted glucose sensors use glucose oxidase, which catalyses the reaction between glucose and water to form gluconic acid and hydrogen peroxide:

$$\text{glucose} + O_2 \rightarrow \text{gluconic acid} + H_2O_2$$

If a voltage is applied to the electrode, the H_2O_2 is oxidized with the release of two electrons:

$$H_2O_2 \rightarrow O_2 + 2H^+ + 2e^-$$

In other words, a current is generated which is proportional to the ambient glucose concentration. This is the same reaction as is used on many of the strips used for finger-prick glucose estimation.

One way to use this technology to give a continuous glucose sensor is the microdialysis technique which has been developed commercially by Menarini (www.menarini.com) as the GlucoDay. The patient wears a small pump which circulates saline through a loop of microdialysis tube implanted under the abdominal skin. As the saline traverses the semipermeable microdialysis tube it picks up glucose in proportion to ambient tissue concentrations. The glucose estimation is performed within the machine itself, ex vivo, and a continuous tracing of tissue glucose levels is recorded.

The main drawbacks are the sheer bulk of the equipment necessary to house the pump and the two reservoirs (for the saline and the waste), the fact that one cannot shower and the fact that the tubing has to be changed in the hospital every couple of days. After each change, it may need many hours to reequilibrate before calibration. The slower the flow through the tubing the better the equilibration with interstitial fluid and hence the accuracy, but the longer the delay which may be as much as 30 min and which causes problems with the response time of the apparatus, especially in the context of closed-loop insulin pumps. A newer model is in clinical trials.

The field of sensor technology has in practice been dominated by the products originally marketed by MiniMed, which became Medtronic in 2001. The first commercially available sensor became available in 1999 and was called the Continuous Glucose Monitoring System (CGMS), although strictly speaking it performs measurements every 10 s which are averaged every 5 min so that it is only near continuous. A hollow plastic tube is introduced into subcutaneous fat using a steel needle in the middle as introducer. The glucose oxidase is around the tip of the tube and is connected via a wire to the 'monitor' on the belt, which applies the necessary voltage to the electrode and records the resultant current (Figure 5-4).

As with all sensors, calibration is a potential problem. Ideally one wants to calibrate at time points which give a wide range of glucose values. At the same time, there is a delay between blood and tissue glucose levels of some 10–15 min so that one also wants the glucose level to be stable at the time the calibration is done. In practice, these conditions are hard to meet but, clinically, absolute precision may be less important than the ability to detect trends in changes in glucose concentrations. The accuracy may break down at low glucose levels, when tissue glucose uptake reduces local concentrations more than blood levels, but in other circumstances tissue glucose is a sufficiently accurate guide to blood levels.

The original Minimed CGMS could store data over a 3-day period, but it then had to be downloaded through a PC to find out what glucose levels had been doing over the past 72 h. When it was first marketed, the hope was that it would revolutionize the management of Type 1 diabetes by identifying where the problems lay with the insulin doses being used. In practice, consistent patterns in diurnal glucose profiles can usually be identified with old-fashioned finger-pricks and what the sensors usually did was to demonstrate, if one did not already know it, that no 2 days are the same for the patient with Type 1 diabetes and that it is not their fault that they cannot achieve perfect control.

The thinking behind the CGMS was not to use it on its own but to develop it to the point that it could be used to drive an insulin pump. Indeed, there was a certain symmetry to a patient wearing a pump on one side of their belt and a CGMS monitor on the other. However, when Medtronic went forward to clinical trials, they chose instead to go for a fully implanted system using the intraperitoneal pump described above, driven via a subcutaneous wire by an intravenous sensor inserted through the subclavian vein and suspended in the superior vena cava just above the right atrium to give an intravenous/intraperitoneal (iv/ip) system.

Clinical trials with this system began in 2001 and very promising results were reported, particularly from Eric Renard's group in Montpelier. However, although it proved possible to use the system quite successfully to control overnight and inter-prandial glucose levels, the response time of the sensor was not quick enough to respond to the rapid changes in insulin requirements encountered immediately after a meal or, just as importantly, to reduce insulin infusion rates when glucose levels fell. This in turn resulted from the fact that there had been problems with the fragility of the sensors in the turbulence of vena caval blood flow. The sensor had had to be strengthened and the price paid for greater rigidity had been a slower response time.

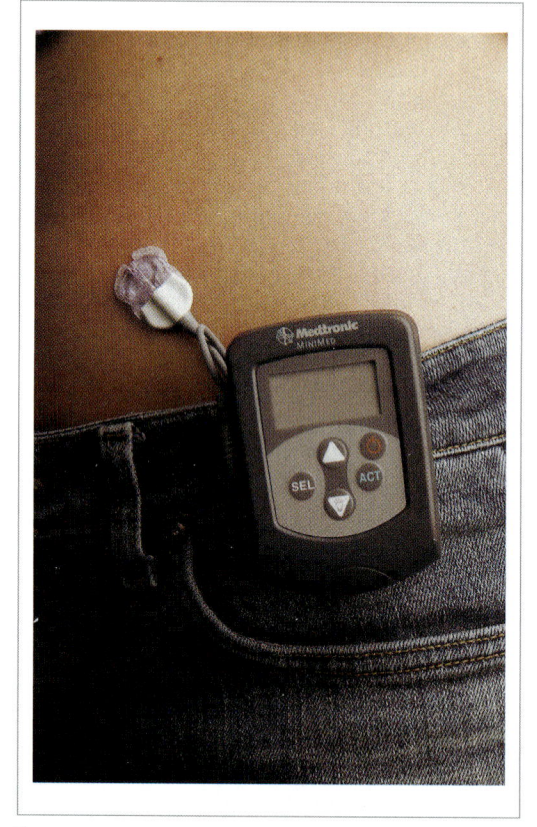

Figure 5-4. Minimed's original Continuous Glucose Monitoring System (CGMS). The 'monitor' on the belt applies a voltage to the subcutaneous sensor and collects output current from the electrode. In this version, data were downloaded onto a PC at the end of the 3-day monitoring period and related to insulin doses, meals, activity, etc. retrospectively. Reproduced by kind permission of Medtronic Ltd.

This highlighted the whole question of what one was trying to achieve. As indicated in the introduction, insulin effectively behaves as two separate hormones. When we eat, we 'tell' the pancreas that we are going to do so and the β-cells are primed in terms of insulin secretion increasing even before food has been ingested. Furthermore, secretion of incretins, released from the gut in response to food, changes the algorithm regulating the amount of insulin secreted such that more insulin is secreted at a given glucose level. While it is perfectly possible with a system of 'meal announcement' to tell an insulin pump that a meal is imminent and the algorithms need to change, the goal of the project was a fully automatic system which did not need any input from the patient and was not therefore at risk from human error.

If this was the goal, then the trial was a failure. Even though intraperitoneal insulin delivery has clear advantages, the fully implanted artificial pancreas has, at least for the time being, been abandoned in favor of the tried and tested subcutaneous sensor driving an external pump giving insulin subcutaneously (an sc/sc system).

Current State of Play

Pumps

It is the 30th anniversary of the first insulin pumps. During this time, much effort has gone into their development. Although new generations of pump continue to evolve, conventional pumps have now become sophisticated and reliable machines.

The major pump manufacturers and their pumps are (alphabetically):

1. Animas
   http://www.animascorp.com/
2. Cozmo
   http://www.delteccozmo.com/
3. Minimed Paradigm
   http://www.minimed.com/
4. Roche Accu-Chek (and they continue to market the Disetronic D-tron Plus, which has the advantage of pre-filled insulin syringes)
   http://www.disetronic-usa.com/

The websites all have a pronounced North American slant, which is appropriate given the fact that more than 20% of patients with Type 1 diabetes are on pumps in the United States compared to less than 5% in Britain (with other European countries somewhere in between). This in turn represents the historical fact that pumps have only recently been financed in the United Kingdom. Pumps currently cost between £2,300 and £2,700 plus roughly £1,000/year for consumables.

Those interested in future developments in insulin pumps may wish also to visit the websites of Omnipod, made by Insulet (http://www.myomnipod.com/), which does away with tubing but is not yet approved in Europe, the h-Patch from Valeritas (http://www.valeritas.com/h_patch.shtml), which is primarily aimed at Type 2 diabetes, and the tiny nanopump developed by Debiotech, recently acquired by Animas (http://www.debiotech.com/debiotech.html).

Sensors

In 1982, when the first closed-loop artificial pancreas paper was published, the limiting factor to its long-term success was perceived to be one of biocompatibility. Twenty-five years on, this has not been solved but the potential need to replace sensors has been accepted and the focus has switched elsewhere.

Recently, real-time sensors have become available so that the patient can see at a glance what their glucose level is at any one time and, just as importantly, how fast it is changing and in what direction. Three companies currently have real-time continuous glucose sensors approved by the FDA. They are (alphabetically):

1. Abbott FreeStyle Navigator (Figure 5-5)
   http://www.continuousmonitor.com/
2. DexCom Seven (so called because it is approved for use for 7 days)
   http://www.dexcom.com/html/dexcom_products.html
3. Medtronic MiniMed Guardian Real-time (Figure 5-6)
   http://www.minimed.com/products/insulinpumps/index.html

A detailed table comparing the respective products can be found at
http://www.childrenwithdiabetes.com/continu-ous.htm.

All do essentially the same thing. They differ slightly in the size of the electrode and the frequency with which it is suggested they should be changed. All incorporate a small transmitter and a receiver with a screen and can be used as hypo-/hyper-glycemia alarms. This latter

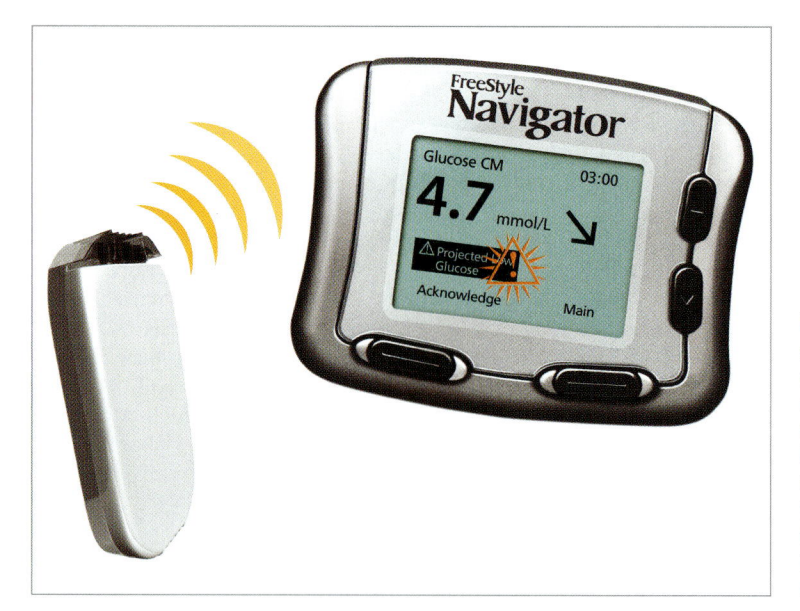

Figure 5-5. Abbott FreeStyle Navigator. The small unit on the left is attached to the skin and covers the electrode itself. The tissue glucose concentration is transmitted to a hand-held unit which displays not only the actual glucose level but also the fact that it is falling and displays an alarm for a risk of impending hypoglycemia. Reproduced by kind permission of Abbott Diabetes Care.

function is not perfect, however, because if you set the alarm to go off when glucose levels fall below, say, 4 mmol/l, the sensor delay may mean that you are not given enough warning and are already confused by the time you are being told to take action. If on the other hand, you set the alarm threshold higher, it is constantly going off at normal glucose levels. The sound of the warning beeps from glucose sensors has already become commonplace at gatherings of scientists working in the field! Nevertheless, the important point is that these sensors give the patient an idea not only of what their blood glucose levels is but also of whether it is rising or falling.

Although links between sensor manufacturers and pump manufacturers are in the offing, Minimed is currently the only manufacturer to appear in both lists. In fact, they have recently developed the Paradigm Real-Time system, in which it is the pump which collects and displays the glucose data transmitted from the sensor, obviating the need for a second 'box' (Figure 5-6). Although the pump is not driven by the sensor, this represents a step toward a fully integrated artificial pancreas. For those patients not using sensors, they have also now developed (in collaboration with Bayer) the Contour Link, a glucose meter able to transmit finger-prick glucose data to the Paradigm pump for recording and trend analysis.

While every diabetes meeting currently includes a favorable presentation on the benefits of real-time glucose monitoring, it remains to be seen whether in due course drawbacks will also become apparent. The past year has seen many presentations on the benefits to the patient but for every patient who can respond appropriately to a given change in glucose level there may be at least one other patient who reacts inappropriately and for whom a real-time sensor could potentially cause as many problems as it solves. A clinical trial of outcomes is currently in progress.

There are also, of course, major cost implications. MiniMed's current UK costs are £2,200 for the system plus £375 per 10 sensors. Because it is so expensive, we currently have approval to use real-time sensors only on a small number of patients with particularly unstable diabetes and frequent hypoglycemia though the use of one for a few days may also be useful in chosen cases to identify unrecognized problems.

Once sensors are used to drive pumps, the safety issues will become even more important and far more data will be needed on the accuracy and reliability of the sensors. Clearly if a sensor tells a pump that the glucose level is 12 mmol/l when it is in fact only 6 the consequences for the patient could be extremely dangerous. Exactly what safety measures will need to be taken, or whether a pump will need more than one sensor (so that if they disagree with each other an alarm is triggered), remains to be seen.

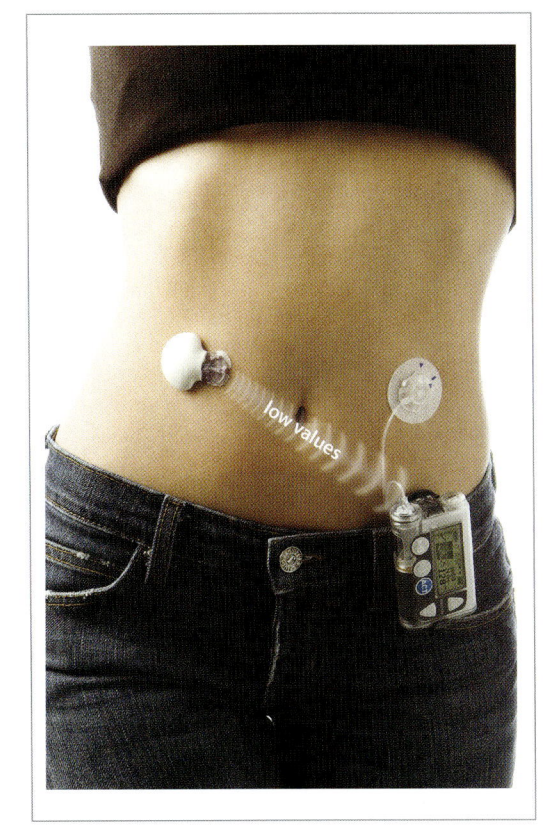

Figure 5-6. Medtronic MiniMed Paradigm Real-time monitor with MiniLink. The sensor has been inserted into the subcutaneous tissue in the right iliac fossa. This patient is also wearing a paradigm insulin pump infusing insulin continuously via the tubing and a cannula into the subcutaneous tissue of the left iliac fossa. Tissue glucose levels, transmitted from the sensor via the MiniLink, are collected in the pump which displays not only the actual tissue glucose levels but also the rate of change. At this stage, insulin delivery rates cannot be regulated by sensor glucose data. Reproduced by kind permission of Medtronic Ltd.

Control Algorithms

While the manufacturers cited above can now provide the hardware both for the sensors and for the pumps, the attention now turns to the software connecting the two and the necessary control algorithms.

Although many systems have been explored, the two which have been most thoroughly studied are the Model Predictive Control (MPC), an adaptive system capable of 'learning' to some extent, and the Proportional-Integral-Derivative (PID) system which adds together functions reflecting the current glucose level, how far it is from the desired target and how fast it is changing. Whereas the PID system is essentially retrospective, looking back over previous glucose levels to come up with a suggested insulin infusion rate, the MPC system is more forward looking, basing its recommendations for insulin infusion rates on the patient's own responses to given insulin infusion rates in the past. It is said to have advantages in systems with long delays and at extremes of glucose levels. A detailed review of this highly specialized area can be found in Roman Hovorka's excellent recent review.[12]

One of the major issues with feedback loops is the effect of a delay at any point in the system. Hovorka has estimated that an iv sensor linked to an ip pump has a delay of about 70 min between the glucose sensing and the insulin effect (compared to a delay of only 30 min with a native pancreas) and this rises to almost 100 min with an sc sensor and sc insulin delivery. Delays in a feedback loop tend to cause oscillation and the question is whether it will ever be possible to achieve good enough control with a single programme with such a long delay.

Clinical experience with closed-loop pumps remains very limited with only about 100 patient days at this point. Good glycemic control has been shown to be possible with a closed-loop so long as the subject does not eat, because the variation in the amount of insulin needed is modest, but problems arise following a meal when, if insulin levels do not increase promptly as soon as food is ingested, an unacceptably large hyperglycemic excursion results. More importantly, if insulin levels do not fall fast enough when glucose levels start to fall, the patient runs a real risk of overshooting into hypoglycemia.

It is theoretically possible to circumvent this problem with a hybrid, semi-automatic system involving 'meal announcement' whereby the patient gives the pump a signal that they are about to eat which changes the computer algorithm. This mimics the physiological situation in which the pancreatic β-cells do not operate with a single control algorithm. When you eat, the K cells in the stomach and upper small bowel secrete GIP (glucose sensitive insulinotropic polypeptide), while the L-cells further down the gut secrete GLP-1 (glucagon-like peptide, Type 1). These incretins 'tell' the β-cells that you have eaten and change the algorithm so that, at a given glucose level, the β-cells secrete more insulin. In fact, even before you eat, neural signals lead to an increase in insulin secretion before blood glucose levels begin to rise.

The idea of making an artificial pancreas which is more independent than the native pancreas and needs only a single algorithm seems somewhat ambitious. With hybrid systems, it will be necessary to persuade the regulatory authorities that an artificial pancreas which is not fully automatic and which relies on human input will still prove to be safe. The Yale group has successfully used a system whereby there is only one algorithm but the patient gives a pre-meal priming dose of insulin 15 min before the meal to raise insulin levels more quickly than would otherwise occur.[13]

Although the control algorithms are the piece of the puzzle that there is least experience of, one feels quite positive because serious mathematicians are now putting a lot of thought and effort into the design of appropriate software. One important new advance is that, in contrast to the old physiological 'gray box' mathematical modeling, the FDA has just given approval for an in silico metabolic simulator which makes it possible to compare different control algorithms without the need for animal trials.

Closed Loop Pumps and the JDRF Artificial Pancreas (AP) Project

In 1982, with open-loop pumps already available and the publication of the first closed-loop paper, one felt that closed-loop pumps might only be 5 years away. Yet it took until 1999 before satisfactory glucose sensors became available. In 2001, when Minimed began trials of their fully implanted closed loop system, one again felt that closed-loop pumps were only a few years away. These studies were able to achieve good control, at least so long as the patients did not eat, but were abandoned due to problems with the sensor.

Against this background, the announcement in late 2005 by the Juvenile Diabetes Research Foundation (JDRF), whose mission statement is a cure for Type 1 diabetes, of major support for its Artificial Pancreas Project is a major cause for optimism. Not only will this ensure long-term funding and support for the project but, just as importantly, since it is now a charity rather than a pharmaceutical company making the running, it will also provide great help to clear the legal and regulatory hurdles which an artificial pancreas necessarily entails.

Conclusion

The fact that we have reached this stage owes a lot to Mr. Al Mann, who founded Minimed in 1980 and who personally financed the project for many years at a time when other companies were giving up. As we reach the 30th anniversary of insulin pumps, we have several manufacturers making portable, sophisticated, and reliable pumps.

Glucose sensors have proved much more difficult and it took all of the 1980s and 1990s until the first glucose sensor was approved. Even now, there remain problems both with their accuracy and, more particularly, with their reliability. The early attempt at a trial for a closed-loop pump in 2001 used an intravenous sensor (and intra-peritoneal insulin delivery) but reliability problems have meant that intravenous sensors are no longer available. The delay inherent in a closed-loop system which uses subcutaneous sensors and subcutaneous insulin delivery currently being developed for an artificial pancreas introduces additional problems because it introduces such a long delay into the feedback loop. If such a system is to work, it seems likely that it will have to be semi-automatic. That is to say, the pump is automatic through the night and between meals but relies on patient intervention to deal with meal boluses. Such an approach is looking really very promising.[13]

By the time a safe and successful artificial pancreas becomes a reality, countless millions will have been spent on the project and it will be hard to recoup these development costs. One hopes that companies will not even try to do so. The recent setting up by the JDRF of its AP (Artificial Pancreas) project has revitalized the whole field. The hope is that within the next 5–10 years the artificial pancreas will provide the solution which gives all patients with Type 1 diabetes the prospect of near-normal glucose control and hence the best possible quality of life and a greatly reduced risk of diabetic complications.

References

1. Kerr D, James J, Nicholls H. Technologies as therapeutic devices. What do we expect from users of insulin pump therapy? *Infusystems Int.* 2008;7:1–4.
2. Pickup JC, Keen H, Parsons JA, Alberti KGMM: Continuous subcutaneous insulin infusion: an approach to achieving normoglycaemia. *BMJ.* 1978;i:204–207.
3. Juice: The Creative Fuel that drives Today's World Class Inventors. Evan I Schwartz. Harvard Business School Press; 2004.
4. Sönksen PH, Judd SL, Lowy C. Home monitoring of blood-glucose. Method for improving diabetic control. *Lancet.* 1978;i:729–32.
5. Pickup J, Mattock M, Kerry S: Glycaemic control with continuous subcutaneous insulin infusion compared with intensive insulin injections in patients with Type 1 diabetes: meta-analysis of randomised controlled trials. *BMJ* 324:705, 2002.
6. *The Diabetes Control and Complications Trial Research Group.* The Effect of Intensive Treatment of Diabetes on the Development and Progression of Long-Term Complications in Insulin-Dependent Diabetes Mellitus *N Engl J Med.* 1993;329(14):977–86.
7. Bode BW, Stubbs HA, Schwartz S, Block JE. Glycemic characteristics in continuously monitored patients with Tye 1 and Typ2 diabetes. *Diabetes Care.* 2005; 28:2361–2366.
8. Albisser AM, Leibel BS, Ewart TG et al. An artificial endocrine pancreas. *Diabetes.* 1974;23:389–96.
9. Pfeiffer E-F, Kerner W. The artificial endocrine pancreas: its impact on the pathophysiology and treatment of diabetes mellitus. *Diabetes Care.* 1981;4:11–26.
10. Shichiri M, Kawamori R, Yamasaki Y, Hakui N, Abe H. Wearable artificial endocrine pancreas with needle-type glucose sensor. *Lancet.* 1982;2:1129–1131.
11. Textbook of Diabetes, ed. Pickup JC and Willams G. Chapter 34. Third edition, Blackwell, 2003.
12. Hovorka R. Continuous glucose monitoring and closed-loop systems. *Diabet Med..* 2006;23:1–12.
13. Weinzimer SA, Steil GM, Swan KL, Dziura J, Kurtz N, Tamborlane WV. Fully Automated Closed-Loop Insulin Delivery Versus Semiautomated Hybrid Control in Pediatric Patients With Type 1 Diabetes Using an Artificial Pancreas. *Diabet Care.* 2008;31:934–939.

6

From Basic Wound Healing to Modern Skin Engineering

L.C. Andersson, H.C. Nettelblad and G. Kratz

Introduction

The skin is our largest organ and it simultaneously fulfills many functions required in everyday life. The most important function of the skin is to act as a barrier between the body and the external environment. Many immune cells are also present in the skin to provide protection against invading micro-organisms. The skin is in addition an important participant in the physiological water homeostasis and it is one of the main ways the body regulates its temperature. Normal skin has sensation with protective value; a physical tensile capacity allowing for body mobility and it provides the external contour as well as the texture and the color of the exterior.

Over the millennia mankind has been fascinated by the body's ability to heal itself. Throughout history the main goal has always been to cover skin defects and to close wounds in order to protect the human body. Skin grafting and flap surgical procedures have been used in order to facilitate wound healing for thousands of years. Due to the advances in critical care and resuscitation, patients who, in the past, would have died in the acute phase are now surviving. Consequently there is a much greater need for high-quality skin substitutes. The clinical demand has driven newer technologies, building upon principles learned using cadaver and autografts, to the creation of engineered skin substitutes using living allograft cells as well as the combining of technologies to create composites – the most advanced products and at present the closest products to living skin. An autologous split thickness skin graft currently still remains superior to all commercially available skin substitutes with regards to its unique qualities. There are, however, situations where we prefer to use non-autologous substitutes, either because the patient may be too fragile for the added surgical trauma of harvesting split-skin grafts or due to the fact that there is not enough skin which could be harvested, for example, post-burn.

Structure of the Skin

The skin consists of two principal layers: the epidermis and the dermis. The epidermis consists of a keratinized layer with no vital cells and cell layers of keratinocytes which produce keratin. The epidermis provides protection against micro-organisms and loss of fluids. The epidermis within the basal cell layer contains melanocytes that produce melanin, our skin pigmentation. The dermis mainly consists of fibroblasts and interstitial connective tissue. The fibroblasts produce collagen and elastine, which provide the tensile strength of the skin composite. The dermis also harbors hair follicles, which are lined by epidermal cells and are localized adjacent to sebaceous glands, which produce sebum. There are also sweat glands, blood vessels, and nerves in the dermis (Figure 6-1). The dermis provides the tensile strength and elasticity that allows mobility of the skin.[1]

Historical Overview

Our ancestors struggled to treat wounds and defects inflicted either by nature or by acts of man. Skin substitutes in the form of xenografts

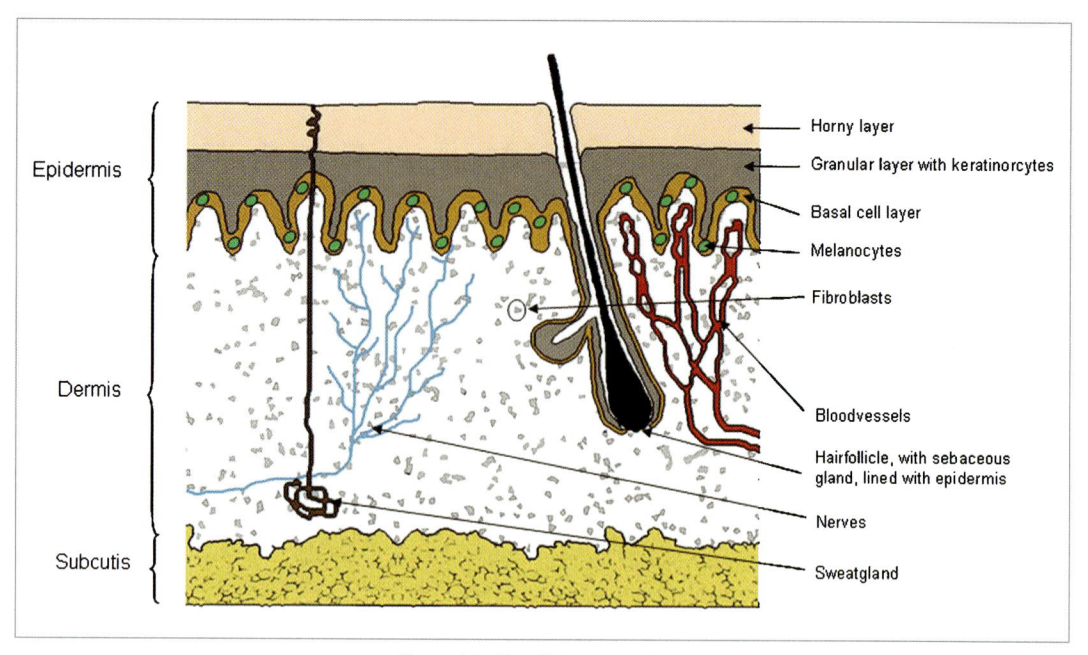

Figure 6-1. The skin in cross section.

were first used to provide wound coverage as far back as 1500 BC (frog skin). In the 1600s, lizard skin was used in western cultures and this progressed to the use of mammalian skins as well as cadaver skin during the twentieth century, including dog and rabbit skin and the still-used pigskin products.[2-4] Facial deformities such as defects after the amputation of the nose were the type of problems that received the most attention. A famed practitioner, Sushruta (circa 600 BC), described operations for reconstruction of the nose without any form of anesthesia. Tissue from the forehead was dissected but remained attached to the area between the eyebrows and was then turned down in order to reconstruct a nose and left intact for 3-4 weeks. The nasal bridge was then divided and the nose was improved in its shape. It was further described that the donor defect in the forehead healed rather well and left very little deformity.[5] During the Roman Empire, Celsus (25 BC-50 AD) raised smaller flaps which involved the skin and the fat (pieces of skin and fat, with blood circulation still attached to the body in at least one area) in order to reconstruct skin defects in facial areas.[6] Over the years, many others have contributed to new techniques and variations involving different types of flaps in order to correct defects with, but it was not until the beginning of the nineteenth century that the concept of skin grafting (auto grafting: a skin piece from one part of the body was cut loose with no attachment and no circulation, then grafted onto a well-vascularized wound on the same individual) became clinically used. Sir Astley Cooper removed skin from an amputated thumb and used it to cover the stump defect with as a full-thickness skin graft in 1817.[7] Nevertheless, skin grafting was not fully recognized and accepted for clinical use until the last quarter of the nineteenth century. In 1869, Reverdin reported that the healing of granulating wounds was improved by so-called "epidermic grafts".[8] In 1874, Thiersch advocated the use of larger sheets of epidermal grafts to cover wounds with and also emphasized the importance of an epidermal component in the graft with a small amount of dermis (Figure 6-2). The grafts used were thin split thickness skin grafts containing both the epidermis and the parts of the dermis and these pieces of skin were tangentially excised and grafted onto wounds and skin defects. The actual donor sites were then left to heal spontaneously through epithelialization from the depth and from the sides of the donor defect, which was itself superficial enough and the healing would be achieved in approximately 2 weeks.[9] Xenografts gave way to homografts in

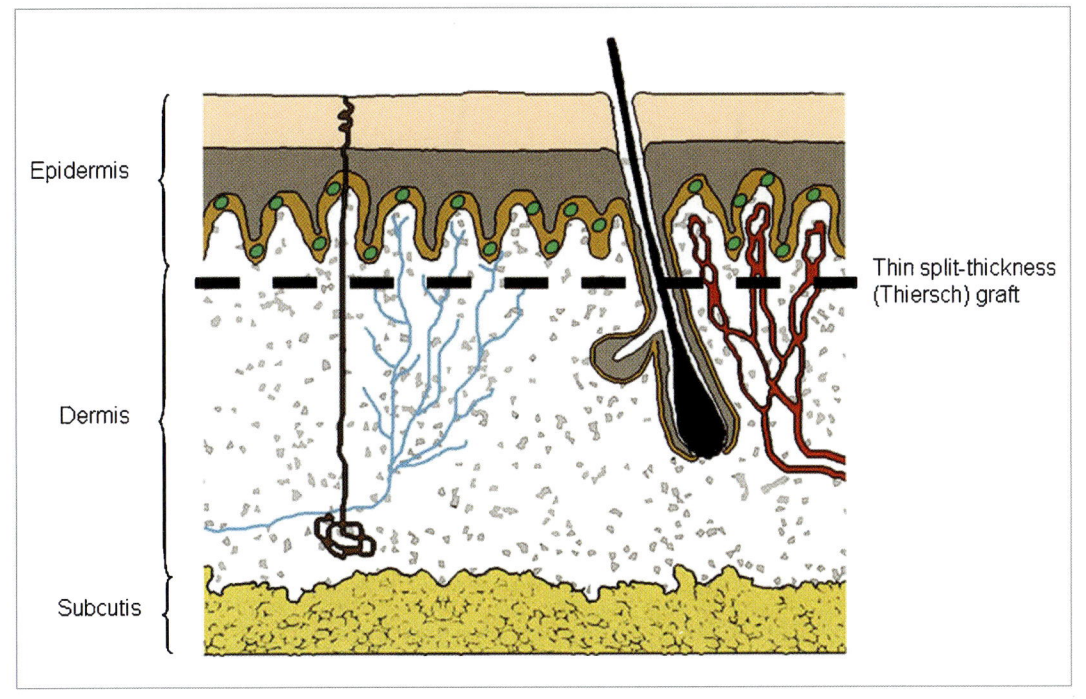

Figure 6-2. The skin in cross section - indicating the depth of a Thiersch graft.

the form of allograft (cadaveric graft) and autograft. The modern development of intensive care and improved surgical techniques enabled skin and fat flaps to be developed further into tissue flaps involving, e.g., skin, fat, tendon, muscle, and bone tissue. The tissue could be harvested in one part of the body and transferred to another body region in order to cover wounds with. The blood supply after having been disconnected at the original site was re-established via microsurgery. Many other developments in modern medicine also contributed to the overall need for larger wound areas to be covered with skin, e.g., burns and trauma[10] Our increased understanding of immunology and wound healing has also been a contributing factor of great importance in modern wound management. The clinical demand of skin has driven the bio-engineering of skin, in the form of skin substitutes and skin cultivation, which will be integrated, more and more into clinical practice in the future.[11]

Wound Healing

The body will immediately respond with an acute inflammation if the skin is acutely damaged. Many physiological substances are released at this stage in order to initiate the normal wound-healing process. Granulation tissue of fibroblasts and new capillaries will grow into the wound. Collagen will be produced to provide stability and strength and an epithelialization from the wound edges will start. There are many factors that contribute to a normal wound-healing process and many others, which disturb this important process. An acute wound may not progress in the normal wound-healing process and instead become chronic. The understanding of wound healing constantly increases and many new treatments which facilitate wound healing are continuously being developed.[9]

Epidermal Wound Healing

The epidermal cells divide and migrate if damage to the epidermis has occurred. A wound no deeper than after the harvest of a split-skin graft (Figure 6-3) will heal spontaneously (epithelialization) if no infection arises, usually within 2–3 weeks with the correct type of wound dressing which protects from external bacteria, viruses, and particles. Damage to the epidermis does not normally result in

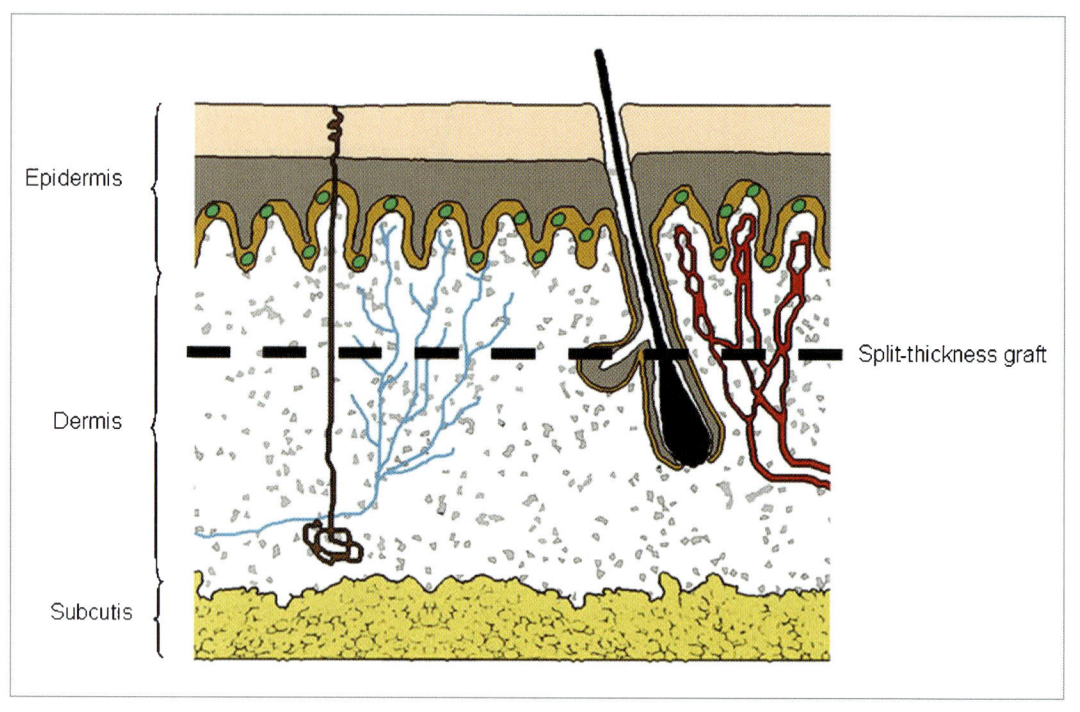

Figure 6-3. The skin in cross section -indicating the depth of a split-thickness graft.

contractive scarring but some pigmentation variation may be seen as a long-term result. The healing of the epidermis will proceed both from the wound edges as well as from the underlying tissues since there are keratinocytes which line the hair follicles. It can take several years for the basal cell membrane to remodel and for the melanocytes to migrate into the damaged area.[9]

Dermal Wound Healing

The healing of a wound, which extends deep down into the dermis, at the same depth as when a full-thickness skin graft is harvested, will take a lot longer than the healing of an epidermal superficial wound (Figure 6-4). There will be no epithelialization from the deeper tissues due to lack of keratinocytes in these planes, but healing takes place solely from the wound edges. Before the epithelialization from the wound edges can take place, a layer of granulation tissue consisting of fibroblasts and capillaries will form in order to reinstitute the dermis. The actual epithelialization from the wound edges will then spontaneously start on top of the granulation tissue. The wound should decrease by 10–15% of the original size per week in order to represent normal wound healing.[12] The actual healing time of deep dermal or deeper tissue wounds will vary, all depending on the size of the wound and external interfering factors, e.g., foreign bodies, micro-organisms, and the patients' general condition. Large dermal wounds may need surgical intervention with debridements and skin grafting in order to heal. The dermal fibroblasts will produce collagen and scar tissue will form. The scar tissue in the dermis will over time be remodeled, but the scarred skin will contract and become less flexible and smoother than normal skin is. The dermal tensile strength may also be reduced in scarred skin. The skin mobility in scarred skin after dermal healing will be reduced and skin scar contractions may have to be surgically "released" or corrected in order to improve the function of a specific area of the body. The scarred skin after damage to the dermis also appears different in pigmentation than an individual's normal skin. The whole maturing process of a dermal scar can take several years and surgical interventions may be necessary during parts of this process in order to improve a patient's function and appearance.[9] These

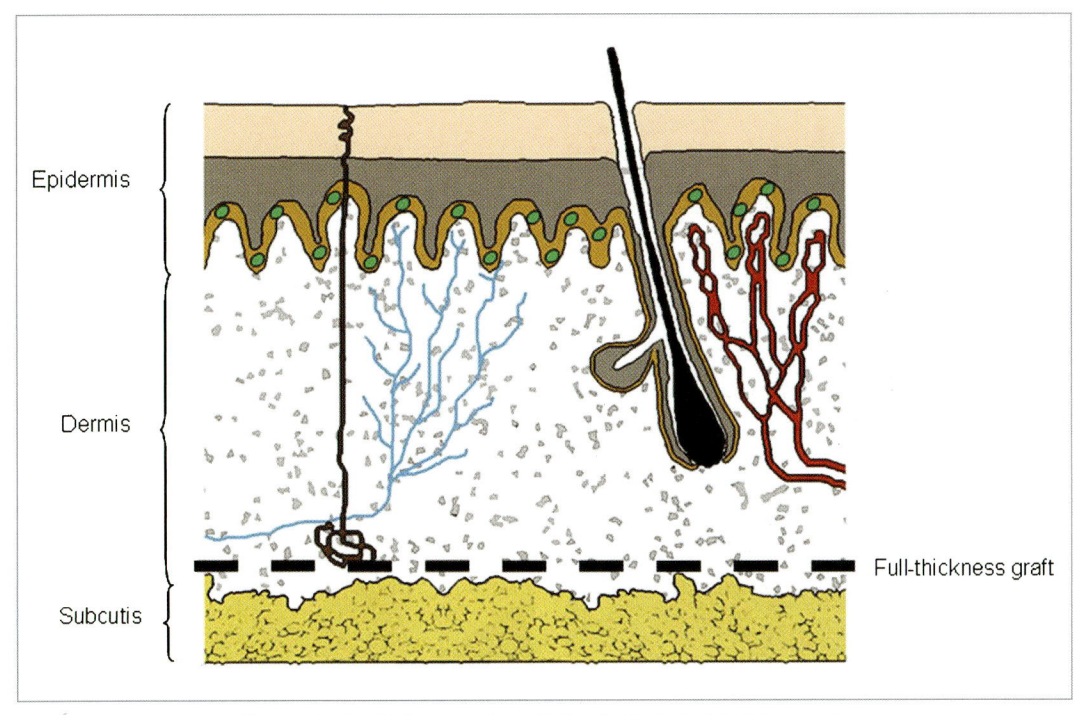

Figure 6-4. The skin in cross section indicating the depth of a full-thickness graft.

types of clinical problems can especially be seen in burn injuries to the hands, due to the large flexibility and mobility of the hand. It is often initially necessary to debride and excise deeper hand-burns and to cover the healthy bleeding wounds with superficial skin grafts in order to avoid secondary infections and contractive scarring with reduced hand function. Further corrective surgery may still be required later, but the early excision of the dead tissue is very important as it significantly enhances the chances of good hand function (Figure 6-5).[13]

Clinical Management of Wounds

Modern wound-healing treatments consist of debridement, negative pressure wound therapy, topical growth factors, the use of bio-engineered tissue, reconstructive wound-closure techniques (skin grafts, local flaps, pedicle flaps and microsurgical free flaps), and hyperbaric oxygen. It is important to have at least one of the physicians on the multidisciplinary wound team familiar with modern wound-care techniques. Debridement is the basis of all wound-healing strategies. Debriding a wound is defined as removing necrotic tissue, foreign material, and bacteria from an acute or chronic wound, all of which inhibits the wound healing.[12] An acute wound has yet to progress through the sequential stages, a chronic wound has become "stuck" in one of the wound-healing stages. The advent of negative pressure wound therapy has reduced the number of non-healing wounds. The negative pressure device can provide rapid formation of granulation tissues and its ability to decrease edema helps prepare the wound for simple wound-closure techniques.[14]

Pre-debridement Assessment

The goal of treating any type of wound is to create an environment that is conductive to normal and timely healing. The process begins with the identification of a correct diagnosis of the wounds' etiology and continues with optimizing the patient's medical condition, including blood flow to the wound site. A proper wound assessment before debridement is essential, the origin and age of the wound should be determined, the patient's general condition (nutrition, smoking, local circulation, etc.) must also be taken into

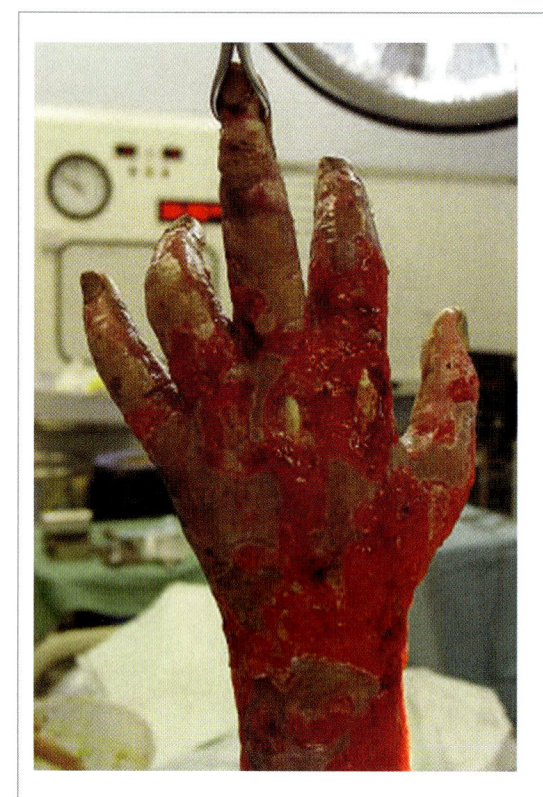

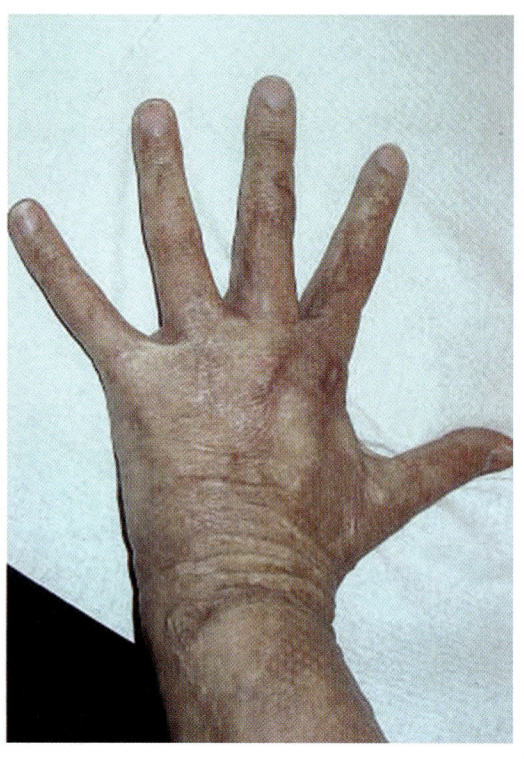

Figure 6-5. Deeply burnt hand (left) with exposed tendons before debridment and six months later after excision and skin grafting with meshed split-skin grafts.

account and a careful medical history should be obtained to identify any possible wound-healing inhibiting medical conditions. It is also clearly important to understand the extent of a wound, specifically with regards to wound depth and the involvement of deeper tissue, e.g., tendons and bone. An underlying osteomyelitis could feed a wound with bacteria if undiscovered.[15] Magnetic resonance imaging (MRI) is today the gold standard way to diagnose osteomyelitis. An infected tendon and fascia can, in the same way, be a focus of infection. The wound-healing process and the take of a skin graft may be disturbed if the bacterial concentration on a wound is higher than 10^5 per gram of tissue. A further increase of the bacterial load could spread from a local superficial infection to a systemic one which leads to septicemia. The application of topical antibiotics such as silver sulfadiazine, mafenide acetate, and silver nitrate all help to lower the bacterial count and reduce the risk of sepsis and can these be used before wound debridement.[16,17]

Debridement

Different debridement techniques include surgery, topical agents, and bio-surgery. The most important surgical step in treating any wound is to perform adequate debridement to remove all foreign material and unhealthy or non-viable tissue until the wound edges and base consist only of normal, soft, well-vascularized healthy tissue.[12] Only an atraumatic surgical technique (sharp dissection, skin hooks, bipolar cautery, etc.) should be used in order to avoid damaging the underlying healthy tissue.[18] This underlying healthy tissue will become the basis for the wound-healing progression. A chronic wound has to be converted by debridement to an acute wound so that it can then proceed through the normal healing phases. Frequent debridements remove the inhibitors of wound healing such as metalloproteases, including the collagenase matrix metalloproteinase 1 and 8 and elastase and it allows the growth factors to function more effectively.[19] An immediate debridement is necessary when a necrotizing fasciatis or an ascending cellulitis occurs in conjunction with a wound. No other treatment could achieve bacterial control in such a wound status. Biological debriding agents such as maggots are an effective alternative to surgical debridement in patients who cannot go to the operating theatre for medical reasons. The maggots secrete enzymes that dissolve necrotic tissue and the biofilm that surrounds bacteria. This forms a nutrient-rich liquid that larvae can feed on. They are placed on wounds and covered with a semipermeable dressing. Debridement by maggots is painless but the sensate patient can feel the larvae moving. Importantly maggots help to sterilize wounds because they consume all bacteria regardless of their resistance to antibiotics including methicillin-resistant *Staphylococcus aureus* (MRSA).[20–23]

Post-debridement Treatment

After debridement a clear, well-vascularized wound should be kept in the optimal environment for healing (moist, clean, and vascularized) in order to enable the use of growth factors. Moist healing has been shown to be far more rapid than healing under an eschar or in other dry conditions. In this environment, the wound base can support and promote successful collagen deposition, angiogenesis, epithelialization, and wound contracture; the result should be the formation of healthy red granulation tissue with neoepithelialization at the borders. Epithelializing wounds are characterized by a pink neoepithelium that usually creeps in from the edges.[12] A well-vascularized wound should, after debridement, heal by secondary intention or accept a skin graft.[24–26] Other surgical wound-closure techniques may also be required, e.g., flaps, all depending on the wound's location and extent. Exposed bone should if possible be covered with vascularized tissue, which is transferred into the wound in conjunction with the debridement. Preferably should a muscle–fat–skin flap be used in order to heal the wound defect, as well as to help the bone tissue "fight" a threatening osteomyelitis (Figure 6-6).

Dressings of Wounds

There is no single dressing suitable for all types of wounds and often a number of different dressing types will be needed throughout the healing process. Dressings containing silver have returned in advanced wound care and are found used in conjunction with many products.[27,28] Silver ions kill a broad spectrum of bacteria including methicillin-resistant *Staphylococcus aureus* (MRSA), Vancomycin-resistant *Enterococcus*, and *Pseudomonas aeruginosa*.[12]

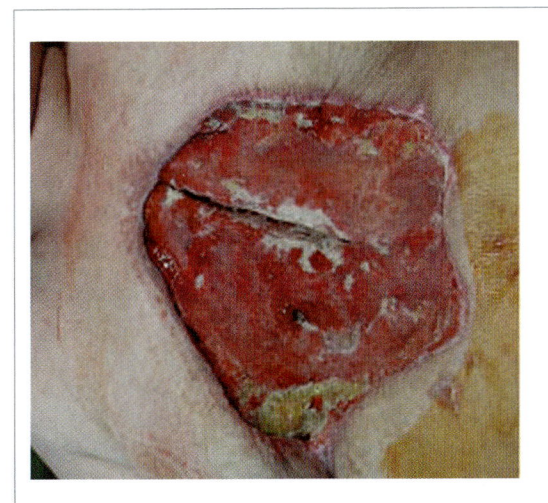

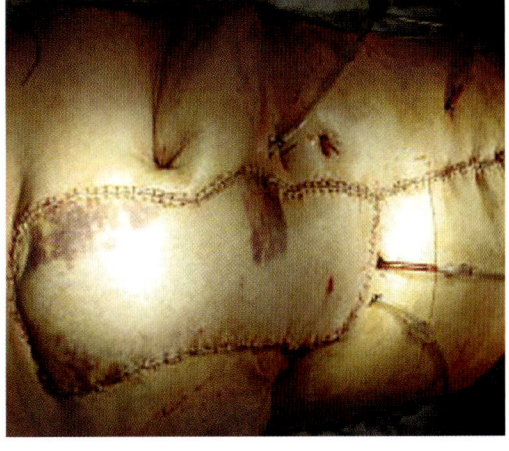

Figure 6-6. Chronic wound with osteomyelitis and exposed bone (sternum) after heart surgery (left). Debridement and wound closure with a pedicled musculo-cutaneus rectus abdominis flap (right).

Modern Skin Engineering

Tissue engineering is an interdisciplinary scientific field that combines the principles of life science and engineering toward the development of biologic substitutes that will serve to restore, maintain, or improve tissue function.[29] First, specific cells must be harvested, isolated, and expanded in tissue culture. The second component of tissue engineering focuses on the scaffold for tissue structure. Collaboration with biomedical engineers is critical for the development of novel scaffolds that will have the optimal combination of immunological compatibility, sufficient mechanical strength, and biodegradability (Figure 6-7). Third, the implanted construct should be incorporated into the healing tissue helping to restore structure and function.[10] Various tissues have been engineered but the most developed are skin substitutes and a number of these produces have US/FDA approval and are currently available.[2] The need for skin grafting has been the driving force behind the development of these skin substitutes.[11] The skin is the largest single organ of the human body and although composed of only two specialized tissue layers, it remains a reconstructive challenge in many cases when compromised. The philosophy of replacing like with like has contributed to the development of the treatment strategies used today. The simplest treatment is secondary closure, which is when a wound is left to heal spontaneously. This does not always lead to a good functional and esthetic result and more complex tissue reconstruction may be necessary. Advanced type of tissue reconstruction in the form of distant-free tissue transfer can lead to superior functional results, but sets large demands on the patient and the surgical team. A large wound area due to its size may not be possible to treat with the patients' own tissue. A layer of tissue, which is mechanically similar to the original skin over a reconstruction site, has to be used in order to complete the reconstruction and to avoid failure. This has made bioengineered skin substitutes a solution that has received much attention lately. Skin substitutes are a heterogeneous group of substances that aid in the temporary or permanent closure of many types of wounds. Depending on wound and product characteristics, different skin substitutes may be chosen. Artificial skin substitutes, products of tissue engineering, consist of microengineered, biocompatible, polymer matrix in combination with cellular, and/or extracellular elements such as collagen.[30] An ideal skin substitute should possess the physical characteristics and function of normal skin while healing takes place. However, no perfect or ideal skin substitute yet exists.[2]

Characteristics and Clinical Use of Skin Substitutes

Skin substitutes are a heterogeneous class of therapeutic devices that vary in their biology and application. Although there is no single perfect skin substitute, certain characteristics can be considered when evaluating alternatives. A long shelf-life and easy storage makes the product readily available. The substitute should be easy to prepare and apply without intensive training. Flexibility of thickness allows the product to be tailored to every type of wound. The product should be able to withstand a hypoxic wound bed and have a degree of resistance to infection in order to allow relatively ischemic tissues to be candidates for application. The ideal skin substitute should have resistance to tensile forces and provide permanent and long-term wound stability. It should reproduce both components of the skin (epidermis and dermis) and provide no antigenicity that could compromise the graft or host or present difficulties with future applications.[2] Because no single product meets all these criteria, each patient case requires careful evaluation before choosing the appropriate treatment. Although many acute and chronic wounds may benefit from a tailored

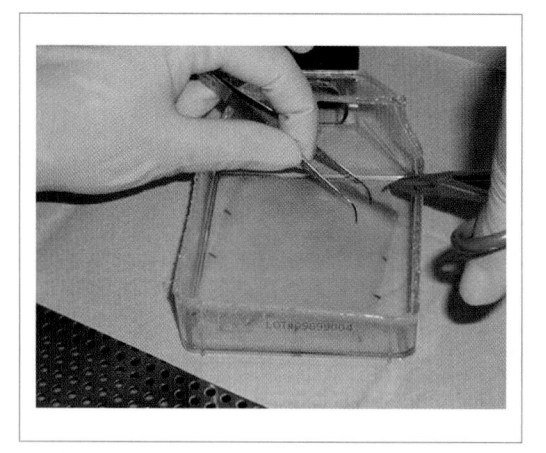

Figure 6-7. Preparation of a bio-engineered skin substitute.

multidisciplinary approach that utilizes one or more of the products mentioned, each patient should be evaluated for other possible therapies before the use of skin substitutes. Adequate assessment of patient-related factors, surgical debridement, and infection control will first have to be performed. Different techniques such as local or regional flaps or microvascular (free tissue) transplantation should be considered and the incorporation of a skin substitute can be included in the patient's treatment plan. If a patient is not considered a candidate for wound or defect reconstruction, creative applications of skin substitute technologies may not only significantly benefit a patient, but also be the only option for wound closure.[2]

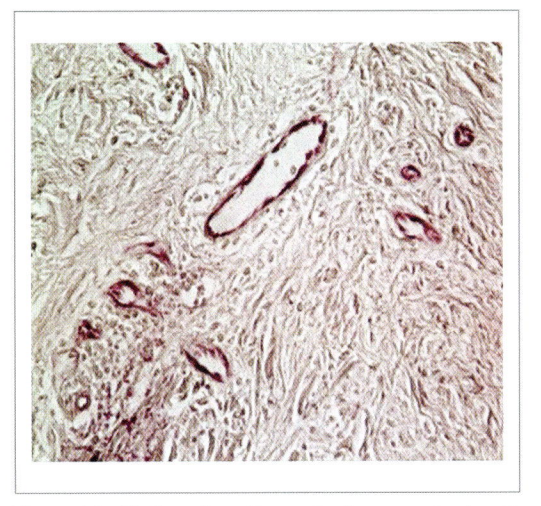

Figure 6-8. Histology from biopsy showing a neodermis with ingrowth of capillaries, collagen, and fibroblasts after use of a cell free dermal substitute.

Types of Skin Substitutes

Xenografts are tissues transplanted from one species onto another species, used as a temporary graft (e.g., frog skin and lizard skin). Porcine products are the most commonly used xenografts today.[3,4] *Permacol* and *OASIS* are among the currently available products.[31,32]

Allografts are grafts transplanted between genetically non-identical individuals of the same species. Most human skin substitute allografts come from cadaveric sources. Allografts fall into three categories: epithelial/epidermal, dermal, and composite (epidermal and dermal). Within these three categories, they may be acellular, cellular/living, or cellular/nonliving. *AlloDerm* is a commercial available acellular dermal allograft that was initially developed for skin defects, but it has also been used on burns and soft tissue replacement.[33–35] This product retains dermal elements and the basement membrane allowed keratinocytes to migrate into the material. A subsequent split-thickness graft or cultured keratinocyte graft is added after neovascularization of the neodermis (Figure 6-8) for epidermal cover. Clinical use of acellularized human cadaveric dermis and ultra-thin skin grafts has shown good clinical results in face, hand, and foot burns.[33–35] *Graftjacket*, *Neoform*, and *DermaMatrix* are further acellular dermal allografts available.[36,37] *ICX-SKN, TransCyte* (also known as *Dermagraft-TC*) and *Dermagraft* are cellular dermal allografts which use a scaffold of dermal collagen that is seeded with neonatal fibroblasts to stimulate cells within the host's wound to promote healing.[38–44]

Composite allograft products are the most advanced and closest products to living skin that are currently commercially available. *Apligraft* and *Orcelare* are the currently available products. *Apligraf* has been used in the treatment of epidermolysis bullosa (EB). In a study of nine patients with 96 sites of skin loss, 90–100% healing was observed by 5–7 days with clinically normal appearing skin in place by days 10–14.[45,46] *OrCel*, a composite bilayer produce with neonatal keratinocytes impregnated onto a coated non-porous sponge composed of type I bovine collagen has also been used for wound coverage after contracture release in EB patients.[47,48] The FDA has approved its use for reconstruction or treatment of recessive dystrophic EB of the hands and skin graft donor sites in these patients. Studies evaluating its use in chronic venous and diabetic lower extremity ulcers are ongoing.

Autografts are tissues grafted to a new position on the same individual. They are commonly divided into three main categories:[2]

(1) *Split-thickness skin grafts (STSGs)* which contain the epidermis and a variable thickness of the upper layers of dermis, leaving the remaining layers of dermis in place to heal by secondary epithelialization from the wound edges and keratinocytes within the adnexa of the deeper dermis.

(2) *Full-thickness skin grafts (FTSGs)* which contain the epidermis and the entire dermis.[49] These types of grafts are preferred in areas

where significant scarring or contracture of the grafts would provide harmful esthetic or functional consequences. Because of the limited supply of FTSG donor sites they are usually reserved for reconstructing wounds of the head, neck, hands, and genitals.

(3) *Cultured autologous skin substitutes* which are frequently referred to as cultured epidermal autografts (CEAs). This nomenclature includes epidermal grafts and excludes dermal/epidermal grafts. The CEAs are grafted onto a wound and the healing of the new epidermis is initiated (Figure 6-9). *Epicel* and *Laserskin* are among the currently available products.[50,51] *Cultured skin substitute (CASS)* is a CEA with the addition of a cultured autologous dermal layer, making it a more anatomically correct skin substitute. This product is still in clinical trials but it does in theory represent the most advanced autologous skin substitute available. The product is created by culturing autologous fibroblasts and keratinocytes with collagen and glycosaminoglycan substrates.[52,53]

A synthetic monolayer substitute Suprathel is a monolayer acellular synthetic dressing which has proven to decrease pain when used on donor sites.[54,55]

Synthetic biolayer substitutes are acellular products engineered without allogenic cells, they function as dermal templates and promote in growth of host tissues to repair defects or create a neodermis. After in growth, skin grafting can be performed on top of the new dermis. They also contain a removable silicone epidermal layer to help protect the wound from moisture loss and contamination. Commercially available products are *Biobrane* and *Integra*. *Biobrane* is a biosynthetic skin substitute consisting of a bilaminate membrane of nylon mesh bonded to a thin layer of silicone, which is, coated with porcine type 1 collagen-derived peptides (dermal analogue). The silicone layer functions as temporary epidermis.[56–58] *Integra Bilayer Matrix Wound Dressing* is a synthetic bilayer acellular skin substitute composed of an outer silastic sheet (epidermal analogue) with a matrix composed of bovine collagen and glycosaminoglycan (dermal analogue).[59–67] The silastic sheet provides temporary cover before skin grafting is performed.

What Does the Future Hold in Modern Skin Engineering?

The wound-healing treatments with debridement remain very important. Infection control is vital for any healing. None of the available skin substitutes has been shown to be superior to autologous split-skin grafting (Figure 6-10). Existing substitutes do also have problems which include graft take, infection, immune and allergic reactions, and the need for a second procedure. We can today cultivate keratinocytes, fibroblasts as well as melanocytes in vitro and the cultivated cells are transplanted onto patients in different ways and in combination with skin substitutes, in order to facilitate wound healing and to provide patients with better esthetic and functional results (Figures 6-11, 6-12). The skin cannot regenerate itself and it

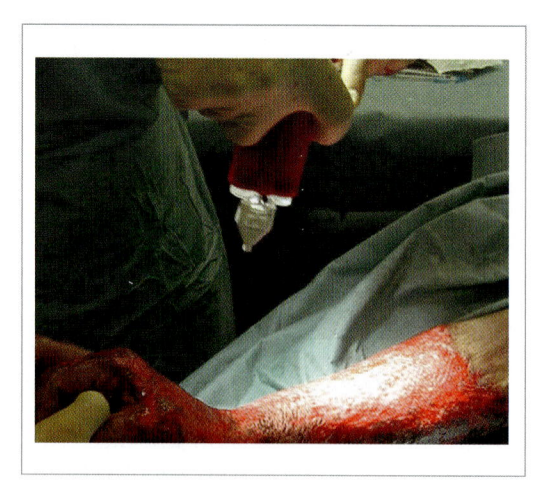

Figure 6-9. Spraying of cultivated cells onto dermal skin.

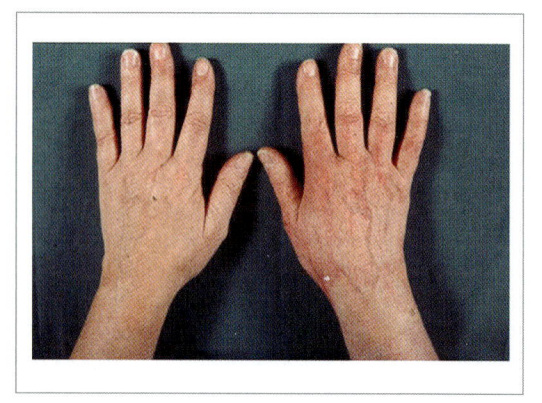

Figure 6-10. Late result of skin-grafted right hand compared to non-injured left hand.

From Basic Wound Healing to Modern Skin Engineering 103

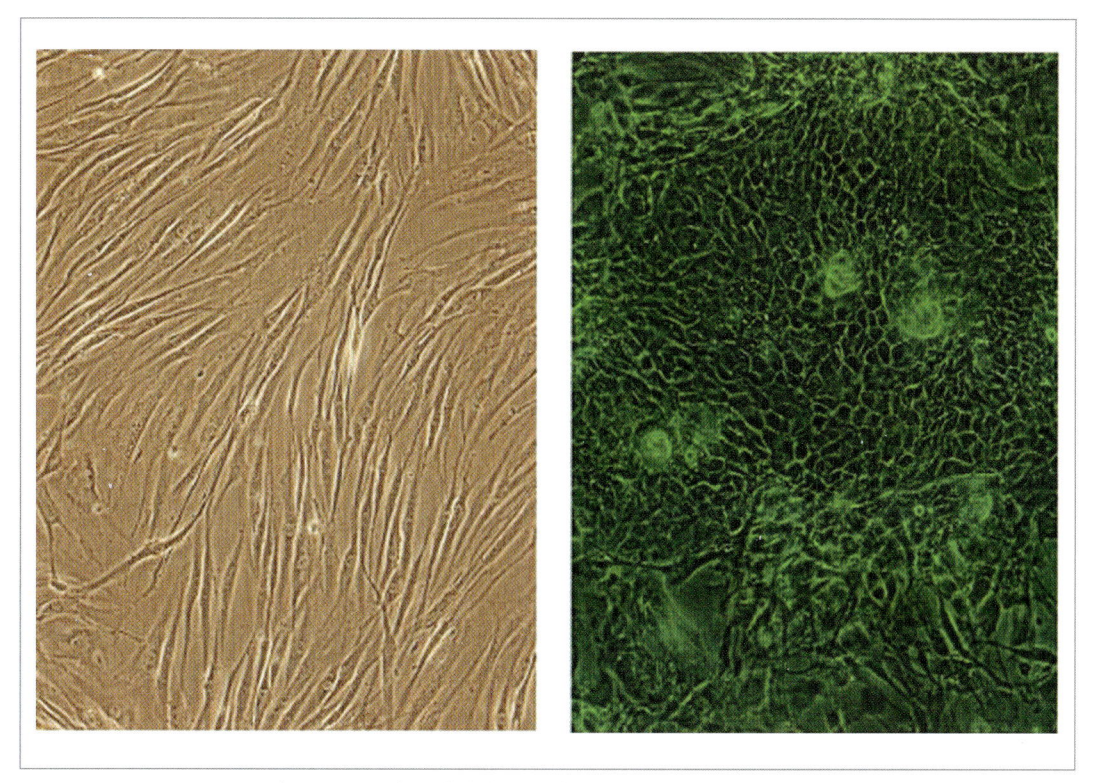

Figure 6-11. Cultivated Fibroblasts (left) and Keratinocytes (right) in vitro.

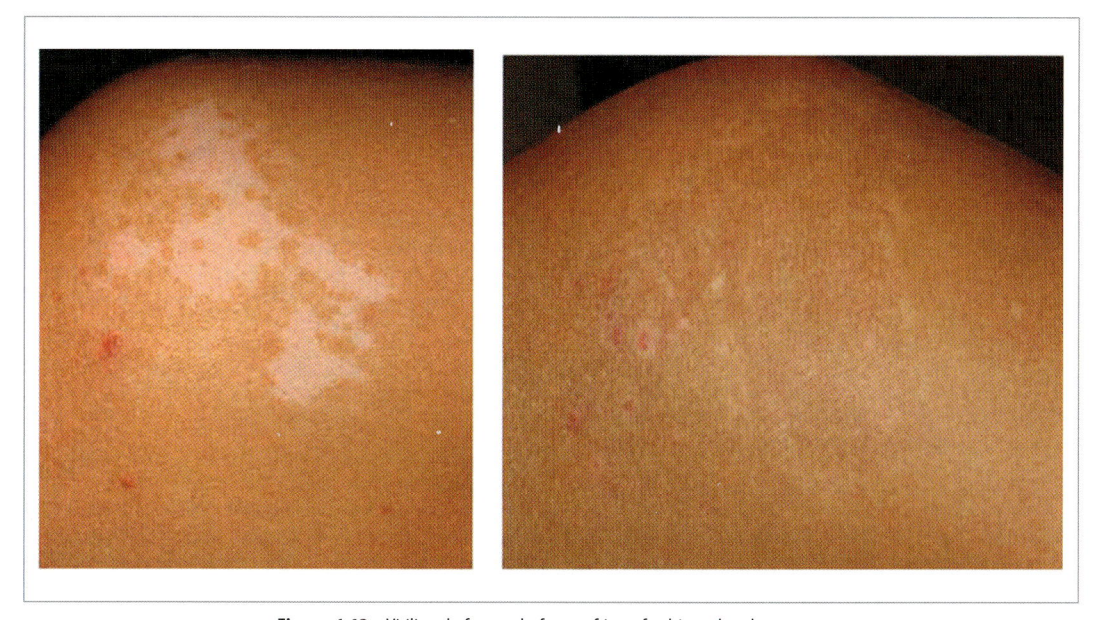

Figure 6-12. Vitiligo, before and after grafting of cultivated melanocytes.

does heal with scarring which sometimes contracts severely. The future involves further understanding of the wound-healing mechanisms as well as further discoveries of the different functions of the different skin cells. The discovery of plasticity of cells (cells ability to transdifferentiate) may also influence the development of new types of skin substitute products with no antigenicity.[68–73] The "key" to the stimulation of regeneration of the skin could reduce/eliminate skin scarring and provide us with better protection against micro-organisms which continue to threaten our existence.

References

1. Rudolph R, Ballantyne DL. Skin grafts. In: McCarthy J (ed). Plastic Surgery: Vol 1 General Principles. Philadelphia, PA: WB Saunders, 1990;221–25.
2. Shores JT, Gabriel A, Gupta S. Skin substitutes and alternatives: a review. *Adv Skin Wound Care*. September 2007; Vol. 20 No. 9. PP. 493–508.
3. Piccolo N, Piccolo-Lobo M, and Piccolo-Daher M. Use of frogskin as a temporary biological dressing, *Proc Am Burn Assoc*. 1992;24.
4. Chiu T, Burd A. "Xenograft" dressing in the treatment of burns. *Clin Dermatol*. 2005;23:419–23.
5. Bhishagratna K. The Sushruta Samhita: An English Translation Based on Original Texts. Cosmo Publications 2006.
6. Spencer WG. Celsus De Medicina, with English translation. Vol. 3. Cambridge, MA: Harward University press. 1938.
7. Balch CM, Marzoni FA. Skin transplantation during the pre-Reverdin era, 1804–1869. *Surg Gynecol Obstet*. 1977;144:766.
8. Reverdin JL. Greffes epidermiques; experience faite dans le service de M. le docteur Guyon, a l'Hopital Necker, pendant 1869. Bull Soc. Imperiale Chir. Paris Series 2, Vol.10, published in 1870.
9. Peacock EE, Cohen IK. Wound healing. In: McCarthy J (ed). Plastic Surgery: Vol 1 General Principles. Philadelphia, PA: WB Saunders, 1990;161–178.
10. Chong AKS, Chang J. Tissue Engineering for the Hand Surgeon. A Clinical Perspective. *J Hand Surg*. March 2006;31A:3.
11. Mooney DJ, Mikos AG. Growing new organs. *Sci Am*. 1999;280:60–65.
12. Attinger CE, Janis JE, Steinberg J, Schwartz J, Al-Attar A, Couch K. Clinic approach to Wounds: Debridement and Wound Bed Preparation Including the Use of Dressings and Wound-Healing Adjuvants. Plastic and Reconstructive Surgery. *Clinical Approach to Wounds*. June Supplement 2006;117:7S.
13. Zellweger G. Die Behandlung Der Verbrennungen. 1985;118:121.
14. Defranzo AJ, Argenta LC, Marks M, et al. The use of vacuum-assisted closure therapy for the treatment of lower-extremity wound with exposed bone. *Plast Reconstr Surg*. 2001;108:1184.
15. Grayson ML, Gibbons GW, Balogh K, et al. Probing to bone in infected pedal ulcers: A clinical sign of osteomylitis in diabetic patients. *JAMA*. 1995;273:721.
16. Fox CL. Silver sulfadiazine, a new topical therapy for Pseudomonas in burns. *Arch Surg*. 1968;96:184.
17. Kucan JO, Robson MC, Heggers JP, et al. Comparison of silver sulfadiazine, povidone-iodine and physiological saline in the treatment of chronic pressure ulcers. *J Am Geriatr Soc*. 1981;29:232.
18. Edgerton MT. The Art of Surgical Technique, Baltimore: Williams & Wilkins; 1988.
19. Trentgrove NJ, Stacey MC, Macauley S, et al. Analysis of the acute and chronic wound environments: The role of proteases and their inhibitors. *Wound Repair Regen*. 1999;7:442.
20. Courtenay M, Church JC, Ryan TJ. Larva therapy in wound management. *J R Soc Med*. 2000;93:394.
21. Sherman RA, Hall MJ, Thomas S. Medicinal maggots: An ancient remedy for some contemporary afflictions. *Ann Rev Entomol*. 2000;45:55.
22. Wollina U, Karte K, Herold C. Biosurgery in wound healing: The renaissance of maggot therapy. *J Eur Acad Dermatol Venerol*. 2000;14:285.
23. Sherman RA, Sherman J, Gilead L, et al. Maggot therapy in outpatients. *Arch Phys Med Rehab*. 2001;81:1226.
24. Krizek TJ, Robson MC. The evolution of quantitative bacteriology in wound management. *Am J Surg*. 1975;130:579.
25. Robson MC, Heggers JP. Delayed wound closure based on bacterial counts. *J Surg Oncol*. 1970;2:379.
26. Robson MC, Heggers JP. Bacterial quantification of open wounds. *Mil Med*. 1969;134:19.
27. Tredget EE, Shankowsky HA, Goeneveld A, et al. A matched-pair, randomised study evaluating the efficacy and safety of Acticoat silver coated dressing for treatment of burn wounds. *J Burn Care Rehabil*. 1998;19:531.
28. Yin HQ, Langford R, Burrell RE. Comparative evaluation of the antimicrobial activity of Acticoat antimicrobial dressing. *J Burn Care Rehabil*. 1999;20:195.
29. Langer R, Vacanti JP. Tissue engineering. *Science*. 1993;260:920–926.
30. Enoch S, Grey JE, Harding KG. ABC of wound healing. Recent advances and emerging treatments. *BMJ*. 22 April 2006;332:962–965.
31. Harper C. Permacol: clinical experience with a new biomaterial. *Hosp Med*. 2001;62:90–5.
32. Hodde JP, Ernst DM, Hiles MC. An investigation of the long-term bioactivity of endogenous growth factor in OASIS Wound Matrix. *J Wound Care*. 2005;14:23–5.
33. Wainwright DJ. Use of an acellular allograft dermal matrix (Alloderm) in the management of full-thickness burns. *Burns*. 1995;21:243–8.
34. Munster AM, Smith-Meek M, Shalom A. Acellular allograft dermal matrix: immediate or delayed epidermal coverage? *Burns*. 2001;27:150–3.
35. Sheridan R, Choucair R, Donelan M, Lydon M, Petras L, Tomkins R. Acellular allodermis in burns surgery: 1-year results of a pilot trial. *J Burn Care Rehabil*. 1998;19:528–30.
36. Brigido SA, Boc SF, Lopez RC. Effective management of major lower extremity wounds using an acellular regenerative tissue matrix: a pilot study. *Orthopedics*. 2004;27(Suppl):s145–9.
37. Schoepf C. Allograft safety: efficacy of the tutoplast process. *Implants- Int Magazine Oral Implant*. 2006;7.
38. Lukish JR, Eichelberger MR, Newman KD, et al. The use of a bioactive skin substitute decreases length of stay for pediatric burn patients. *J Pediatr Surg*. 2001;36:1118–21.

39. Demling RH, Desanti L. Management of partial thickness facial burns (comparison of topical antibiotics and bio-engineered skin substitutes) *Burns.* 1999;25:256–61.
40. Mansbridge J, Liu K, Patch R, Symons K, Pinney E. Three-dimensional fibroblast culture implant for the treatment of diabetic foot ulcers: metabolic activity and therapeutic range. *Tissue Eng.* 1998;4:403–14.
41. Harding KG, Moore K, Phillips TJ. Wound chronicity and fibroblast senescence-implications for treatment. *Int Wound J.* 2005;2:364–8.
42. Boyd M, Flasza M, Johnson PA, Roberts JS, Kemp P. Integration and Persistence of an investigational human living skin equivalent (1CX-SKN) in human surgical wounds. *Regen Med.* 2007;2:369–76.
43. Bello YM, Falabella AF, Eaglstein WH. Tissue-engineered skin. Current status in wound healing. *Am J Clin Dermatol.* 2001;2:305–13.
44. Purdue GF, Hunt JL, Still JM Jr. et al. A mulitcenter clinical trial of a biosynthetic skin replacement, Dermagraft-TC, compared with cryopreserved human cadaver skin for temporary coverage of excised burn wounds. *J Burn Care Rehabil.* 1997;18(1 Pt 1):52–7.
45. Fivenson DP, Scherschun L, Cohen LV. Apligraft in the treatment of severe mitten deformity associated with recessive dystrophic epidermolysis bullosa. *Plast Reconstr Surg.* 2003;112:584–8.
46. Fivenson DP, Scherschun L, Choucair M, Kukuruga D, Young J, Shwayder T. Graftskin therapy in epidermolysis Bullosa. *J Am Acad Dermatol.* 2003;48:886–92.
47. Still J, Glat P, Silverstein P, Griswold J, Mozingo D. The use of a collagen sponge/living cell composite material to treat donor sites in burn patients. *Burns.* 2003;29:837–41.
48. Sibbald RG, Zuker R, Coutts P, Coelho S, Williamson D, Queen D. Using a dermal skin substitute in the treatment of chronic wounds secondary to recessive dystrophic epidermolysis bullosa: a case series. *Ostomy Wound Manage.* 2005;51(11):22–46.
49. Wright KA, Nadire KB, Busto P, Tubo R, McPherson JM, Wentworth BM, Alternative delivery of keratinocytes using a polyurethane membrane and the implications for its use in the treatment of full-thickness burn injury. *Burns.* 1998;24:7–17.
50. Carsin H, Ainaud P, Le Bever H, et al. Cultured epithelial autografts in extensive burn coverage of severely traumatized patients: a five year single- centre experience with 30 patients. *Burns.* 2000;26:379–87.
51. Lobmann R, Pittasch D, Muhlen I, Lehnert H. Autologous human keratinocytes cultured on membranes composed of benzyl ester of hyaluronic acid for grafting in nonhealing diabetic foot lesions: a pilot study. *J Diabetes Complications.* 2003;17:199–204.
52. Harriger MD, Warden GD, Greenhalgh DG, Kagan RJ, Boyce ST. Pigmentation and microanatomy of skin regenerated from composite grafts of cultured cells and biopolymers applied to full-thickness burn wounds. *Transplantation.* 1995;59:702–7.
53. Boyce ST, Goretsky MJ, Greenhalgh DG, Kagan RJ, Rieman MT, Warden GD. Comparative assessment of cultured skin substitutes and native skin autograft for treatment of full-thickness burns. *Ann Surg.* 1995;222:743–52.
54. Schwarze H, Kuntscher M, Uhlig C, et al. Suprathel, a new skin substitute, in the management of donor sites of split-thickness skin grafts: Results of a clinical study. *Burns.* 2007; E-pub:doi: 10.1016/j.burns. 2006. 10.393.
55. Banes AJ, Compton DW, Bomhoeft J, et al. Biologic, biosynthetic, and synthetic dressings a temporary wound covers: a biochemical comparison. *J Burn Care Rehabil.* 1986;7:96–104.
56. McHugh TP, Robson MC, Heggars JP, Phillips LG, Smith DJ Jr, McCollum MC. Therapeutic efficacy of Biobrane in partial- and full-thickness thermal injury. *Surgery.* 1986;100:661–4.
57. Feldman DL, Rogers A, Karpinski RH. A prospective trial comparing Biobrane DuoDERM and Xeroform for skin graft donor sites. *Surg Gynecol Obstet.* 1991;173:1–5.
58. Prasad JK, Feller I, Thomson PD. A Prospective controlled trial of Biobrane versus scarlet red on skin graft donor areas. *J Burn Care Rehabil.* 1987;8:384–6.
59. Grzesiak JJ, Pierschbacher MD, Amodeo MF, Malaney TI, Glass JR. Enhancement of cell interactions with collagen/gylcosaminoglycan matrices by RGD derivatization. *Biomaterials.* 1997;18:1625–32.
60. Stern R, McPherson M, Longaker MT.Histologic study of artifical skin used in the treatment of full-thickness thermal injury. *J Burn Care Rehabil.* 1990;11:7–13.
61. Komorowska-Timek E, Gabriel A, Bennett DC, et al. Artificial dermis as an alternative for coverage of complex scalp defects following excision of malignant tumours. *Plast Reconstr Surg.* 2005;115:1010–7.
62. Machens HG, Berger AC, Mailaender P, Bioartificial skin. *Cells Tissue Organs.* 2000;167:88–94.
63. Orgill DP, Straus FH 2nd, Lee RC. The use of collagen-GAG membranes in reconstructive surgery. *Ann NY Acad Sci.* 1999;888:233–48.
64. Fitton AR, Drew P, Dickson WA. The use of a bilaminate artificial skin substitute (Integra) in acute resurfacing of burns: an early experience. *Br J Plast Surg.* 2001; 54:208–12.
65. Klein MB, Engrav LH, Holmes JH, et al. Management of facial burns with a collagen/glycosaminoglycan skin substitute-prospective experience with 12 consecutive patients with large, deep facial burns. *Burns.* 2005;31: 257–61.
66. Groos N, Guillot M, Zilliox R, Braye FM. Use of an artificial dermis (integra) for the reconstruction of extensive burn scars in children. About 22 grafts. *Eur J Paediatr Surg.* 2005;15:187–92.
67. Jeschke MG, Rose C, Angele P, Fuchtmeier B, Nerlich MN, Bolder U. Development of new reconstructive techniques: use of Integra in combination with fibrin glue and negative-pressure therapy for reconstruction of acute and chronic wounds. *Plast Reconstr Surg.* 2004;113:525–30.
68. Brazelton TR, Rossi FM., Kesher, GI, Blau, HM. From marrow to brain: expression of neuronal phenotypes in adult mice. *Science.* 2000;290:1775–1779.
69. Mezey E, Chandross KJ, Harta G, Maki RA, McKercher SR. Turning blood into brain: cells bearing neuronal antigens generated in vivo from bone marrow. *Science.* 2000;290:1779–1782.
71. Orlic D, Kajstura J, Chimenti S, Jakoniuk I, Anderson SM, Li B, et al. Bone marrow cells regenerate infracted myocardium. *Nature.* 2001;410:701–705.
72. Sigurjonsson OE, Perreault MC, Egeland T, Glover JC. Adult human hematopoietic stem cells produce neurons efficiently in the regenerating chicken embryo spinal cord. *Proc Natl Acad Sci USA.* 2005;102:5227–5232.
73. Wurmser AE, Nakashima, K, Summers RG, Toni N, D, Amour KA, Lie DC, et al. Cell fusion-independent differentiation of neural stem cells to the endothelial lineage. *Nature.* 2004;430:350–356.

Artificial Sphincters

Austin Obichere and Ibnauf Suliman

Introduction

Sphincters in broad term refer to circular muscles within the gastrointestinal or urogenital tract that regulate the release of bowel contents or urine to the outside. Incontinence (fecal or urinary) is due to inability to control stool or urine expulsion as a result of disease, accident, or injury to the anal and sphincter urethrae muscles, respectively. The concept of artificial sphincter use in surgery is not new and was first conceived over 50 years ago to restore continence either by surgically fashioning/transposing muscle or by implanting prosthetic materials to achieve normal bowel or urinary action.

This chapter will review the origin and evolution of artificial sphincters in colorectal surgery. Its role in the clinical management of end-stage fecal incontinence and as an alternative to abdominal wall colostomies will be discussed, and promising future strategies for restoring normal anal defecation examined. A detailed account of the artificial urinary sphincter is outside the scope of this chapter and will be discussed elsewhere.

Origin of Artificial Sphincters

The emergence of artificial sphincters in surgery followed attempts to either surgically fashion or implant prosthesis to achieve urinary or bowel control and avoid diverting urinary tubes/catheters and abdominal wall stomas. The evolution of the artificial bowel sphincter arguably takes it origin from the work of 'M. Pillore', a French surgeon who successfully performed a caecostomy for complete bowel obstruction caused by rectal carcinoma in 1776. Unfortunately, the patient died 20 days after the operation and an autopsy revealed gangrene of the small bowel due to two pounds of mercury he had ingested, believing this would overcome his obstruction. However, the birth of a left iliac colostomy was conceived nearly two decades later in 1793 by Duret – in a desperate attempt to relieve intestinal obstruction in an infant 3 days old with imperforate anus. He had initially performed lumbar colostomy upon the dead body of a baby 2 weeks old, but abandoned this approach as he feared leakage of meconium into the peritoneum. We are told that the operation was a success and that the infant lived to a ripe old age of 45 years. Other notable achievements of this remarkable pioneer surgeon include anchoring the mesocolon with suture to prevent stoma retraction. He recognized the occurrence of stomal prolapse and initiated a crude form of continence through bowel cleansing of stool via the 'artificial anus' using plain water containing two drops of syrup of rhubarb.

The contribution of these pioneer surgeons firmly established the colostomy as a successful treatment strategy for managing malignant or end-stage benign colorectal disorders that has not needed to change for over 200 years. However, despite much progress in surgical technique, stoma design, and management, fecal incontinence and perceived abnormal body image remain major pitfalls impairing patient quality of life and has resulted in a relentless quest for better fecal effluent control with surgically fashioned or prosthetic bowel sphincters.

Surgically Fashioned Bowel Sphincters

In selected patients, construction of an artificial or neo-anal sphincter can be achieved by transposing preserved fascia or skeletal muscle in close proximity to the anal canal. The resulting neo-sphincter constitutes an acceptable alternative to a permanent colostomy, thus avoiding the psychological issues relating to perceived abnormal body image of a stoma. Such a neo-sphincter may be described as passive, dynamic, or physiological.

Passive Neo-sphincter

Harvey Stone conceived the idea of using preserved fascia as a subcutaneous purse string suture that was drawn up snugly around the anus for treating anal incontinence of operative or traumatic origin. Several years later in 1929, he modified this procedure, anchoring the two loops of fascia to the gluteus maximus muscle on opposite sides so that the anus could be tightened by contraction of the muscle.[1] It is of interest that much earlier, at the turn of the 20th century, Chetwood described a technique whereby the gluteus maximus muscle was transposed for sphincter reconstruction while Chittenden in 1930 promoted another variety of the passive neo-sphincter utilizing bilateral gluteus maximus flaps that were sutured anterior to the rectum thus suspending it in a hammock of muscle.[2,3]

The gluteus maximus muscle gained further popularity in reconstructive surgery for anal incontinence when Bistrom (1944) described a method of detaching a part of the origin of the muscle and fashioning an opening through which the rectum was pulled through to create a sphincter mechanism.[4] It soon became evident that the direct pull of the parallel muscle bundles even at normal resting tone provided some degree of continence that could be reinforced voluntarily and that the normal physiological length tension relationship was re-established. Furthermore, the muscle is well innervated and vascularized, which permits transfer of a segment with little risk of developing ischemia.

More recently, construction of an anal sphincter mechanism using either the origin or the insertion of the gluteus maximus muscle has been reported.[5,6] The former being a modification of the original technique described by Bistrom, involved creation of bilateral muscular slings that were split to encircle the rectum in order to stabilize each other at a proper resting tension and fiber length. In the case of the latter, muscle was detached from its insertion on the linear aspera of the femur to create a double scissor-like diaphragm around the rectum which was then anchored to the ischial tuberosities. However, despite reported claims of improved anal continence by proponents of these two methods, they have failed to gain widespread acceptance and have so far been restricted to isolated cases.

Utilization of the gracilis muscle to create a continent neo-anal sphincter in four children with end-stage anal incontinence was described by Pickrell in 1952 and emerged as the favored operation because the muscle was not bulky and did not impair certain motor functions such as climbing stairs. In his original article, Pickrell described transposition of a single gracilis muscle in a clockwise fashion 360° surrounding the rectum and fixed to the contra-lateral ischial tuberosity with suture.[7] Modifications of this technique now include a bilateral muscle wrap which adopts either one of two configurations; a complete circumferential wrap using both muscles or the creation of a sling behind the rectum with a single gracilis muscle reminiscent of the puborectalis, while the other was rotated in a clockwise fashion to encircle the rectum.

These operations were designed primarily for the management of end-stage fecal incontinence due to defective anal sphincter function as opposed to attempts in restoring anal continence after abdomino-perineal excision of the rectum. However, passive transposition of a single gracilis after surgical ablation of the rectum has also been reported, whereby an opening was created in the muscle through which the colon was pulled through and anchored to the perineum. The transposed gracilis was secured to adjacent deep perineal muscles, the presacral aponeurosis, and the contralateral ischial tuberosity.[8] In one series, use of adductor longus muscle to create a neo-anal sphincter after rectal excision has also been described.[9]

Indications

Passive artificial muscle sphincters were originally designed for the treatment of fecal incontinence, but have recently been added to the armamentarium at the disposal of colo-proctologist where total anorectal reconstruction may be required for the following conditions;

- End-stage fecal incontinence
- Abdomino-perineal excision of rectum
- Congenital anorectal disorder (Imperforate anus/Spina bifida)
- Sphincter injury/trauma.

Types of Passive Neo-sphincters

A variety of skeletal muscles have so far been successfully transposed to create a passive neo-anus. The common denominator in all cases is that the muscle utilized in the creation of a passive artificial anus must carry its own neurovascular supply and lie in close proximity to the anal canal. Skeletal muscles harboring these characteristics are as follows;

- Gracilis (unilateral or bilateral)
- Gluteus maximus (unilateral or bilateral)
- Adductor longus (unilateral)
- Satorius (unilateral)
- Rectus femoris (unilateral)

Complications

A major drawback of passive anal sphincter reconstructive techniques is that fecal continence is short-lived because striated skeletal muscle fatigue easily and cannot sustain prolonged voluntary contraction. This led to attempts by others to discover new techniques and strategies designed to create fatigue resistant-striated skeletal muscles and resulted in electrically stimulated neo-sphincters (fatigue resistant muscles).[10,11]

Reports of muscle necrosis of the harvested neo-sphincter have largely been attributed to poor muscle quality or surgical technique. The gracilis which is by far the most commonly used muscle, receives its neurovascular supply in the upper third of the muscle thereby allowing transposition around its proximal pedicle. Ischemic injury therefore occurs as a result of direct trauma to the neurovascular bundle during muscle harvesting or indirectly, due to excessive pedicle tension from re-routing, peri-operative hematoma formation, or tissue edema.

Infection remains the main harbinger of failure of passive neo-sphincters requiring revisional surgery where initial conservative treatment with antibiotics with or without wound lavage/debridement fails. A variety of organisms both gut-derived and skin microbes have been identified but colononization by methicillin-resistant Staphylococcus aureus (MRSA) means that failure is near irreversible. Sometimes due to overwhelming sepsis such as necrotizing fascitis and associated muscle necrosis, salvage is not possible and neo-sphincter reconstruction using the contra-lateral muscle should be considered and re-scheduled to a later date.

Poor-quality muscle either inherent or due to atrophy from fatigue will result in poor outcome and incontinence. Most patients therefore require self medication with constipating agents to attain acceptable continence followed by the assistance of self-administered enema to evacuate stool. Understandably, achieving the right balance can be difficult and tiresome for many patients.

Dynamic/Electrically Stimulated Neo-sphincters

It was discovered in animal experiments and in humans that repeated electrical stimulation of skeletal muscle from external sources resulted in conversion from type 2 (easily fatigued) to type 1 (fatigue-resistant) muscle fibers.[12,13] This adaptive response to a generated electrical pulse allows sustained voluntary contraction of the neo-anal sphincter, enhancing the fecal continence achieved by a passive muscle wrap.

A significant advance in this technique was pioneered by Cor Baeten and Norman Williams who independently developed different types of implantable device to induce this vital change in muscle property, thereby improving neo-sphincter function and making this sort of surgery a practical reality.[10,11] Baeten developed an intra-muscular (albeit perineural) mode of muscle stimulation, whereas Williams directly stimulated the nerve trunk to the gracilis. The former technique has proved more robust in most surgeon's hands as it avoids problems with electrode displacement which seems commoner when the nerve trunk is stimulated directly (Figure 7-1).

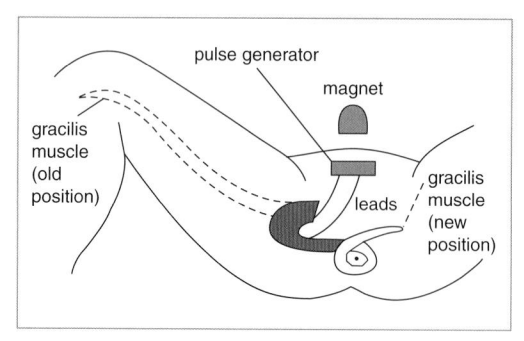

Figure 7-1. Electrically stimulated neo-sphincter.

Indications

The electrically stimulated neo-sphincter has been shown to be more effective than the passive muscle wraps in terms of continence control and quality of life. It is more likely to produce higher resting anal pressures than the non unstimulated neo-sphincter, and hence improve continence. Despite sharing similar indications with its predecessor (see above), dynamic neo-sphincters have gained popularity particularly among highly motivated young adults with sphincter injury from trauma or accident, who are determined to avoid an abdominal wall stoma.

Types of Dynamic Neo-sphincters

The two skeletal muscles most frequently utilized in the construction of surgically fashioned neo-sphincters are the gracilis and gluteus maximus. The former is generally preferred because it is less bulky, easier to transpose, and does not impair motor function like walking up stairs. On the other hand, dissection and separation of the gluteus into two parts with careful preservation of the inferior gluteal neurovascular supply to the distal half, is more challenging and has deterred widespread use of this muscle.

Five different configurations of gracilo-plasty (alpha, gamma, epsilon, split sling, and double wrap) have been described and in one study that compared the first three types, it emerged that the alpha wrap generates lower neo-anal pressures than gamma and epsilon.[14]

Dynamic Neo-sphincter Following Abdomino-perineal Excision of Rectum

The last decade has seen attempts by surgeons to construct a dynamic neo-sphincter following surgical excision of the rectum for carcinoma, with some degree of success.[12,14–17] All authors adopt chronic low-frequency electrical stimulation for muscle conversion even though the timing of its onset and duration vary among investigators. Most experts favor construction of the neo-sphincter with double gracilis muscle wrap at the same time as perineal stoma formation, usually without a defunctioning stoma presumably because it allows early stimulation of the transposed muscle.[12,16,18] But Williams and colleagues employed a three-staged approach that included perineal colostomy formation with vascular delay of the distal gracilis muscle, creation of a stimulated graciloplasty, and closure of the defunctioning stoma.[15]

The gracilis vascular delay procedure, whereby the distal perforating vessels to the muscle are ligated, allows new channels to form from the proximal major vessel and was thought to reduce the risk of distal muscle ischemia after transposition.[19] However, the emergence of direct anatomical and physiological evidence from experimental studies showing only one arterial system within the gracilis muscle questions previous practice involving an additional operation for vascular delay, implying that this approach may now be redundant.[12]

The main indication for rectal excision and neo-sphincter reconstruction in these circumstances has been in the treatment of distal rectal cancer. Initial concerns regarding the risk of jeopardizing the possible cure of the patient in return for avoiding a colostomy have so far been refuted by some studies which have shown that it is an oncologically safe operation. One study reviewed 20 patients who had abdomino-perineal reconstruction with a double dynamic gracilo-plasty after rectal excision for low rectal cancer found no local recurrence, but revealed four patients who developed distant metastasis.[12] In another report of 12 patients who had electrically stimulated graciloplasty after abdomino-perineal excision of the rectum, 10 had rectal adenocarcinoma of which 6 were Dukes stage A, 3 were B, and only 1 was stage C.[14,20] There was no local recurrence at a median follow-up of 54 months (range, 3–79), but pulmonary metastases developed in the patient with Dukes C rectal cancer. Furthermore, in a personal series of 81 patients over a 10-year period of which 37 surviving patients were followed for a mean period of 79 months, the study concluded that restorative perineal graciloplasty did not reduce the effectiveness of abdomino-perineal resection in the cure of cancer.[17]

Functional Outcome of Dynamic Graciloplasty

Total anorectal reconstruction with electrically stimulated graciloplasty after abdomino-perineal excision of the rectum may be primary (reconstruction of the neo-anus in the same operation as the abdomino-perineal resection) or secondary (neo-sphincter reconstruction several years after a Miles resection). The former method is by far the most frequently performed, perhaps due to the anticipated increased morbidity with the latter. In seven patients who had a secondary procedure a mean of 8.5 years after a Miles resection, it was found that although continence was regained in five patients, they suffered numerous complications, additional operations, long hospital stay, and subsequent re-admissions.[21]

The reported functional results following reconstruction of a neo-anorectum with graciloplasty (stimulated or unstimulated) after excision of the rectum for cancer, vary considerably in the literature. One series evaluated 26 out of 31 patients for continence at a mean follow-up of 40 months, revealing continence to liquid and solid stool in 22 patients or 85%.[18] Mercati and colleagues found that all seven patients who had unstimulated graciloplasties in their series were satisfied with the level of continence achieved with the neo-anus, although they acknowledged that these patients suffered a slight-to-moderate fecal incontinence causing a persistently wet anus that required the use of pads.[16] In another study, 'successful' functional outcome was reported in 8 of 15 patients (53%) who were continent to solid and liquid stool, but continence in these circumstances included occasional fecal soiling.[12]

Contrary to the above findings which support a favorable functional outcome, others have reported episodes of incontinence to solid stool, persistent soiling due to liquid stool necessitating wearing of sanitary pads at all times, and difficulty with stool evacuation requiring the aid of regular enemas.[14] This disparity in reported continence may be attributed to differing techniques employed by investigators as exemplified by Williams and colleagues, who favored a staged approach with a single gracilis muscle wrap, while others constructed the neo-sphincter with a double gracilis wrap at the same time as formation of a perineal colostomy.[12,15,16,18] In addition, there is no standardized or validated tool available to measure functional outcome after anorectal reconstruction with the dynamic graciloplasty, thereby encouraging comparison of studies in this area.

It is of interest that amalgamation of data from the literature would appear to suggest that the double gracilis neo-anus gives better functional results compared to the single muscle wrap. However, the contrasting methods employed in these studies in determining the patients' level of continence with a neo-sphincter has been overlooked, and obvious failure in taking account of the effect of observer bias. Moreover, one group recently reviewed morbidity and functional outcome in 15 patients with a mean follow-up of 28 months who had undergone double dynamic graciloplasty after abdomino-perineal resection. They found that of 12 patients available for assessment, five out of six cases without neo-sphincter stenosis, had 'good continence', indicating that the double dynamic graciloplasty was associated with a high rate of stenosis which compromised functional outcome.[22] The reason why this is so has been attributed to the forces generated by asymmetrical contraction of both gracilis muscles. Given these conflicting reports in the literature, it is clear that there are areas of significant variation amongst experts pertaining to graciloplasty configuration, timing of surgery, and implantation of the electrical device and function. Unquestionably, it would seem that the true functional outcome of these procedures remain uncertain.

Complications

The dynamic neo-sphincter operation is technically demanding has a long-learning curve and carries considerable morbidity. It has therefore been recommended this type of surgery be confined to specialist colorectal centers. Complications may also be due to the technical challenges encountered during harvesting and creation of the neo-anus or device related.

As with the passive neo-sphincter, muscle necrosis from direct and indirect causes of ischemia along with reports of infection are also encountered following construction of the dynamic neo-sphincter. Neo-sphincter stenosis is a problem that was described recently and is associated with the double gracilis wrap that appears to generate asymmetrical pressure forces around the neo-anus.[22,23]

The device-related complications are numerous and range from mechanical failure which is frequently the result of complete battery discharge to the local effects of the device itself. Localized pain or discomfort, device or lead migration, and erosion of skin lead disconnection or fracture are some of the well-documented problems of the device. Repeated operations and ultimately explantation of the device are sometimes necessary to address some of these drawbacks contributing to further overall morbidity in these patients.

Inability to evacuate stool is commoner following neo-anal reconstruction with dynamic graciloplasty than with the passive neo-sphincter, presumably because the former has been shown to generate higher neo-anal pressures on manometry. Nonetheless, it is a problem that leaves the patient entirely reliant on enemas to achieve stool expulsion despite terminating electrical discharges from the pulse generator to the neo-sphincter by interrupting the established electrical circuit with a magnet. Given the high morbidity associated with neo-sphincter reconstruction, all patients are likely to benefit from a centralized service with the necessary expertise on site, along with a plan that incorporates pre-operative counseling and a selective approach.

Physiological Neo-sphincter

The passive and dynamic neo-sphincters offer little or no body image disturbance unlike an abdominal wall stoma. They also provide added benefit in terms of continence control via the neo-anus, albeit an effective biological 'thirsch' wire. Unfortunately, these patients rely on regular enemas or irrigation of the neo-anus for the evacuation of 'formed' stool and are incontinent to liquid fecal discharge. Furthermore, the loss of normal reservoir capacity provided by the excised rectum and lack of a sensory component either through disease or surgery means that these types of neo-sphincters will always fall short of normal physiological function.[24]

Recent reports from animal experiments describe a new generation of neo-sphincter reconstruction capable of voluntary action following cross-innervation of the nerve supplying the transplanted muscle and the pudendal nerve. Sato and colleagues created a neo-sphincter with the biceps femoris muscle (equivalent of the human gracilis muscle) in 22 dogs after rectal extirpation and performed anastomosis between the nerve to the muscle and the pudendal nerve.[25] Following nerve regeneration, they demonstrated successful muscle conversion from type 2 to type 1 fibers with apparent satisfactory defecatory function. Similarly, Congiliosi and others rendered three groups of 10 dogs incontinent and compared passive, dynamic, and a physiological neo-anal wrap with pudendal nerve anastomosis.[26] They observed that the physiological group produced a functional anal sphincter superior to the other two methods. More recently one novel study showed experimentally that it was possible to reconstruct a functional external anal sphincter using a free latissumus dorsi flap with pudendal neuromicrovascular anastomoses in nine mongrel dogs rendered fecally incontinent.[27] What these studies seem to imply is that the pudendal nerve potentially has a crucial role in attempts to restore native innervation and voluntary anal sphincter function.

Preliminary studies in human cadavers have shown that it is possible to create a physiological neo-sphincter using the gluteus maximus muscle – inferior half of the muscle supplied by the inferior gluteal neurovascular bundle.[28] Another group also demonstrated in human cadavers that it was possible to technically reconstruct a physiological neo-sphincter using the gracils muscle with pudendal nerve anastomosis.[29] The first clinical case of the 'voluntary' neo-sphincter after abdomino-perineal resection of the rectum has shown encouraging early results for a technique which may signal a new more efficient alternative to the dynamic neo-sphincter[28] (Figure 7-2). Long-term data in 10 out of a series of 19 patients from a single center over an 8-year period indicate that voluntary defecation was achieved in all 10 patients without the need for enemas or irrigation. In addition, better continence scores and quality of life were demonstrated in this group when

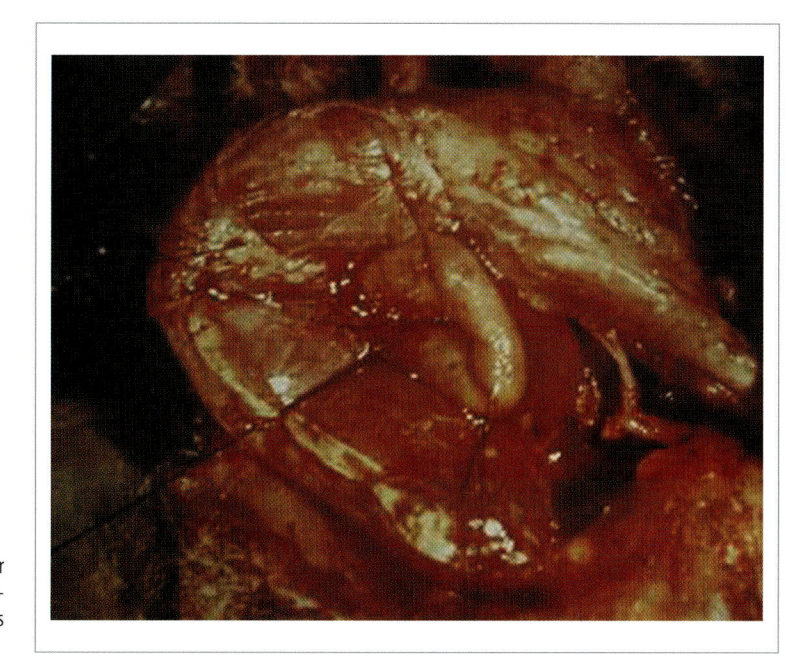

Figure 7-2. Physiological neo-sphincter illustrating pudendal and inferior gluteal nerve anastomosis and gluteus muscle wrap around the colon.

compared to 27 historical controls who had abdomino-perineal excision of the rectum and end colostomy formation.[30] Sato and his colleagues proposed that the resulting restoration of sensitivity after pudendal nerve anastomosis, allows recognition of the need to defecate and might explain the promising results so far reported following construction of the physiological neo-anus.

Indications

Physiological neo-sphincters share similar indications to passive and dynamic types and in common with the other two rely on skeletal muscle that can be transposed along with their own neuro-vascular bundle. The main contraindication, therefore, would include patients with impaired nerve or muscular function from neuromuscular disorders. So far, all 19 patients who have undergone physiological neo-sphincter reconstruction have been diagnosed with low rectal cancer treated by abdomino-perineal excision of the rectum.[30] It is foreseeable that this approach may play a role in the surgical management of end-stage fecal incontinence due to other benign conditions provided that further data confirm the efficacy of this promising technique.

Types

A single center experience utilizing the lower half of the gluteus maximus muscle with its own inferior gluteal neuro-vascular bundle account for all the patients in the literature who have had anal continence restored by physiological neo-sphincter reconstruction. However, use of the gracilis muscle and free latissimus dorsi flaps with pudendal neuromicrovascular anastomoses hold future promise.[27,29] It is expected that other skeletal muscles with their own neurovascular supply may be adopted in the future or perhaps preferred to the gluteus muscle so long as more studies concur that the technique is feasible and is a superior alternative to other types of neo-sphincters.

Complications

With the exception of device-related complications, the physiological neo-sphincters present similar problems encountered with the dynamic neo-anus.

Muscle ischemia and necrosis resulting from infection, intrinsic skeletal muscle characteristics, or poor harvesting techniques are other complications that occur without exception in all neo-sphincters. However, the physiological neo-sphincter whose function is dependent on pudendal nerve growth to re-connect with the muscle, presents a potentially unique problem of disuse muscle atrophy. This phenomenon commonly occurs during the period required for adequate nerve regeneration. Given that the estimated peripheral nerve regeneration rate is 1 mm/day, recovery of muscle function may fail or be delayed, depending on the distance between the site of nerve anastomosis and the muscle end-plate. To overcome this potential drawback of muscle atrophy, it has been suggested that direct electrical stimulation of the muscle during the time required for nerve growth may reverse this process.[30] The evidence supporting the prevention of disuse muscle atrophy in the physiological neo-sphincter has been extrapolated from data demonstrating continued neo-sphincter muscle activity by programmed electrical stimulation using an external device.

Experimental Organ Transplantation

The quest for anal continence after abdominoperineal excision of the rectum has led a number of surgeons to create a neo-anus reconstructed from muscle, or even an anal artificial sphincter.[31] However, clinical results have not been altogether satisfactory, partly because these methods were intended to deal with the strength of the anal sphincter alone, reminiscent of a biological Thiersch.

Anal continence is not just the result of contractile activity in the anal sphincter, but also depends on good sensation, reasonable capacity, and a colon and rectum that are neither too active nor too inert. Furthermore, the ability to be continent and the ability to evacuate are to some extent mutually antagonistic. This means that many of the above surgical attempts to restore continence have been bedeviled by defecatory problems because the patient has no idea when the rectum is full and because contractile rectal activity and deactivation of whatever device is being used to control continence are not coordinated.

Anorectal transplantation should have the potential to solve a number of the above problems. Parts designed for a specialized purpose would seem on first principles to have a better chance of restoring best function compared to transposed muscle or implanted plastics, and the pudendal nerve, being a mixed motor and sensory nerve, should be able to restore sensation, motor function, and perhaps reflexes.

What has been most exciting about novel techniques employing pudendal nerve anastomosis is the prospect of restoring a sensory component. Many of the clinical problems of the dynamic neo-sphincters relate to the lack of knowledge of the need to defecate through loss of a normal sensory pathway. Anorectal transplantation with pudendal nerve anastomosis therefore holds out the prospect of potentially normal anorectal function. But it is beset by its own difficulties, not least the apparent extreme technical difficulty involved surgically, added to which are the issues of returning physiological function and immunological considerations.

Evolution of Organ Transplantation: Essential or for Quality of Life?

Organ transplantation has traditionally been aimed at restoring life to patients who would otherwise face imminent death from fatal disease or failure of a vital organ. This concept was reinforced by transplantation of the heart, lungs, liver – and to a lesser extent kidneys and small intestine, where imminent demise from organ failure might be avoided with long-term dialysis and total parenteral nutrition, respectively. There is no doubt that organ transplantation not only saves lives but might also provide the recipient with a new lease of life and freedom to perform normal daily activities with improved quality of life.

The last two decades have seen patient quality of well-being increasingly recognized as an important outcome measure of surgical practice and it is not in the least surprising why some investigators have now been prepared to consider transplantation of a non-essential organ primarily to improve quality of life – as exemplified by recent clinical transplantation of the larynx, womb, hand, and face.[32–35]

Permanent colostomies following anorectal amputation for cancer can be devastating for some people who would rather contemplate suicide than accept life passing bowel contents through an artificial opening on their abdominal wall.[36–38] It remains debatable whether current alternative surgical techniques such as the perineal stoma and neo-sphincters, which avoid a colostomy, might reasonably be considered a sufficient answer because of persisting defecatory problems which impair quality of life. The physiological neo-sphincters using pudendal nerve anastomosis may be an advance because the pudendal nerve might not only permit reflex sphincter function but also allow the patient to sense the need to defecate.

It is envisaged that anorectal transplantation is a possible strategy that would replace the anorectal structural unit after abdominoperineal resection, if it were technically and biologically feasible. The resulting preservation of body image and potential return of normal anal defecation might improve patient quality of life far beyond currently available methods, thereby reinforcing calls that transplantation of a non-essential organ can be performed for quality of life reasons alone.[39]

Assessing the Feasibility of Anorectal Transplantation

Anatomy and Function of the Pudendal Nerve. The pudendal nerve is a mixed nerve carrying sensory, motor, and autonomic fibers from three roots derived from the second, third, and fourth (S2–S4) ventral rami of the sacral plexus. Normally the three roots unite to form two cords, which unify to create a main trunk, commencing at the upper border of the ischial spine and carrying sensory fibers to genitalia, muscular branches to the sphincter urethrae, perineum, and external anal sphincter. The pudendal nerve trunk passes back between the piriformis and the coccygeus muscle and curls around the sacrospinous ligament before running forward to lie within the pudendal canal (Alcock's) on the inferior lateral wall of the ischiorectal fossa.[40]

The pudendal nerve has three main branches: inferior rectal, which constitutes the motor supply to the external anal sphincter and controls voluntary sphincter action; dorsal nerve of the penis/clitoris, which innervates the genitals; and the common perineal nerve, giving muscular branches to the perineal muscles and sphincter urethrae. The inferior rectal nerve branch emerges from the posterior end of Alcock's canal, before division of the pudendal trunk into its terminal branches (dorsal nerve of penis/clitoris and common perineal) which occurs within the canal itself[41] (Figure 7-3).

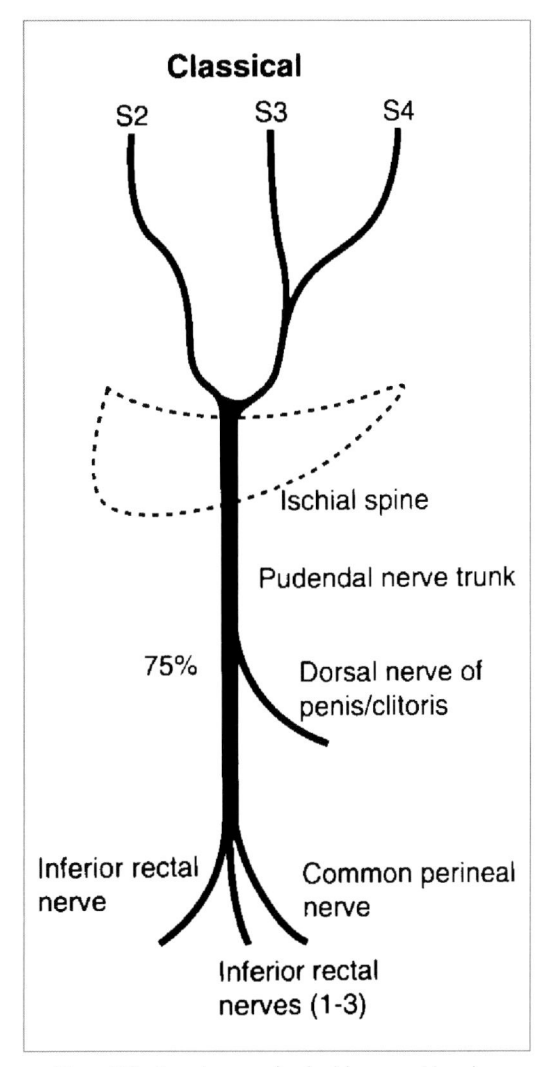

Figure 7-3. Normal course of pudendal nerve and branches.

Like all anatomical structures, the pudendal nerve is not exempt from anomalies involving any part of its entire course. A thorough understanding of variations of the main nerve trunk and its branches is vital for accurate nerve selection in any attempt to reconstruct the 'physiological' anorectum following rectal excision.

Surgical Approach. Most surgeons are unfamiliar with pudendal nerve anatomy because its exposure is infrequently encountered in clinical practice. When access is attempted, the surgeon may find it difficult, with risk of injury to the nerve and its branches. Moreover, interest to date in the pudendal nerve has largely focused

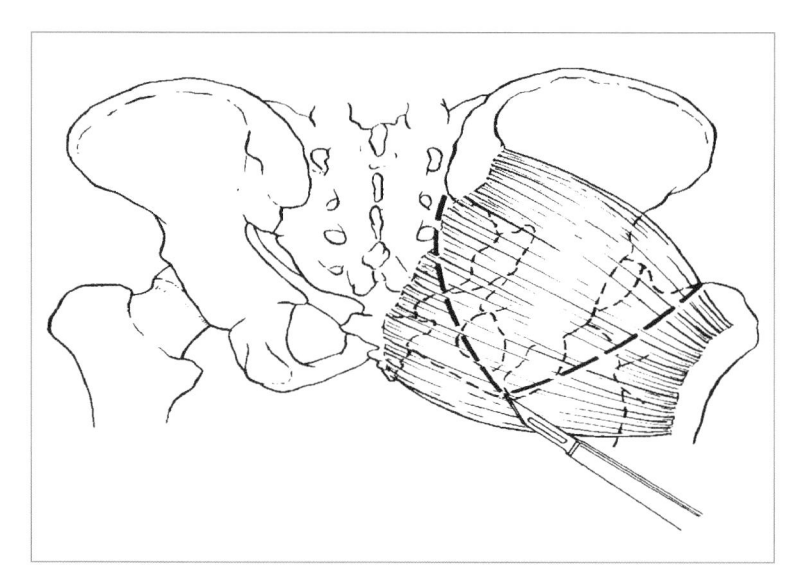

Figure 7-4. Surface landmarks for pudendal nerve exposure in human cadaver.

on the successful application of non- and minimally invasive techniques for the diagnosis and treatment of pudendal neuropathy, a recognized cause of pelvic floor, rectal, and anal sphincter disorders, rather than surgery.[42]

Surgical access to the pudendal nerve in humans has mostly been limited to cadaveric studies and occasional attempts at pudendal nerve decompression for cases of unexplained anal or perineal pain. Pudendal nerve trunk anomalies have been demonstrated, but surgeons wishing to develop a reproducible surgical approach have little to guide them.[43] Indeed, some investigators acknowledge that optimal exposure of the pudendal nerve and its branches without injury is a potential obstacle to attempts to reconstruct a functional anal sphincter complex after rectal extirpation.[26]

One study examined pudendal nerve anatomy in cadavers seeking to identify potential anomalies of clinical significance and to describe a new, simple, reproducible approach for maximal exposure of the nerve and its branches that might contribute to improved access for functional reconstructive procedures.[44] They found that a simple four step surgical approach was not only simple but also reproducible and gave maximal pudendal nerve exposure as follows

Step 1: The mid-point of the lateral border of the sacrum, the ischial tuberosity, and the ipsilateral greater trochanter of the femur were identified and marked with indelible ink (Figure 7-4). These surface landmarks were chosen because they were easily identifiable and define the anatomical region of interest.

Step 2: A vertical incision through skin and subcutaneous tissue was extended from the mid sacrum to the ischial tuberosity, then curved upward and laterally to the greater trochanter to create a flap that was reflected to reveal oblique fibers of the distal half of gluteus maximus arising from its sacral origin and directed downward (Figure 7-5).

Step 3: A longitudinal incision was made through the exposed gluteus maximus onto the sacrum and extended distally to the ischial tuberosity so that lateral retraction of this muscle exposed the glistening fibers of the sacrotuberous

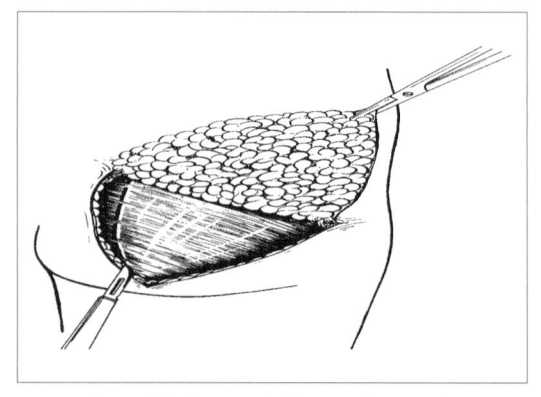

Figure 7-5. Exposure of gluteus maximus muscle.

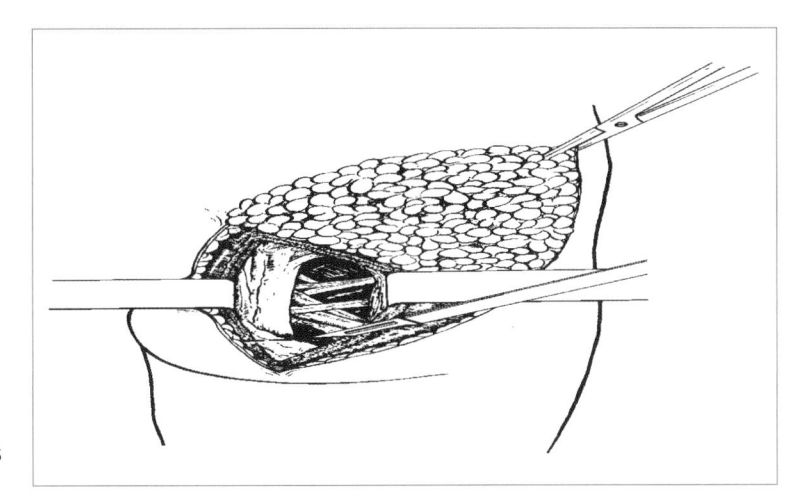

Figure 7-6. Exposure of sacrotuberous ligament.

ligament and inferior gluteal neurovascular bundle arising from its free edge (Figure 7-6).

Step 4: The sacrotuberous ligament was then divided at its distal attachment and drawn outward along its free border to reveal the pudendal neurovascular bundle in a connective tissue tunnel (Alcock's canal) (Figure 7-7).

The study concluded that the aforementioned four-step approach, permitted optimal exposure of the pudendal nerve and its branches thereby facilitating restoration of neural innervation to anal sphincter reconstructive procedures. Similarly, another group explored the anatomic bases of the functional graciloplasty with pudendal nerve anastomoses in seven adult human cadavers.[45] They showed that re-innervation of the gracilis muscle transposed around the anus with pudendal end-to-side anastomoses was feasible and predicted eventual clinical application.

Nerve Regeneration and Attainment of Restored Function. Peripheral nerve regeneration and the return of normal physiological function after transection or injury have been the subject of numerous experimental and clinical studies. Promising experimental results in large animals suggest that a mixed peripheral nerve like the pudendal nerve following controlled injury, as in transection, can regenerate to innervate the target organ and potentially restore automatic function.[25,26] This return in function is almost universally assessed by qualitative techniques as accurate quantitative tests are impossible to interpret in animals, despite their crucial role in the clinical assessment of regeneration. However, more recently, quantitative methods utilizing qol tools and radiological imaging to assess defecatory function have been adopted in patients who have undergone anorectal

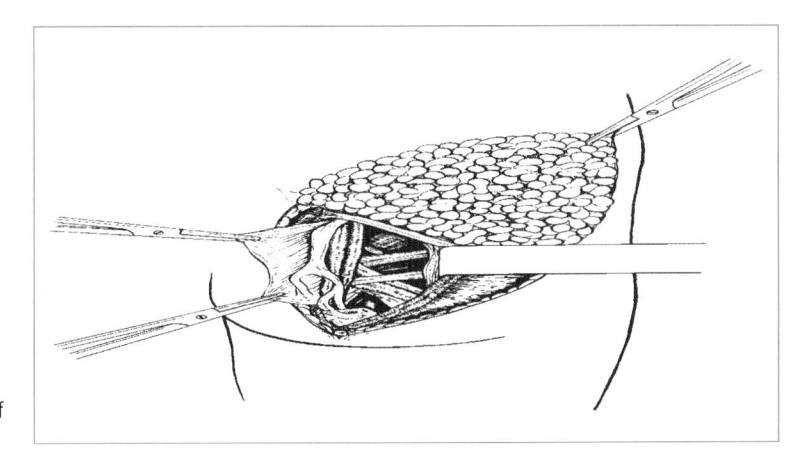

Figure 7-7. Maximal exposure of pudendal neurovascular bundle.

reconstruction with the physiological neosphincter after rectal excision for cancer.

The pathophysiology of nerve injury has not been fully elucidated but current knowledge would seem to implicate diminished viability or death of Schwann cells, axonal degeneration, depletion of nerve or target-derived neurotrophic factors, and the loss of primary sensory (dorsal root ganglia) and motor neurons.[46] Predictably, attempts to improve nerve regeneration would therefore have to rely on the successful manipulation of the aforementioned pathophysiological processes triggered by nerve injury.[47]

Nerve growth factor (NGF), neuropetide-3 (NT-3), and neuropeptide-Y (NT-Y) are just a few of the neurotrophic factors that have been shown to play a role in the maintenance and survival of nerve cells, in addition to mimicking the effect of target organ-derived trophic factors on neuronal cells.[48] Convincing evidence of neuronal regeneration using exogenous neurotrophic factors has been demonstrated, largely in small laboratory animals, although equally encouraging results employing similar techniques have been reported in non-human primates.[49] The outcome of ongoing clinical trials is awaited.

Most investigators recognize that the specificity of re-innervation is the most important determinant of successful nerve regeneration, but there is controversy whether the regenerating axons are physically guided by basal laminar tubes or are drawn directly by neurotrophic factors originating from the distal nerve stump and targets which influence the sorting of regenerating axons.[46] However, it appears that both factors come into play following injury of the peripheral nervous system. A major drawback encountered after nerve injury is the frequent retraction of fibers resulting in a shortfall in length which must be accommodated to allow successful reinnervation of target or end organs. To this end, the use of nerve autograft to fill a significant gap remains the gold standard,[47] but where an autograft is not possible, an allograft or autogenous biodegradable nerve conduits have so far shown promise in experimental studies.[50–52]

Where anorectal transplantation with pudendal nerve anastomosis following surgical ablation of the rectum is shown to be technically and biologically feasible, regeneration of the recipient's pudendal nerve and reinnervation of the graft with the attendant immunological challenges will become the key to success. It is also anticipated that ongoing research leading to better understanding of the host rejection response, advances in immunotherapy, and the development of neurotrophic factors will ultimately transform application of allogenic nerve grafts from the laboratory into the clinical setting.

Technological Advances Which Make Anorectal Transplantation Feasible

Tremendous technological advances over the last 30 years have made organ transplantation a feasible alternative treatment for end-stage organ failure. In many cases, it is considered a less expensive form of treatment for a failed or diseased organ, which adds to the human and clinical interests among investigators and has resulted in remarkable progress in terms of graft survival and recipient well-being. This improved outcome owes much to better surgical techniques and in particular microsurgery which allows anastomosis of vessels and nerve repair of structures measuring less than 1 mm in diameter.

Improvements in graft survival and function have also resulted from better matching at the DR site of HLA locus of the major histocompatibility complex (MHC), coupled with advances in harvested graft preservation techniques.

Perhaps the greatest stride forward in terms of graft survival has been in the area of immune therapy and modulation of the host response to foreign antigen. In 1978, the clinical advent of a novel immunosuppressive agent, cyclosporin A, transformed organ transplantation with improved outcome.[53] Further progress soon followed with the introduction of Tacrolimus (Prograf, FK506), a fungal metabolite which acts in a similar way to Cyclosporin A by inhibiting the earliest steps of T-cell activation.[54]

Randomized clinical trials now indicate that Tacrolimus in comparison to Cyclosporin A results in a further decrease in the incidence of rejection.[55–57] The development of newer drugs in this area offers even greater prospects of achieving one of the ultimate goals in organ transplantation: to protect the transplanted graft and recipient from rejection and adverse effects so well that transplantation for quality of life indications becomes widely accepted.

Anorectal Transplantation

Despite the arguments in favor of anorectal transplantation as an alternative to abdominal wall colostomy after excision of the rectum, there are no data in the literature that have examined the feasibility of this new concept in humans. However, one study explored the technical feasibility of orthotopic allotransplantation of the anorectum and assessed graft viability after abdomino-perineal excision of the rectum in an animal model.[57]

Pre-operative Preparation. Large White Landrace pigs were selected for this study because preliminary cadaveric dissection had shown that females had a well-developed external sphincter muscle complex surrounding the anal canal and vagina, in contrast to males, in which the muscle was less bulky and encircled the anal canal only. In view of this peculiar anatomy, and ease of operation, four females (22–42 kg) provided donor anorectum to four recipient males (29–39 kg) having received pre-medication (xylazine 1 mg/kg and ketamine 5 mg/kg) 1 h before standard general anesthesia (1–2% halothane in 4 L oxygen and 1 L nitric oxide per minute) (Figure 7-8). Intravenous access was established in each recipient and 4.3% dextrose/saline given at a rate of 100 ml/h, during and after transplantation.

Donor Operation. Commencing in the left lateral position, a circumano-vaginal incision was extended on both sides in a posterior lateral direction (Figure 7-9). Preliminary cadaveric dissections had shown that mobilization between the rectum and the coccyx, with detachment of the gluteus maximus muscle along the incision margin, provided optimal exposure of the pudendal neurovascular bundle arising from the lateral pelvic wall.

The external anal sphincter around both anus and vagina was dissected free and detached from the pubic bone (Figure 7-10).

The animal was then placed in the supine position and laparotomy with division of the symphysis pubis performed. The inferior mesenteric artery and vein were prepared for division and the operation was suspended while the recipient was prepared. When this was accomplished, intravenous heparin 200 units per kg body weight was given, and the pudendal structures divided as far proximal as possible to facilitate subsequent re-anastomosis in the recipient. The colon was then transected, followed by division of the inferior mesenteric artery and vein, releasing the specimen. Bench dissection was then performed to detach the vagina from the donor specimen (Figure 7-11). The mesenteric artery was cannulated and perfused with 200 ml heparinized saline (5000 units heparin in 1000 ml normal saline) and preserved at 0–4°C to await transplantation.

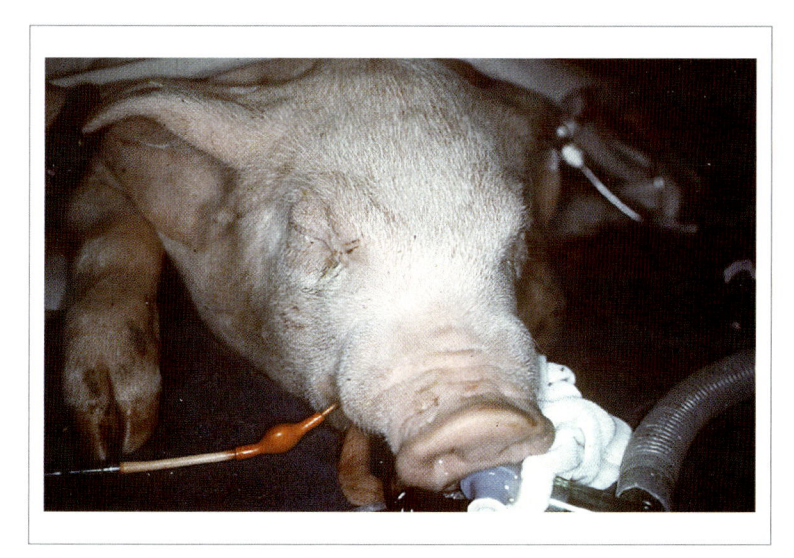

Figure 7-8. Illustration of pig under standard general anesthesia.

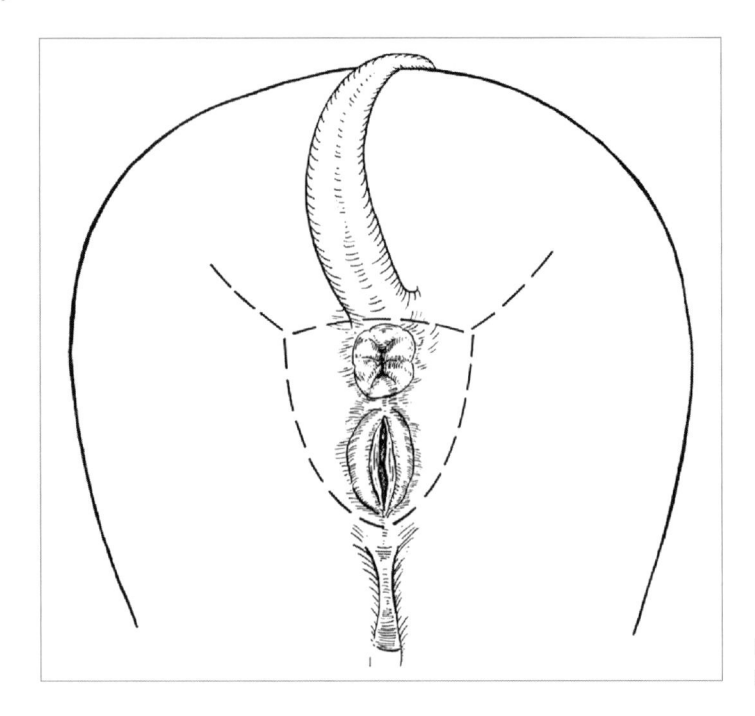

Figure 7-9. Exposure of perineum in pig and circumano-vaginal incision.

Recipient Operation. The perineal phase was similar to the donor operation, except instead of dealing with vagina, these pigs being male, the external anal sphincter encircling the anal canal was stripped free from the cavernosum muscle which was preserved. The abdominal phase omitted division of the pubic symphysis. The next steps were heparinization of recipient (200 units/kg); transperineal introduction of the anorectal graft; rectal anastomosis at the proximal end (single layer of interrupted 3/0 polyglactin) to stabilize the graft before microsurgical anastomosis of inferior mesenteric artery and vein (10/0 nylon in all pigs); laparotomy wound closure; microsurgical pudendal artery anastomosis (10/0 nylon in 2 pigs); bilateral pudendal nerve anastomosis (10/0 nylon by epineural technique in three pigs) (Figure 7-12); and closure of the perineum (3/0 prolene) (Figure 7-13). After transplantation, all recipient animals were given intramuscular analgesia (carpofen 4 mg/kg) every 4 h.

Recorded Variables Post Transplantation. The duration in minutes of the operation and ischemic times were recorded by an observer and various parameters of anastomosed structures (vein, artery and nerve) were measured with a millimeter grid scale using a microscope at ×10 magnification. Orthotopic allotransplantation of the anorectum was attempted in four short-term live pig models, and before they were sacrificed 24 h later, observation at laparotomy revealed two pink grafts, one slightly dusky but healthy graft and one outright failure, reflecting the state of the mesenteric vessels, which were patent in three and thrombosed in one. Histological examination of these observed findings showed no difference between the control biopsies and the three cases with satisfactory mesenteric flow. However, gross ischemia was present histologically in the failed case.

The study concluded that anorectal transplantation was technically feasible in a short-term pig model and called for further long-term studies to assess the return of normal defecation, prevention of sepsis, and overcome rejection issues before it can be considered in humans. It is of interest that in this model, the animals did not receive antibiotic or immuno-suppressive therapy, a reasonable strategy given that the earliest signs of acute rejection may take up to 1 week to develop in the colon.[58] One possible explanation for this delayed large bowel antigenicity compared to the small intestine is the relative paucity of lymphoid tissue in the colon.[59] This

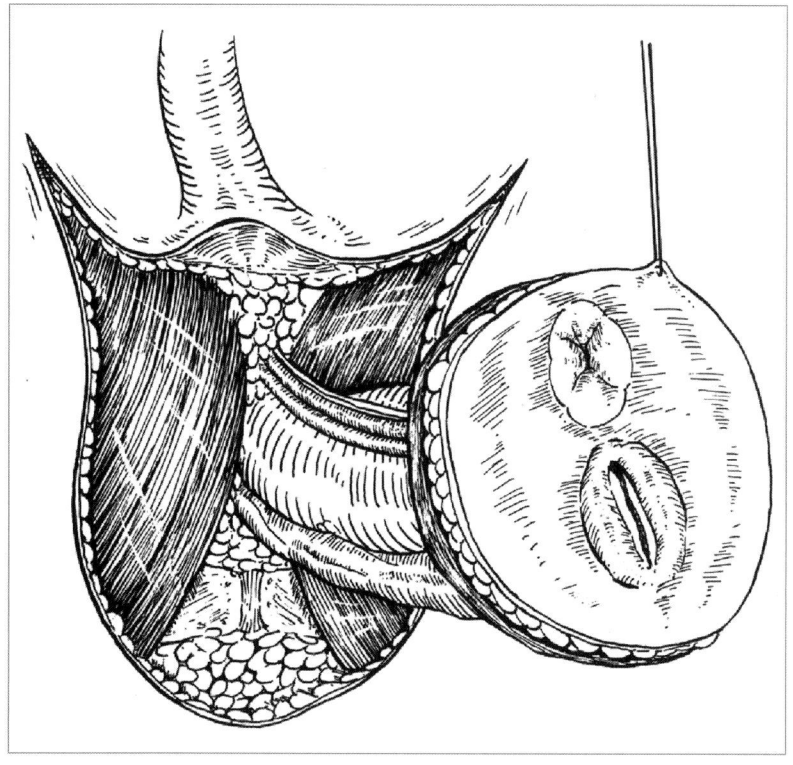

Figure 7-10. Dissection en bloc of the anorectum, pudendal neurovascular bundle, vagina, and uterus.

phenomena may facilitate a good outcome of future attempts at anorectal transplantation, perhaps because fewer immunological challenges are encountered.

Indications

Although clinically unproven, anorectal transplantation would be a reasonable alternative strategy in people requiring rectal extirpation for cancer, trauma, or end-stage benign disease. This novel approach is beset with numerous obstacles not least the technical, immunological, and biological challenges which to date are untested in humans. However, it is foreseen that over the next decade the expected expansion in organ transplantation for quality of life reasons alone as opposed to saving life will drive renewed interest in this area as investigators continue in their quest to restore normal defecation albeit physiological, following surgical excision of the rectum.

Complications

The drawbacks of anorectal transplantation can broadly be divided into problems related to the technique (organ harvesting/preservation, donor/recipient operations) and the immunological and biological challenges.

The technique for anorectal transplantation has yet to be elucidated in humans but knowledge of the normal immune response to foreign protein is fundamental to our understanding of the complex immune-biological events triggered by organ transplantation; that must be conquered not only to prevent rejection but also to improve survival and function of allogenic graft. This immune-biological challenge may take the form of immune response to foreign antigen, allograft rejection, and major histocompatibility complex (MHC).

Immune Response to Foreign Antigen. Allotransplantation induces an immune response in the

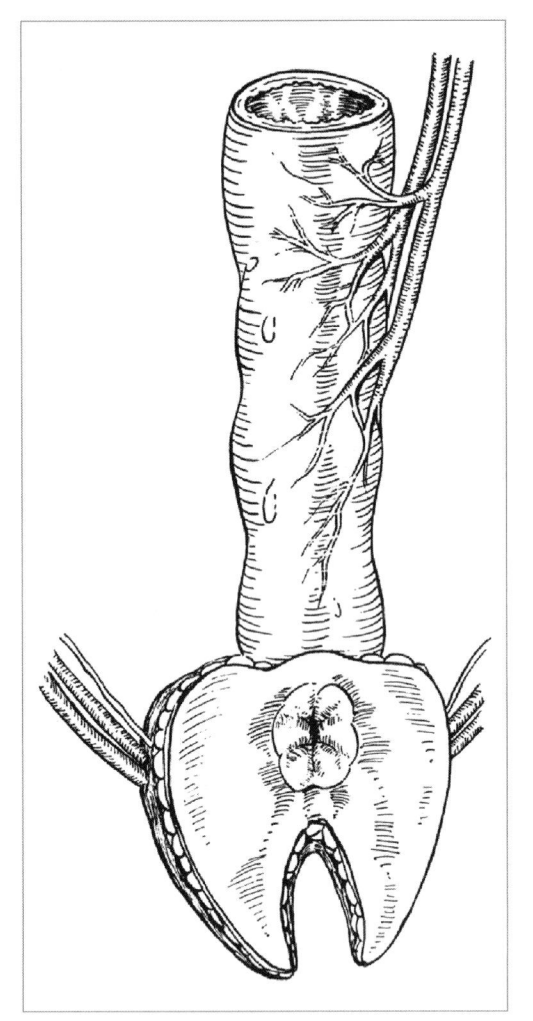

Figure 7-11. Donor anorectal graft.

effector function results in proliferation and differentiation to plasma cells which secrete specific antibody resulting in complement fixation or antibody-mediated cytotoxicity. On the other hand, the non-specific immune response involves the activation and recruitment of macrophages, cytokines, and other non-specific effector cells by their interaction with T cells which causes direct damage of grafts.

Allograft Rejection. The rejection of allograft may occur by one of three mechanisms: cell-mediated, which is orchestrated by circulating T cells; antibody mediated following activation of plasma cells; and other mechanisms which remain poorly understood but are believed to involve cytokines such as tumor necrosis factor (TNF). Based on extensive work in human renal allografts, the speed of organ rejection following transplantation can be classified into three:

- Hyperacute: occurring within minutes to several hours after transplantation due to preformed circulating antibodies.
- Acute: occurring within days to a few months after transplantation and may be the result of cell-mediated immunity
- Chronic: occurring more than 6 months after transplantation and is due to persistent immune response or the long-term side effects of drugs.[60]

Because rejection can be seen to occur at varying intervals after transplantation it is generally assumed to be the result of the different mechanisms outlined above, but it is more likely that all three events are simultaneously activated, albeit to varying degrees. It is reasonable to predict that virtually any cell, cytokine, or chemical mediator that is capable of tissue destruction may play an important role in the ensuing immunological sequelae after organ transplantation, which might explain why it has so far proved difficult completely to control the immune response. Attempts to improve graft survival and function which entail suppression of the entire immune system in recipients might impede activation of those agents which seek to destroy the transplanted organ, but would leave the patient fatally exposed to infectious diseases and oncogenic viruses.

Major Histocompatibility Complex (MHC). A donor graft carries on its surface transplantation antigens known as major histocompatibility

recipient which may be antigen specific (T and B cell mediated) or non-specific (macrophage and cytokine mediated), but frequently involves a combination of these two mechanisms. Antigens are presented to recipient T cells either directly (antigen delivered by donor antigen presenting cell) or indirectly (antigen delivered by recipient antigen presenting cell). The activated T cell via chemical messengers recruits other T and B cells to proliferate, differentiate, and develop effector function which then causes damage in an antigen-specific manner. The effector function of T cells arises through enhanced cytotoxic activity of natural killer cells, interleukin and interferon, while B cell

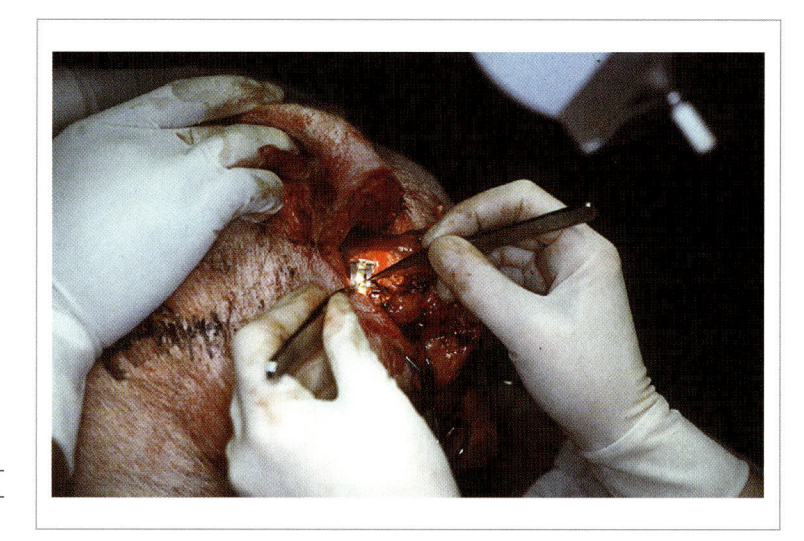

Figure 7-12. Illustration of anastomoses of pudendal neurovascular bundle by microsurgery.

complex (molecules which present antigens to T lymphocytes, MHC) located on the short arm of chromosome six. In humans, these antigens which govern rejection are known as human leucocyte antigens (HLA). The human leocoyte antigen contains three regions which encode for type I, II, and III antigens. Types I and II are highly polymorphic or variable and trigger specific T cell response, while the less polymorphic type III antigen has no role in initiating specific T cell responses, but nonetheless plays an important part in immunity through induction of cytokines and the complement system. The relevance of HLA compatibility between donor and recipient is that when patients are well matched particularly at the DR site of the HLA II locus of the major histocompatibility complex, outcome in terms of graft survival and function fare better than those mismatched.[60]

Prosthetic Bowel Sphincter

Artificial Bowel Sphincter

The artificial urinary sphincter (AUS) was introduced into clinical practice over three decades ago for the management of genuine stress urinary incontinence. The AMS-721 (American Medical Systems) also known as the Brantley Scott AUS initially consisted of four main components (a reservoir, inflatable occlusive cuff, inflating, and deflating pump mechanism). Further modification of this device resulted in the development of the AMS 800 series in 1982, which had three components (balloon, cuff, and pump) and has retained its role as the 'gold standard' artificial urinary sphincter or prototype from which other types of artificial sphincter devices have evolved.

In 1987, Christiansen and Lorentzen were credited with successfully implanting what was essentially a urological device in a single patient for the management of anal incontinence of neuromuscular origin. The prosthesis consisted of three components – a balloon to regulate pressure, a pump representing the control assembly, and a cuff which mirrored the anal sphincter (Figure 7-15). They demonstrated that the device generated a sufficient pressure (66–74 mmHg) which lay within the normal range of resting sphincter pressure, allowing closure of the anal canal without mechanical failure, infection of the device, or local erosion of tissue.[61]

Other investigators have also utilized the 'AMS 800' artificial urinary sphincter (American Medical Systems) for the management of anal incontinence secondary to benign disease.[62-64]

Description of the AMS 800 Artificial Bowel Sphincter

The device is filled with fluid and is implanted entirely within various parts of the body in

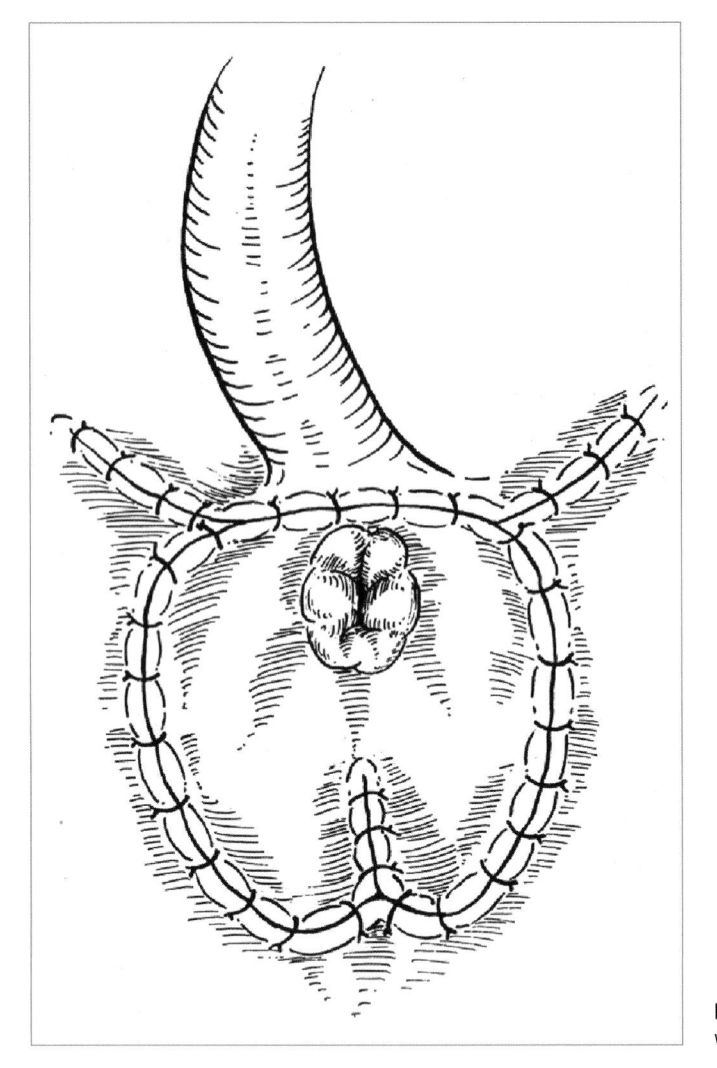

Figure 7-13. Closure of perineal wound in recipient.

either men or women with severe fecal incontinence not amenable to other forms of treatment. It is designed to control stool expulsion and it is claimed to simulate normal sphincter function by opening and closing the anal or neo-anal canal at the control of the patient. The device is made from solid silicone elastomer that is inert and minimizes the risk of rejection by the body. The cuff is implanted around the anal or neo-anal canal, while the pump is placed in the scrotum or labium. The pressure regulating balloon is implanted in the lower abdomen, under the muscle layer, and just above the pubic symphysis. It is normally filled with sterile solution usually saline that can be imaged with plain x-ray.

Device Activation/Deactivation

In the activated or closed position, the cuff is filled with fluid and gently squeezes shut the anal or neo-anal canal to maintain fecal continence. To defecate, the system is deactivated by squeezing and releasing the soft lower part of the pump several times. This leads to the transfer of fluid from the cuff to the balloon, leaving an empty cuff that no longer applies pressure to the bowel and permits expulsion of stool. The fluid that is transferred to the balloon creates pressure within the balloon which pushes the fluid back into the cuff to restore continence. It takes several minutes for the cuff to re-fill, presumably sufficient

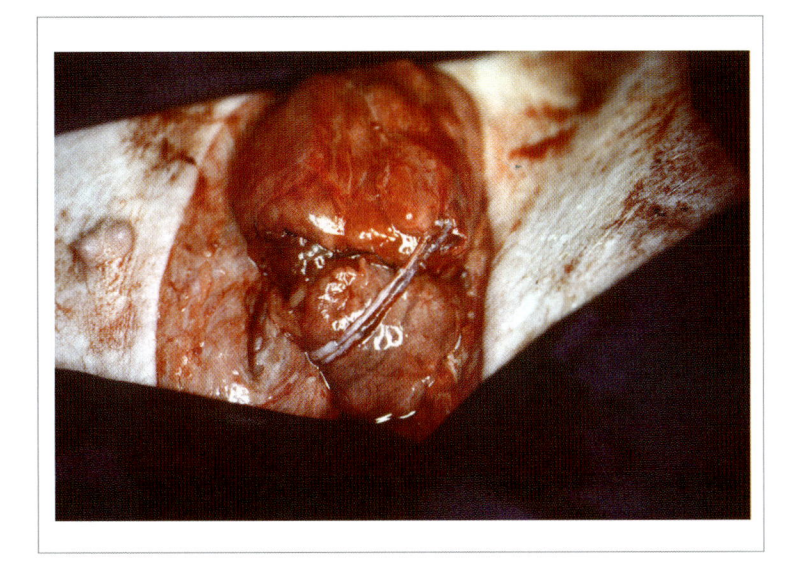

Figure 7-14a. Illustration of technically satisfactory anastomoses of mesenteric vessels before harvesting 24 h post-transplantation.

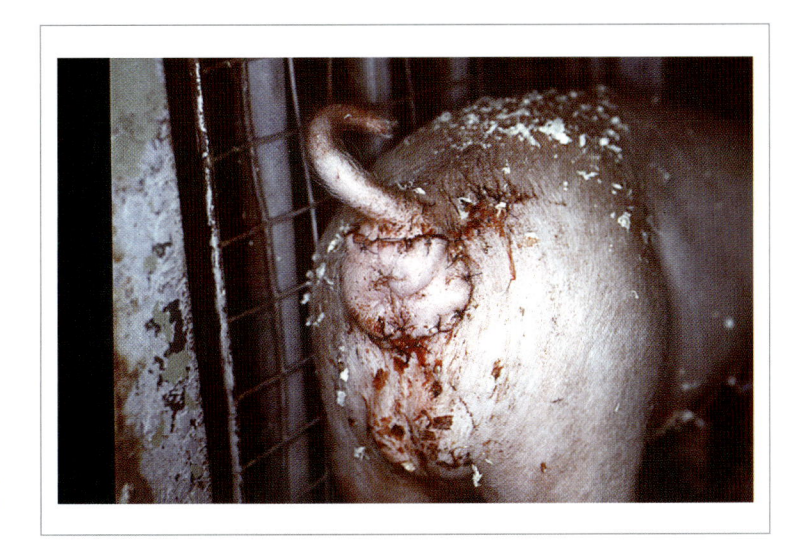

Figure 7-14b. Illustration of healthy looking grafted skin in fully active/alert animal after transplantation.

time for fecal evacuation to take place before the anal canal is squeezed shut again by the filled cuff.

Functional Outcome of the Artificial Bowel Sphincter

In a large personal series of 53 patients Devesa et al. evaluated the technique, and functional results following implantation of the Acticon artificial bowel sphincter for total anal continence not amenable to sphinteroplasty or failed sphincter repair.[65] They reported that the artificial anal sphincter restores continence to solid stool in almost all patients with preceding severe incontinence and that two-thirds of these patients achieved normal continence. Another study evaluated experience with the device in a single institution over an 8-year period. Thirty-seven consecutive patients were prospectively evaluated, the majority of whom had either sphincter disruption or neurologic disease (35/37), while only two patients had hereditary malformation. They concluded that satisfactory continence was achieved following assessment

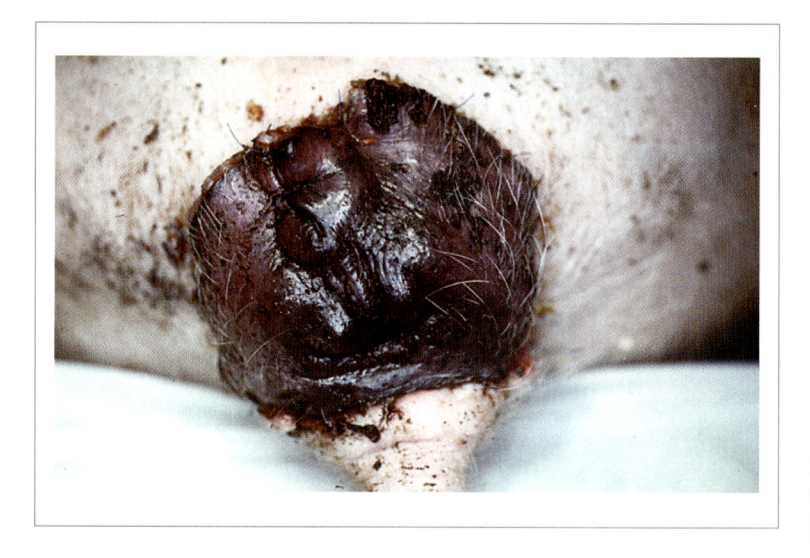

Figure 7-14c. Illustration of outright failure of graft before harvesting 24 h post-transplantation.

with physical examination (anal continence and rectal emptying) and manometry.⁶⁶ One randomized clinical trial compared implantation of the artificial bowel sphincter versus a program of supportive therapy in 14 severely incontinent adults. Using continence (Cleveland Continence Score) and quality of life (SF-36) outcome measures, they found that despite device explantation in one patient (14%), the artificial bowel sphincter was easy to use, effective in restoring

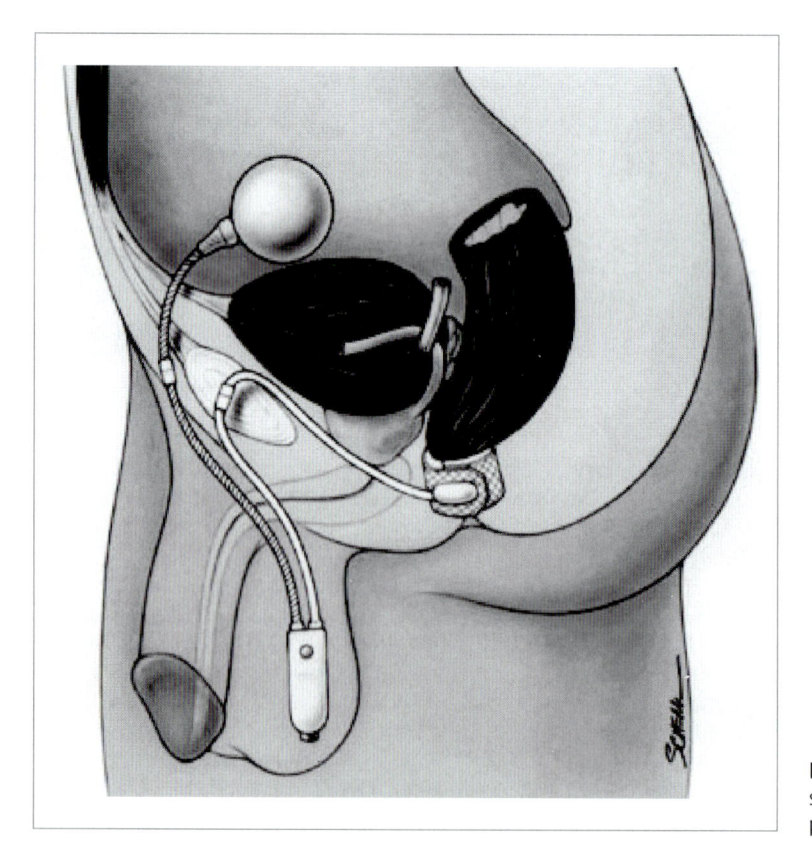

Figure 7-15. Acticon artificial bowel sphincter (AMS) consisting of a cuff, pump, and balloon.

continence and improved quality of life superior to supportive therapy.[67] On the other hand, in a smaller series of 12 patients with implanted artificial neo-sphincter devices for end-stage anal incontinence, Wong et al. found less convincing data in support of the artificial bowel sphincter.[63] They reported complications in a third of their patients which resulted in poor clinical outcome. Furthermore, a systematic review of the safety and effectiveness of the bowel sphincter for fecal incontinence revealed that its implantation is of uncertain benefit and may possibly harm many patients because of high morbidity.[68]

Surprisingly, despite the relative success of these artificial bowel sphincters in the management of end-stage fecal incontinence (neurological disorder or irreparable sphincter defect), there is limited data in the literature evaluating their use after abdomino-perineal excision of the rectum for malignant disease, even though data from experimental studies had shown much promise for future clinical application.[31,69,70] One plausible explanation why this is so may be due to concerns relating to oncological clearance, given that most clinicians would elect to delay neo-anal reconstruction until tumor clearance has been confirmed histologically. For this reason, it is therefore not surprising why currently there are only a few reports of case or personal series that describe implantation of the device after Miles' operation[71,72] or as a secondary procedure in the small number of patients who opt for a perineal colostomy at the time of excision of their rectal cancer.[65,73]

Indications

Artificial bowel sphincters may be considered as a feasible and effective management strategy for fecal incontinence due to benign or malignant disease.

Benign Disease. Patients with end-stage fecal incontinence due to sphincter disruption (obstetrics, trauma, anal surgery) or where previous attempts at sphincter repair have failed are the most frequent indications for treatment with the artificial bowel sphincter. Arguably, the artificial bowel sphincter is currently the only surgical option for treatment of anal incontinence in patients with neurologic disease that affects the pelvic floor and muscles of the lower limb.

There are also those patients particularly in the pediatric population with congenital anomalies such as imperforate anus who would benefit from treatment with the artificial bowel sphincter. In these circumstances, implantation of the sphincter device is usually deployed at the time of the 'pull-through' operation or as a secondary procedure many months or years later.

Malignant Disease. Low rectal or anal cancer requiring abdomino-perineal excision of the rectum results in an incontinent abdominal or occasionally perineal colostomy. Implantation of the artificial bowel sphincter either as a primary or as a secondary procedure following a Miles' operation is a feasible and effective treatment option that may restore anal continence, improve quality of life, and avoid a stoma. However, experience on this subject is limited to a handful of case reports or personal series from single institutions possibly because of the general concern regarding the risk of cancer recurrence alluded to above.

Contraindications

The main contraindication to implantation of the artificial bowel sphincter is active ongoing or chronic infection. Patients with pathological problems that affect rectal compliance, result in chronic diarrhea, persistent fecal impaction, or have had previous surgery resulting in scarring or impairment of the vascular supply to the bowel that precludes implantation of the device in the pelvis. Those selected should have no physical disability, must be medically fit to tolerate a major abdominal operation, and should also be determined and highly motivated to operate the device correctly.

Types

The adaptation of the AMS 800 artificial urinary sphincter in 1987 for the management of fecal incontinence by Christensen et al. led to the evolution of the current artificial bowel sphincter which also consists of the same three components (cuff, balloon, and pump) as the AMS 800 prototype.[61] More recently, other types of artificial bowel sphincters have emerged such as the prosthetic artificial sphincter (PAS), a remote controlled artificial bowel sphincter, and the shape memory alloy (SMA). While the PAS has been successfully tested clinically, the remote controlled and the SMA versions are still at the pre-clinical stage.

Prosthetic Anal Sphincter (PAS). The PAS device was introduced almost a decade ago and initial data from animal experiments revealed that it produced fecal continence without causing ischemia at the point of contact with the intestine.[70] It shared a similarity with the AMS 800 in that it also consisted of three parts (pump, balloon, and cuff) but its inventors claimed that PAS simulated normal action and function of the anal canal under the patients' control by occluding the anorectum at an angle reminiscent of the puborectalis. Another unique design is the pump which has two parts; a bulb which when squeezed empties the cuff of occlusive gel permitting defecation, and a button located over the dome which when depressed re-fills the cuff and restores fecal continence. Using this device in 12 patients with severe fecal incontinence, investigators revealed after a median follow-up of 29 months that the device restored continence in 10 of 11 patients, with no device-related infective complications although one patient developed pseudomembranous colitis requiring device explantation.[74]

Remote Controlled Artificial Bowel Sphincter (ABS). One study describes pre-clinical use of a remote-controlled artificial bowel sphincter prototype that effects fecal continence with comfortable control.[75] This device has similar design to the three part AMS 800, but in this case comprises a micropump based on piezo-technology allowing remote transmission of signals enabling cuff inflation and deflation.

Shape Memory Alloy (SMA). This novel device utilizes a solid driving element, a combination of shape memory alloy(SMA), and layered silicon elastomer sheets for the open and close phase of the artificial bowel sphincter.[76] Although still at the pre-clinical development stage, the authors claim that the device has few parts inside the body and therefore can be implanted more easily.

Patient Selection and Assessment

All patients who fulfill the indications for an artificial bowel sphincter outlined above should be considered. A full evaluation of the patient, including a thorough history and complete physical examination, is essential prior to insertion of an artificial bowel sphincter. It is particularly important to establish that the fecal incontinence is sufficiently disabling to warrant surgical intervention and that all other less invasive alternatives have been previously explored. A pre-operative septic screen to ensure sterility must be ascertained prior to device implantation and should include eradication of MRSA organisms colonizing the skin and the nasal region. If there is any clinical evidence of anal sepsis such as a fistula in ano, device implantation should be postponed and the condition should be dealt with and cured.

Implantation of the Artificial Bowel Sphincter

Pre-operative preparation should include full mechanical bowel preparation with antibiotic and deep venous thrombosis prophylaxis. The antibiotics should cover both aerobic and anaerobic organisms and it is advised that the entire device should be soaked in 120 mg of gentamycin solution prior to implantation. A lower midline laparotomy incision gives good access to the rectum and it is customary to enter the mesorectal plane by dividing the pelvic peritoneal reflection on one side. Minimum dissection distally is required while in this plane to reach the anorectal junction at which point a small incision is made in the contralateral peritoneal reflection to enable the sphincter cuff to encircle the upper border of the anal canal just above the pelvic floor muscles. It is important to establish at this point that with the sphincter cuff deflated, evacuation of bowel contents is not impeded and is easily assessed by using the surgeon's index finger. Implantation of the cuff component of the artificial bowel sphincter is concluded by closing the peritoneal reflection to isolate the device from the peritoneal cavity.

A subcutaneous pouch is then created usually in the right iliac fossa for the control pump but it can also be sited either in the scrotum or labia majora. The connecting tubes from the control pump are attached to the cuff and regulating balloon, respectively, and the latter is left to lie free within the pelvic cavity.

The surgeon should ensure that the device is surrounded by generous subcutaneous tissue within the pouch to prevent damage from trauma, device erosion, or migration. It is also the operators' responsibility to test and confirm satisfactory functioning of the artificial bowel sphincter before the abdomen is closed.

Complications

A number of complications are associated with the artificial bowel sphincter, while some are relatively minor, others such as device failure, infection, or erosion present major problems necessitating explantation of the device.

Mechanical Failure. This is nearly always related to the technique employed during device implantation given that less than 3% of all mechanical failures are attributed to the device itself. The vast majority of the technical problems are due to inadvertent blocking or kinking of the tubing system or fluid leakage from accidental damage causing inadequate balloon pressure. Like any other, mechanical device, the artificial bowel sphincter is subject to wear and tear that may include control pump failure, disconnection of its prime components, or even damage from repeated trauma. Either category will impair the normal transmission of fluid to the cuff and prevent the squeezing shut of the intestine to maintain fecal continence. These complications occur almost immediately with failure of continence on activating the device. A non-functioning device is an indication for careful inspection and possible surgical revision where an irremediable problem is identified.

Infection. Uncontrolled infection inevitably results in explantation of the device and the best form of treatment remains unquestionably, prevention. Because infection most frequently occurs after implantation of the device, strict sterile techniques and antibiotic prophylaxis are mandatory, along with regular observation in the postoperative period to detect early signs or symptoms of sepsis. There are of course some people who carry a greater risk of infection such as those with existing stomas, skin conditions, impaired immunity, and diabetes. These patients should be carefully counselled and warned that it may not be possible to re-implant the device after explantation due to infection. The infection rates of these devices range between 20 and 40% and one study which reported experience with the device in the United Kingdom showed that infection with methicillin-resistant *Staphylococcus aureus* (MRSA) was the most common cause of failure.[77]

Erosion. Erosion refers to the wearing away of tissue adjacent to the device. The immediate surrounding organ is at greatest risk and include the anal canal, scrotum, labium, urethra, urinary bladder, and the skin overlying the perineum or lower abdominal wall to name but a few. This occurs because of ongoing sepsis, improper size, or positioning of the device, prior tissue damage from radiation and skin conditions; while pain, erythema, tenderness, or changes in skin texture are the earliest worrying signs. Sometimes the device is visible having broken through the overlying skin in which case revision or explanation is required. In a large personal series of 53 patients who received the artificial sphincter device for fecal incontinence, nearly 20% patients suffered cuff and/or pump erosion as a late complication.[65]

Migration. Any part of the device can migrate to a new location remote from the original site of implantation. Usually poor surgical technique such as improper pump or regulating balloon placement, cuff selection, and tubing length which can either damage adjacent remote tissue or lead to device malfunction. However, early detection will prevent long-term damage and allow revision as opposed to device explantation.

Recurrent Incontinence. While fecal continence achieved with the artificial bowel sphincter is variously reported in the literature as between 60 and 90%, the true rate of recurrent incontinence with the device in situ is not known. First, many of these patients fail to report varying degrees of incontinence because they are highly motivated and determined to avoid a colostomy. Second, the various validated tools that are in use to measure fecal incontinence are subjective, lack uniformity, and measure differing aspects of fecal incontinence. Third, there is no universally agreed definition of recurrent incontinence with the device in situ given that few studies document explantation of the device because of unsatisfactory function compared to its removal as a result of complications. It is also relevant to highlight the fact that the overwhelming majority of studies on this subject are case series or single center experience with their inherent biases. All these factors contribute to the present confusion and the deduction that can be drawn from the literature is that the true incidence of recurrent incontinence is unknown.

Constipation/Fecal Impaction. These are common problems that occur following device implantation but are usually resolved by a combination of dietary modification and use of oral laxatives. Occasionally, regular enemas to evacuate the neo-rectum may be required in those patients who encounter repeated constipation or fecal impaction.

Summary

The use of artificial sphincters in colorectal surgery is an acceptable management strategy to restore anal defecation in patients with end-stage fecal incontinence or following rectal excision for cancer, who would otherwise have to face life with a permanent colostomy. These sphincters may be fashioned surgically or involve implantation of an artificial device. The passive neo-sphincters have largely been superseded by the electrically stimulated variety which is the gold standard in terms of efficacy, but unfortunately, carry considerable morbidity. It is therefore recommended that patients considering anal reconstruction with the electrically stimulated neo-sphincter should be carefully selected and surgery restricted to specialist colorectal centers. However, while data pertaining to the physiological neo-sphincter is currently limited, it has shown promise given the exciting prospects of restoring anal defecation under normal voluntary control.

Anorectal transplantation has been shown to be technically feasible experimentally, but it is beset with formidable obstacles not least the returning physiological function and immunological considerations. Nonetheless, it is foreseen that further interest in this novel method of restoring normal anal defecation will be driven by the quest to restore quality of life by transplantation of none essential organs. The implantable artificial sphincters offer an acceptable alternative with reported continence rates comparable to the neo-sphincters, but device-related complications are frequent and may result in failure or explantation.

References

1. Stone H. Plastic operation for anal incontinence. *Arch Surg.* 1929;18:845.
2. Chetwood CH. Plastic operation for restoration of the sphicter ani with report of a case. *Med Rec.* 1902;61:529.
3. Chittenden A. Reconstruction of anal sphincter by muscle strips from glutei. *Ann Surg.* 1930;92:152.
4. Bistrom O. Plastischer Erzatz das M. sphincter ani. *Acta Chir Scand.* 1944;24:120.
5. Hentz VR. Construction of a rectal sphincter using the origin of the gluteus maximus muscle. *Plast Reconstr Surg.* July 1982;70(1):82–5.
6. Bruining HA, Bos KE, Colthoff EG, Tolhurst DE. Creation of an anal sphincter mechanism by bilateral proximally based gluteal muscle transposition. *Plast Reconstr Surg.* January 1981;67(1):70–3.
7. Pickrell KL, Broadbent TR, Masters FW, Metzger JT. Construction of a rectal sphincter and restoration of anal continence by transplanting the gracilis muscle; a report of four cases in children. *Ann Surg.* June 1952;135(6):853–62.
8. Simonsen OS, Stolf NA, Aun F, Raia A, Habr-Gama A. Rectal sphincter reconstruction in perineal colostomies after abdominoperineal resection for cancer. *Br J Surg.* May 1976;63(5):389–91.
9. Fedorov VD, Shelygin YA. Treatment of patients with rectal cancer. *Dis Colon Rectum.* February 1989;32(2):138–45.
10. Baeten CG, Konsten J, Spaans F, Visser R, Habets AM, Bourgeois IM, et al. Dynamic graciloplasty for treatment of faecal incontinence. *Lancet.* November 9, 1991; 338(8776):1163–5.
11. Williams NS, Patel J, George BD, Hallan RI, Watkins ES. Development of an electrically stimulated neoanal sphincter. *Lancet.* November 9, 1991;338(8776): 1166–9.
12. Geerdes B, Kurvers H, Konsten J, Heineman E, Baeten C. Assessment of ischaemia of the distal part of the gracilis muscle during transposition for anal dynamic gracilo-plasty. *Br J Surg.* 1997;84(8):1127–9.
13. Rosen H, Novi G, Zoech G, Feil W, Urbarz C, Schiessel R. Restoration of anal sphincter function by single-stage dynamic graciloplasty with a modified (split sling)technique. *Am J Surg.* March 1, 1998;175(3):187–93.
14. Mander BJ, Abercrombie JF, George BD, Williams NS. The electrically stimulated gracilis neosphincter incorporated as part of total anorectal reconstruction after abdominoperineal excision of the rectum. *Ann Surg.* December 1996;224(6):702–9.
15. Williams NS, Hallan RI, Koeze TH, Watkins ES. Restoration of gastrointestinal continuity and continence after abdominoperineal excision of the rectum using an electrically stimulated neoanal sphincter. *Dis Colon Rectum.* July 1990;33(7):561–5.
16. Mercati U, Trancanelli V, Castagnoli GP, Mariotti A, Ciaccarini R. Use of the gracilis muscles for sphincteric construction after abdominoperineal resection. Technique and preliminary results. *Dis Colon Rectum.* December 1991;34(12):1085–9.

17. Cavina E. Outcome of restorative perineal graciloplasty with simultaneous excision of the anus and rectum for cancer. A ten-year experience with 81 patients. *Dis Colon Rectum.* February1996;39(2):182–90.
18. Cavina E, Seccia M, Banti P, Zocco G. Anorectal reconstruction after abdominoperineal resection. Experience with double-wrap graciloplasty supported by low-frequency electrostimulation. *Dis Colon Rectum.* August 1998;41(8):1010–6.
19. Patel J, Shanahah D, Riches D. The arterial anatomy and surgical relevance of the human gracilis muscle. *J Anat.* 1991;176:270–272.
20. Mander BJ, Williams NS. The electrically stimulated gracilis neo-anal sphincter. *Eur J Gastroenterol Hepatol.* May 1997;9(5):435–41.
21. Rongen MJ, Dekker FA, Geerdes BP, Heineman E, Baeten CG. Secondary coloperineal pull-through and double dynamic graciloplasty after Miles resection–feasible, but with a high morbidity. *Dis Colon Rectum.* June 1999;42(6):776–80.
22. Rullier E, Zerbib F, Laurent C, Caudry M, Saric J. Morbidity and functional outcome after double dynamic graciloplasty for anorectal reconstruction. *Br J Surg.* July 2000;87(7):909–13.
23. Rullier E, Laurent C, Zerbib F, Garrelon JL, Caudry M, Saric J. [Anorectal reconstruction by coloperineal anastomosis and dynamic double graciloplasty after abdomino-perineal resection]. *Ann Chir.* 1998;52(9):905–12.
24. Abercrombie JF, Rogers J, Williams NS. Total anorectal reconstruction results in complete anorectal sensory loss. *Br J Surg.* January 1996;83(1):57–9.
25. Sato T, Konishi F. Functional perineal colostomy with pudendal nerve anastomosis following anorectal resection: an experimental study. *Surgery.* June 1996;119(6): 641–51.
26. Congilosi SM, Johnson DR, Medot M, Tretinyak A, McCormick SR, Wong WD, et al. Experimental model of pudendal nerve innervation of a skeletal muscle neosphincter for faecal incontinence. *Br J Surg.* September 1997;84(9):1269–73.
27. Schwabegger AH, Kronberger P, Obrist P, Brath E, Miko I. Functional sphincter ani externus reconstruction for treatment of fecal stress incontinence using free latissimus dorsi muscle transfer with coaptation to the pudendal nerve: preliminary experimental study in dogs. *J Reconstr Microsurg.* February 2007; 23(2):79–85.
28. Sato T, Konishi F, Kanazawa K. Anal sphincter reconstruction with a pudendal nerve anastomosis following abdominoperineal resection: report of a case. *Dis Colon Rectum.* December 1997;40(12): 1497–502.
29. Pirro N, Sieleznef I, Malouf A, Ouaissi M, Di M V, Sastre B. Anal sphincter reconstruction using a transposed gracilis muscle with a pudendal nerve anastomosis: a preliminary anatomic study. *Dis Colon Rectum.* November 2005;48(11):2085–9.
30. Sato T, Konishi F, Endoh N, Uda H, Sugawara Y, Nagai H. Long-term outcomes of a neo-anus with a pudendal nerve anastomosis contemporaneously reconstructed with an abdominoperineal excision of the rectum. *Surgery.* January 1, 2005;137(1):8–15.
31. Satava RM, King GE. An artificial anal sphincter. Phase 2: Implantable sphincter with a perineal colostomy. *J Surg Res.* March 1989;46(3):207–11.
32. Affleck J. A sound operation? Docs debate benefits, risks of first larynx transplant. Philadelphia Daily News. January 10, 1998.
33. Grady D. Medical first: a transplant of a uterus. NY Times (Print). March 7, 2002;A1, A11.
34. Cooney WP, Hentz VR. Hand transplantation–primum non nocere. *J Hand Surg [Am].* January 2002;27(1):165–8.
35. Devauchelle B, Badet L, Lengele B, Morelon E, Testelin S, Michallet M, et al. First human face allograft: early report. *Lancet.* July 15, 2006;368(9531):203–9.
36. Orbach CE, Tallent N. Modification of perceived body and of body concepts. *Arch Gen Psychiatry.* February 1965;12:126–35.
37. Devlin HB, Plant JA, Griffin M. Aftermath of surgery for anorectal cancer. *Br Med J.* August 14, 1971;3(5771):413–8.
38. Wade BE. Colostomy patients: psychological adjustment at 10 weeks and 1 year after surgery in districts which employed stoma-care nurses and districts which did not. J Adv Nurs 1990 Nov;15(11):1297-304.
39. Birchall M. Human laryngeal allograft: shift of emphasis in transplantation. *Lancet.* Feb 21, 1998;351(9102):539–40.
40. Sinnatamby C. Last's Anatomy. 10th ed. Edinburgh: Churchill Livingstone; 1998.
41. McMinn R, Peggington J, Abrahams P. A Colour ATlas of Human Anatomy. 5th ed. Churchill Livingstone, 1993.
42. Shafik A. Endoscopic pudendal canal decompression for the treatment of fecal incontinence due to pudendal canal syndrome. *J Laparoendosc Adv Surg Tech A.* August 1997;7(4):227–34.
43. Sikorski A, Olszewski J, Miekos E. Anatomical considerations of selective pudendal neurectomy. *Int Urol Nephrol.* 1987;19(2):159–63.
44. O'Bichere A, Green C, Phillips RK. New, simple approach for maximal pudendal nerve exposure: anomalies and prospects for functional reconstruction. *Dis Colon Rectum.* July 2000;43(7):956–60.
45. Pirro N, Konate I, Sielezneff I, Di MV, Sastre B. Anatomic bases of graciloplasty using end-to-side nerve pudendal anastomosis. *Surg Radiol Anat.* December 2005;27(5): 409–13.
46. Liuzzi FJ, Tedeschi B. Peripheral nerve regeneration. *Neurosurg Clin N Am.* January 1991;2(1):31–42.
47. Flores AJ, Lavernia CJ, Owens PW. Anatomy and physiology of peripheral nerve injury and repair. *Am J Orthop.* March 2000;29(3):167–73.
48. Terenghi G. Peripheral nerve regeneration and neurotrophic factors. *J Anat.* January 1999;194(Pt 1):1–14.
49. Ahmed Z, Brown RA, Ljungberg C, Wiberg M, Terenghi G. Nerve growth factor enhances peripheral nerve regeneration in non-human primates. *Scand J Plast Reconstr Surg Hand Surg.* December 1999;33(4): 393–401.
50. Trumble TE, Shon FG. The physiology of nerve transplantation. *Hand Clin.* February 2000;16(1):105–22.
51. Hazari A, Wiberg M, Johansson-Ruden G, Green C, Terenghi G. A resorbable nerve conduit as an alternative to nerve autograft in nerve gap repair. *Br J Plast Surg.* December 1999;52(8):653–7.
52. Strauch B. Use of nerve conduits in peripheral nerve repair. *Hand Clin.* February 2000;16(1):123–30.
53. Calne RY, White DJ, Thiru S, Evans DB, McMaster P, Dunn DC, et al. Cyclosporin A in patients receiving renal allografts from cadaver donors. *Lancet.* December 23, 1978;2(8104-5):1323–7.
54. Warty V, Diven W, Cadoff E, Todo S, Starzl T, Sanghvi A. FK506: a novel immunosuppressive agent. Characteristics

of binding and uptake by human lymphocytes. *Transplantation.* September 1988;46(3):453-5.
55. Fung JJ, Eliasziw M, Todo S, Jain A, Demetris AJ, McMichael JP, et al. The Pittsburgh randomized trial of tacrolimus compared to cyclosporine for hepatic transplantation. *J Am Coll Surg.* August 1996;183(2): 117-25.
56. Pirsch JD, Miller J, Deierhoi MH, Vincenti F, Filo RS. A comparison of tacrolimus (FK506) and cyclosporine for immunosuppression after cadaveric renal transplantation. FK506 Kidney Transplant Study Group. *Transplantation.* April 15, 1997;63(7):977-83.
57. O'Bichere A, Shurey S, Sibbons P, Green C, Phillips RK. Experimental model of anorectal transplantation. *Br J Surg.* November 2000;87(11):1534-9.
58. Yamauchi T, Taira A, Yoshida H. Rejection of the colon in multi visceral organ transplantation in pigs. *In Vivo.* January 1993;7(1):9-12.
59. Nakhleh RE, Gruessner AC, Pirenne J, Benedetti E, Troppmann C, Uckun F, et al. Rejection of the colon versus ileum in a pig model of total bowel transplantation. *Transplant Proc.* October 1996;28(5):2445-6.
60. Hakim N. Introduction to Organ Transplantation. First ed. London: Imperial College Press; 1997.
61. Christiansen J, Lorentzen M. Implantation of artificial sphincter for anal incontinence. *Lancet.* August 1, 1987;2(8553):244-5.
62. Christiansen J, Sparso B. Treatment of anal incontinence by an implantable prosthetic anal sphincter. *Ann Surg.* April 1992;215(4):383-6.
63. Wong WD, Jensen LL, Bartolo DC, Rothenberger DA. Artificial anal sphincter. *Dis Colon Rectum.* December 1996;39(12):1345-51.
64. Vaizey CJ, Kamm MA, Gold DM, Bartram CI, Halligan S, Nicholls RJ. Clinical, physiological, and radiological study of a new purpose-designed artificial bowel sphincter. *Lancet.* July 11 1998;352(9122):105-9.
65. Devesa JM, Rey A, Hervas PL, Halawa KS, Larranaga I, Svidler L, et al. Artificial anal sphincter: complications and functional results of a large personal series. *Dis Colon Rectum.* September 2002;45(9):1154-63.
66. Michot F, Costaglioli B, Leroi AM, Denis P. Artificial anal sphincter in severe fecal incontinence: outcome of prospective experience with 37 patients in one institution. *Ann Surg.* January 2003;237(1):52-6.
67. O'Brien PE, Dixon JB, Skinner S, Laurie C, Khera A, Fonda D. A prospective, randomized, controlled clinical trial of placement of the artificial bowel sphincter (Acticon Neosphincter) for the control of fecal incontinence. *Dis Colon Rectum.* November 2004;47(11):1852-60.
68. Mundy L, Merlin TL, Maddern GJ, Hiller JE. Systematic review of safety and effectiveness of an artificial bowel sphincter for faecal incontinence. *Br J Surg.* June 2004;91(6):665-72.
69. Sofia CA, Rush BF, Jr., Koziol J, Rocko JM, Seebode JJ. Experiences with an artificial sphincter to establish anal continence in dogs. *Am Surg.* June 1988;54(6):390-4.
70. Hajivassiliou CA, Carter KB, Finlay IG. Assessment of a novel implantable artificial anal sphincter. *Dis Colon Rectum.* June 1997;40(6):711-7.
71. Lirici I, Di P, Ponzano H. Dynamic graciloplasty versus implant of artificial sphincter for continent perineal colostomy after Miles' procedure: Technique and early results. *Minim Invasive Ther Allied Technol.* December 2004;13(5):347-61.
72. La TF, Masoni L, Montori J, Ruggeri E, Montori A. The surgical treatment of fecal incontinence with artificial anal sphincter implant. Preliminary clinical report. *Hepatogastroenterology.* Septmber 2004;51(59): 1358-61.
73. Marchal F, Doucet C, Lechaux D, Lasser P, Lehur PA. Secondary implantation of an artificial sphincter after abdominoperineal resection and pseudocontinent perineal colostomy for rectal cancer. *Gastroenterol Clin Biol.* April 2005;29(4):425-8.
74. Finlay IG, Richardson W, Hajivassiliou CA. Outcome after implantation of a novel prosthetic anal sphincter in humans. *Br J Surg* November 2004;91(11):1485-92.
75. Schrag HJ, Ruthmann O, Doll A, Goldschmidtboing F, Woias P, Hopt UT. Development of a novel, remote-controlled artificial bowel sphincter through microsystems technology. *Artif Organs.* November 2006;30(11): 855-62.
76. Luo Y, Higa M, Amae S, Takagi T, Yambe T, Okuyama T, et al. Preclinical development of SMA artificial anal sphincters. *Minim Invasive Ther Allied Technol.* 2006;15(4):241-5.
77. Malouf AJ, Vaizey CJ, Kamm MA, Nicholls RJ. Reassessing artificial bowel sphincters. *Lancet.* June 24, 2000;355(9222):2219-20.

Cochlear Implant

George Fayad and Behrad Elmiyeh

A cochlear implant is a surgically implanted electronic device which may benefit children and adults with severe to profound sensorineural hearing.

Unlike a hearing aid, which simply makes sounds louder (amplification), the cochlear implant converts sounds into electrical signals and sends those signals directly to the auditory nerve (hearing nerve), bypassing damaged structures of the inner ear (hair cells). The auditory nerve in turn takes the signals to the brain.

A cochlear implant, despite of being an advanced and complex technology, is unable to restore hearing fully. However, it can provide a perception of sound and be a means for communication when conventional hearing aids are inadequate. The extent of hearing improvement varies between patients and is difficult to predict accurately.

A cochlear implant is made up of two parts.

The external part is worn like an external hearing aid and consists of a **microphone**, which picks up sounds, a **speech processor**, which selectively filters sound and converts acoustic signals into electrical signals. These signals are sent through a thin cable to the **transmitter**, which is a magnetic pad placed behind the external ear and transmits the processed sound signals to the internal device by electromagnetic induction.

The internal part is the electronic implant device, which is surgically placed under the skin behind the ear. This internal part has a **receiver**, which converts sound energy to electrical signals and sends them through an internal cable to the **electrode**. The electrode is a transmitter wire with specialized ending, wound through the cochlea, stimulating the cochlear nerve directly, by passing the damaged hair cells. The brain interprets the nerve activity as sound.

Past, Present, and Future of Cochlear Implants

In the 1950s, Djourno and Eyriés reported the first detailed description of direct stimulation of the auditory nerve in order to generate hearing.[1]

In the 1960s, more extensive experiments with electrical stimulation to the cochlea were carried out by researchers such as Doyle[2] and Simmons[3]. During the 1970s, the clinical applications of electrical stimulation of the auditory nerve were refined by House[4] and Michelson.[5] Speech processors were developed and studies explored the single-electrode implants' safety and elicited useful perception of sound. The first objective, scientific assessment of implant performance, was carried out by Bilger et al. The Bilger report showed that the implant improved patients' lip reading scores, speech production, and quality of life.[6]

In the 1980s, the age criteria for use of the implant lowered and several hundred children benefited from this device. During the same period, a multi-channel cochlear device was designed and surgically implanted by Graham Clark, an Australian Otolaryngologist.[7]

In the years that followed, innovations in implant technology resulted in production of commercially viable multi-electrode cochlear prosthesis with sophisticated, yet smaller processors and lower surgical risks.

Over the past three decades about 100,000 adults and children worldwide have received these devices.

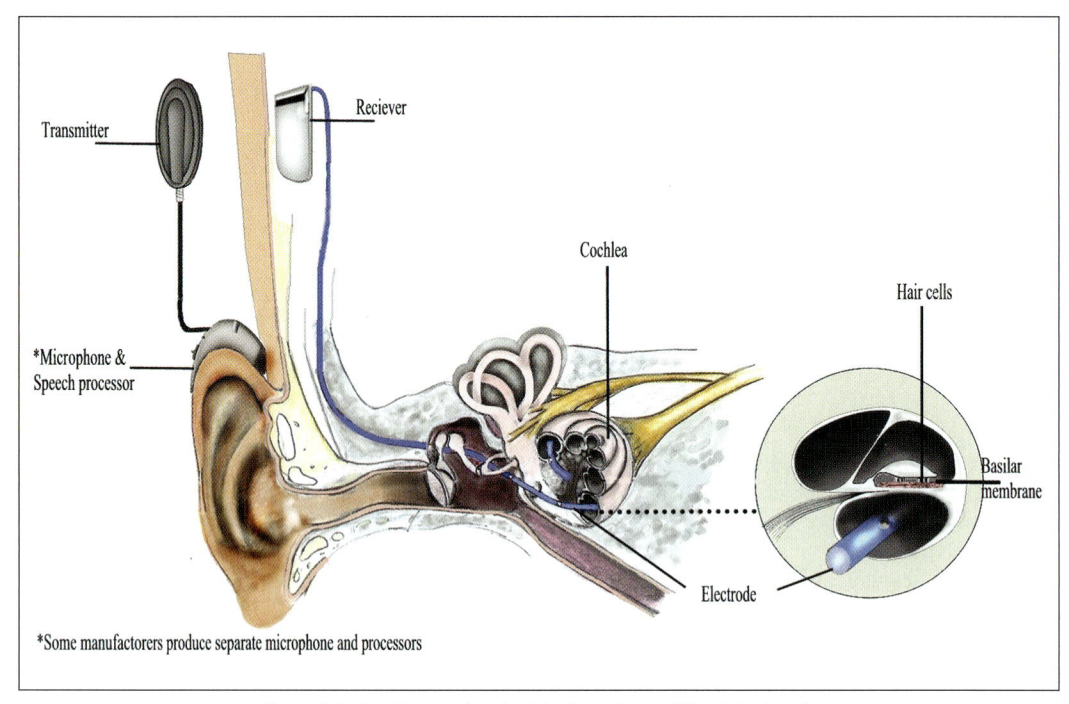

Figure 8-1. A cochlear implant (with kind permission of Mrs. Raha Ansari).

The research and advancement of this significant technological breakthrough continues. In the future, cochlear implants may even be able to restore or provide a normal hearing to deaf individuals. At the same time, cochlear implants might become obsolete if research in molecular and gene therapy succeed to stimulate the growth of new sensory hair cells.

Cochlear Implant Services

Cochlear implant surgery requires a multidisciplinary approach. There are specialized adult and children implant teams, which consist of an Otolaryngologist, Audiological Scientist, Audiologist, Clinical Psychologist, and a Speech and Language Therapist. For adults, the team includes a Hearing Therapist, and for children, a Teacher of the Deaf and Specialist Community Pediatrician. A successful outcome requires collaboration from patients, families, schools, and the implant team.

The implant teams are committed to provide a high-quality and comprehensive services including extensive pre-operative assessment and counseling, time consuming and intensive post-operative speech and hearing therapy, and follow up for adjusting and setting the device. Appreciation and respect to different social, cultural, and linguistic backgrounds make these services accessible to all candidates.

Common Indications for Cochlear implant

- Severe to profound sensory neural hearing loss in both ears with a functioning auditory nerve.
- Little to no benefit from conventional hearing aids.
- Living in or desiring to live in the "hearing world".
- High motivation, strong commitment. and realistic expectations.
- Strong social and educational support.
- Especially in the case of infants and young children having a family willing to work toward speech and language skills with therapy.

Cochlear Implant Suitability

Cochlear implant surgery may be beneficial to children with congenital and or acquired deafness, young, or middle-aged adults with hearing loss due to genetic causes, autoimmune disease, or unknown reasons; and older adults with progressive hearing loss due to aging or noise exposure.

The outcome is more favorable if an implant is fitted at a young age or soon after an acquired hearing loss. This suggests that such a response can be at least partially attributed to plasticity within the auditory system.

However, the suitability of a patient for cochlear implantation can only be evaluated on an individual basis, taking into account a patient's hearing history, cause of hearing loss, amount of residual hearing, speech recognition ability, general health status, and family commitment to the intensive rehabilitation and educational process as well as follow-up testing and monitoring of the cochlear implant. The results of these comprehensive assessments allow the clinicians to advise candidates on the benefits they may gain from the device.

Audiological evaluation includes various tests such as determination of unaided air and bone conduction thresholds, speech discrimination, and auto acoustic emissions.

Auditory brain steam response (ABR) is an electrophysiological testing, particularly important when testing young children in order to rule out the possibility of functional deafness.

Pre-operative Speech and Language evaluation demonstrates developmental language and communicative status. This helps in order to define inappropriate expectations for speech and language skills following the intervention with a cochlear implant.

Psychological evaluation is probably really performed with pediatric patients but may be used in adults who present with concerns regarding cognitive status. Psychological evaluation determines any other factors which may also be hindering the child's auditory development. Accordingly appropriate help and counseling can be provided to the parents.

Computed tomography (CT) of the temporal bone can identify any cochlear anomalies and assess whether it is possible to insert a cochlear implant electrode into the cochlea. The information can also be used in order to choose the most appropriate ear for implantation and the surgical approach. Magnetic resonance image (MRI) examines the soft tissues carefully to establish if the auditory nerve is structurally sound.

Medical evaluation is also necessary to assess patient's general health and suitability for the cochlear implant surgery.

Ethical Issues

Cochlear implants for congenitally deaf children are often considered to be most effective when implanted at a young age; hence they are implanted before the recipients can decide for themselves.

Much of the strongest objection to cochlear implants has come from the deaf community, which consists largely of pre-lingually deaf people whose first language is sign language. Individuals who are deaf and the deaf community do not consider deafness as a disability and indeed celebrate their deaf culture like all languages do. However, there has been a greater acceptance of cochlear implant technology by the deaf communities over the last decade.

Cochlear Implant Surgery

The device is surgically implanted under general anesthesia, and the operation usually takes 1–3 h.

First a small area of hair behind the ear is shaved and an incision is made on the skin around the back the ear. Some of the mastoid bone positioned behind the ear is drilled, with the aid of a surgical microscope, to get into the middle ear through which the cochlea, located in the inner ear, is accessed.

A few millimeters of the bone behind the wound is removed to seat the cochlear device. This is reduced the bump felt under the skin.

Having placed the device, a cochleostomy, a small opening into the cochlea is created; and the electrode is delicately threaded into it.

Prior to closure of the wound, an audiological physicist tests the implant's function.

At the end of the operation, a dressing is applied. Often the patient is kept in the hospital one night for observation.

An x-ray from the site of the operation will be taken within 1 week of the surgery to check the position of the cochlear implant's electrode.

Initial fitting takes place approximately 4-6 weeks after the surgery when the wound has fully healed and the device is switched on for the very first time. Adjustments will be required in the subsequent appointments.

Complications of Cochlear Implant

Cochlear implant surgery is a safe procedure and serious complications are rare. This is due to newer and safer cochlear devices as well as improved surgical techniques. The pre-operative immunization against pnemococcal meningitis reduces the risk of this rare complication even further.

In addition to complications associated with the general anesthesia, there are risks related to the surgery itself, include bleeding, infection, tinnitus, poor hearing outcome, temporary dizziness secondary to the vestibular system damage, numbness in the area of the scar, taste disturbance due to chorda tympani injury, and damage to the facial nerve that can cause muscle weakness, or, in worst cases, disfiguring paralysis.

There are also risks associated with the implant, such as mechanical or electrical failure and rejection. These problems may require removal or replacement of the implant.

References

1. Djourno A, Eyriés C, Vallancien B.De l'excitation electrique du nerf cochleaire chez l'homme, par induction a distance, a l'aide d'un micro-bobinage inclus a demeure. *CR Soc Biol (Paris)*. 1957;151:423–425.
2. Doyle JH, Doyle JB Jr,Turnbull. Electrical stimulation of eight cranial nerve. *Arch Otolaryngol*. October 1964;80: 388–91.
3. Simmons FB. Electrical stimulation of the auditory nerve in man. *Arch Otolaryngol*. July 1966;84(1):2–54.
4. House WF, Urban J. Long term results of electrode implantation and electronic stimulation of the cochlea in man. *Ann Otol Rhinol Laryngol*. July–August 1973;82(4): 504–17.
5. Michelson RP, Merzenich MM, Schindler RA, Schindler DN. Present status and future development of the cochlear prosthesis. *Ann Otol Rhinol Laryngol*. July–August 1975;84(4 Pt 1):494–8.
6. Bilger RC, Black FO. Auditory prostheses in perspective. *Ann Otol Rhinol Laryngol Suppl*. 1977;86(3Pt. 2 Suppl. 38):3–10.
7. Clark GM, Patrick JF, Bailey Q. A cochlear implant round window electrode array. *J Laryngol Otol*. Febraury 1979;93(2):107–9.

9
Stem Cells and Organ Replacement

Nataša Levičar, Ioannis Dimarakis, Catherine Flores, Evangelia I Prodromidi, Myrtle Y Gordon and Nagy A Habib

Introduction

Significant research activities in tissue engineering or regenerative medicine (the term recently used) field started in the 1970s and there is currently a great excitement over the possibility of replacing damaged body parts through regenerative medicine. Potential strategies to replace repair and restore the function of the damaged tissues or organs include stem cell transplantation, transplantation of tissues engineered in the laboratory, and the induction of regeneration by the body's own cells. It is believed that novel cellular therapeutics can perform better than any medical device, recombinant protein, or chemical compound. Possible candidate cells to be used include autologous primary cells, cell lines, and various stem cells including bone marrow (BM) stem cells, cord blood stem cells, fetal cells, and embryonic stem (ES) cells. Stem cells are defined by their capacity for self-renewal and multilineage differentiation, making them uniquely situated as a powerful tool to treat a wide variety of diseases. In recent years, advances in stem cell biology, including embryonic and adult stem cells, have made the prospect of tissue regeneration a potential clinical reality and several studies have shown the great promise that stem cells hold for therapy.[1,2] In this review, we will discuss the use of embryonic and adult stem cells in treatment for liver and kidney failure, diabetes, myocardial infarction, and neuronal disorders.

Embryonic Stem Cells

ES cells are isolated from the inner cell mass of 5-day-old blastocysts.[3] They represent a potential source of cells with remarkable properties: practically unlimited self-renewal and ability to differentiate into many specialized cell types.[4] They are pluripotent and able to give rise to cells belonging to all three germ layers: ectoderm, endoderm, and mesoderm.[5] Neurons and skin have been formed from ES cells, indicating ectodermal differentiation.[5,6] ES cells are able to differentiate to cardiac cells, bone, cartilage, and endothelial cells indicating mesodermal differentiation.[7-9] Moreover, they are able to give rise to pancreatic cells, indicating endodermal differentiation.[10] However, many existing approved ES cell lines have been cultured on mouse feeder cell layers, which can supply many needed growth factors. This has exposed the human ES cells to potential risk of viral transfer between species and has limited their clinical potential.[11] Another major limiting factor for their usefulness in clinical therapy lies in their tumorigenicity when introduced in vivo. The injected ES cells formed teratomas when injected subcutaneously in NOD/SCID mice.[5]

The ability of these cells to potentially differentiate into any cell type has generated great hopes for regenerative medicine. However, since their initial isolation, research on these cells has been hampered or banned in some countries because of ethical concerns about destroying human embryos, and therefore human life, to obtain them.[12] The ethical debate now focuses on defining the stage at which life is considered to begin and from what point the embryo should be protected. These obstacles have generated the search for the alternative sources of cells such as adult stem cells.

Adult Stem Cells

Like ES cells, adult stem cells possess self-renewal capacity and multilineage differentiation potential.[13] Adult stem cells are present in approximately 1–2% of the total cell population within a specific tissue and are vital in the maintenance of local tissue homeostasis by continuously contributing to tissue regeneration, replacing cells lost during apoptosis or direct injury. Adult stem cells are usually quiescent and are held in an undifferentiated state within their niche until they receive a stimulus to differentiate.[14] More recent developments have proved that adult stem cells reside in nearly every tissue, including the BM, brain, digestive system, skin, retina, muscles, pancreas, and liver.[15] However, there is a controversy about whether cells isolated from a particular tissue originated in that tissue or are circulating BM stem cells.[16,17]

The best characterized and most widely understood adult stem cells are hematopoietic stem cells (HSC), which sustain the formation of the blood and immune systems throughout life and were first identified in 1961.[18] The BM compartment is largely made up of HSC and committed progenitor cells, non-circulating stromal cells (called mesenchymal stem cells (MSC)) that have the ability to develop into mesenchymal lineages.[19,20] It was previously thought that adult stem cells were lineage restricted, but recent studies demonstrated that BM-derived progenitors in addition to hematopoiesis also participate in regeneration of ischemic myocardium,[21] damaged skeletal muscle[22] and neurogenesis.[23] MSC can be isolated as a growing adherent cell population and can differentiate into osteoblasts, adipocytes, and chondrocytes.[20]

Renal Failure

The kidney is a complex organ with filtration, reabsorptive, and secretory functions as well as endocrine/metabolic activity. The importance of the kidney as a life-sustaining organ is highlighted in situations in which kidney function is compromised or even lost. Without any functioning kidney, death can occur within a few days. Impaired renal function includes abnormalities of both glomerular filtration and renal tubular reabsorption and secretion. Tubular function tends to be mainly disrupted by metabolic insults to the tubular cells (for example, ischemia or toxins) and could result in tubulointerstitial fibrosis and eventually acute renal failure (ARF). ARF is quite common and affects up to 7% of all hospitalized patients, with a mortality rate that ranges from 20 to 70% depending on the studied population.[24] Glomerular function can be disrupted by diseases that alter glomerular structural arrangements (for example, structural damage to glomerular basement membrane, endothelium, epithelium, or mesangium) and ultimately lead to chronic renal failure (CRF). Chronic injury of the kidney is responsible for the majority of cases of end-stage renal disease. The means by which kidney function can be replaced in humans include dialysis and renal allogeneic transplantation. Dialysis is life saving but often poorly tolerated. Transplantation of human kidneys is limited by the availability of donor organs. In addition, mortality rates still remain high despite the existence of these types of treatment. Therefore, there is clearly need for new replacement therapies for kidney patients.

Stem Cell Therapy for Kidney Diseases

The potential of human ES cells to generate mesodermal tissue is encouraging for renal cell differentiation. Indeed, ES cells have the potential to differentiate into renal progenitor cells. Yamamoto et al.[25] recently showed that murine ES cells had the potential to give rise to mesonephric ducts and ureteric buds in teratomas. In contrast, Steenhard and colleagues[26] reported 50% integration of undifferentiated ES cells (*E12–E13*) into the tubules of embryonic kidneys without evidence for teratomas. Conversely, they found only rare evidence for integration of injected ES cells into the glomerular epithelial tufts that form in organ culture. Kobayashi and co-workers created Wnt-4 transformed murine ES cells and showed in vivo and in vitro that these assembled into tubule-like formations and expressed aquaporin-2.[27]

In addition, cells differentiated from mouse ES cells via embryoid bodies have been shown to express markers of renal lineages in vitro[28] and in vivo.[29] In the presence of nephrogenic factors, such as retinoic acid, activin-A, and bone morphogenetic protein-7 (BMP-7), ES cells can form renal epithelial cells that are capable of integrating into a developing kidney with very high efficiency.[30]

The use of therapeutic cloning for replacement of transplantable kidney tissue in vivo was recently demonstrated by Lanza and colleagues,[31] who employed a nuclear transfer technique to generate cloned bovine fetuses from an adult animal. Renal cells were then isolated from their E56 cloned fetus, passaged and expanded in vitro and seeded onto a collagen-coated polycarbonate membrane that was then subcutaneously implanted into the nuclear donor. The renal cells self-aggregated into "renal units" within the membrane, were subsequently vascularized by the genetically identical host, and ultimately appeared to produce a concentrated urine-like fluid. No evidence of acute rejection of these bioartificial renal units was observed.

Growing research and interest in the use of extra-renal cells for replacing renal structures and functions has been lately described. Cells exogenous to the kidney possess the ability to differentiate into multiple cell lineages and can become incorporated into a number of organs as part of the normal processes of cell turnover or organ repair. The adult BM seems to be the source of extra-renal stem cells. However, it remains unknown whether BM-derived cells invade the kidney and differentiate into renal cell types, remain in the kidney and are induced to differentiate following tissue injury, or whether they first home to the BM and are then recruited to the damaged kidney. Most studies investigating BM plasticity have used human patients or experimental animals that have received a kidney or BM transplant. However, different injury models used, different methods of detecting engrafted cells, and different populations of BM transplanted are some of the reasons for controversial observations in this field. Moreover, the exact mechanism of BM contribution to renal tissues is not clear with the scientific community being divided between transdifferentiation of BM cells to kidney cells or fusion of BM cells with terminally differentiated renal cells.[32]

Endothelium

In the kidney, endothelial cells are present in large vessels and in the abundant network of peritubular capillaries. In addition, a lymphatic network, thought to increase with renal damage, is lined by endothelial cells. Highly differentiated endothelial cells are also found in the glomerulus. During vascular rejection, donor endothelial cells become the predominant focus of the immune attack since the blood vessels of a transplanted organ are the interface between donor and recipient. Endothelial damage is also an important feature of chronic allograft nephropathy, the most common cause of long-term graft loss. High numbers of circulating endothelial cells are found in renal transplant patients, indicating ongoing damage of the endothelium.[33] Repair of damaged endothelium in renal allografts by circulating recipient cells was reported over 30 years ago.[34] Sinclair[35] also showed that extensive acute damage of the renal vasculature in an allograft may be repaired by host cells, while less severely damaged grafts could be restored by proliferating neighboring donor endothelial cells. This was confirmed many years later by Lagaaij and co-workers,[36] who showed that endothelial cells of the recipient could replace those of the donor in human kidney grafts severely damaged by vascular rejection. The number of recipient cells decreased with lesser degrees of tissue damage. Studies of renal transplantation in rats indicated that endothelial chimerism could be induced also by ischemia or toxicity caused by immunosuppressive treatment.[37] Recently, it was shown in human renal transplants that potential lymphatic progenitor cells derive from the circulation and incorporate into the growing lymphatic vessel.[38] Rookmaaker and colleagues[39] first reported that endothelial cells, contributing to renal vessels in a female patient with thrombotic microangiopathy, were derived from the BM of a male donor. Dekel et al.[40] recently showed that transplantation of adult CD34$^+$-enriched HSC into ischemic and growing human kidneys had a role in vasculogenesis.

The origin of the glomerular endothelium in transplanted human kidneys is less clear, although in rodents there is firm evidence that BM contributes to glomerular endothelium. Cornacchia and co-workers[41] showed that glomerular endothelial progenitor cells were derived from the BM in mice. Furthermore,

BM-derived cells were shown to participate in glomerular endothelial repair and contribute to microvascular repair after induction of reversible anti-Thy 1.1 glomerulonephritis in a rat allogeneic BM transplant model.[42] Conversely, other groups did not find any evidence for BM-derived endothelial cells in rats with or without specific glomerular injury, when they stained engrafted cells with endothelial markers.[43,44] Later, it was shown that intrarenal administration of culture-modified BM mononuclear cells reduced endothelial injury in Thy-1 nephritis, presumably due to incorporation of BM-derived endothelial cells into the glomerular lining and production of angiogenic factors.[45]

In the context of severe irreversible glomerular damage induced by anti-Thy-1.1 antibody followed by unilateral nephrectomy in the rat, BM cell infusion improved renal function and glomerular hemodynamics and reduced mortality in chimeric animals with this type of disease.[46,47] In addition, BM-derived cells differentiated into glomerular endothelial cells during glomerular healing after the induction of mouse Habu-snake venom nephritis.[48]

Interstitium

The renal interstitium consists of extracellular matrix (ECM), fibroblasts, vascular pericytes, and inflammatory cells. Normally, fibroblasts have a role in wound healing and repair through the ECM molecules and other proteins they produce. Activated fibroblasts or myofibroblasts, also express alpha-smooth muscle actin (α-SMA) and intermediate filaments, desmin, and vimentin. In the kidney, interstitial fibrosis is a common feature of both tubular and glomerular injury and high numbers of interstitial myofibroblasts are usually strong predictors of progressive renal fibrosis and kidney failure.

Fibroblasts may also originate from the BM and migrate via the peripheral blood to populate the kidney. Recipient circulating smooth muscle precursor cells have been found in vascular and interstitial compartments of renal allografts undergoing chronic rejection.[49] Such cells appear transiently attached to the tubular basement membrane in mice after uranyl acetate-induced ARF, suggesting that they might be involved in promoting cellular recovery in association with monocytes or macrophages.[50] Direkze et al.[51] found evidence for BM-derived (myo)fibroblasts in kidneys of sex-mismatched BM-transplanted mice following paracetamol administration at a toxic dosage. In a mouse model of ARF induced by ischemia reperfusion, it was shown that about 6.5% of α-SMA-positive interstitial cells came from donor BM, suggesting a role for BM-derived cells in renal interstitial fibrosis.[52] Conversely, BM-derived interstitial cells did not make a significant contribution to collagen I synthesis in mice transplanted with BM from transgenic donors, in which the transgene was under the control of a promoter for the $\alpha 2$ chain of collagen I and injured by unilateral ureteric obstruction.[53]

Tubular Epithelium

Each part of the tubular system has important functions, which are dependent upon normal cellular function of tubular epithelial cells (TEC). Proximal tubules in the cortex are mainly involved in the selective reabsorption of various useful components of the glomerular filtrate to the bloodstream. The adult tubular epithelium has the potential to regenerate following acute damage induced by ischemic or toxic insults. Cells from outside the kidney, for instance cells originating from the BM, can potentially home to the injured epithelium and be triggered to differentiate.

In humans, observations of BM participation in tubular repair are mainly limited to renal transplantation studies, as very rarely can renal biopsies of a BM-transplanted patient be obtained. Extra-renal cells possible of BM origin have been shown to participate in tubular regeneration after ARF in human renal transplants. Two groups have detected between 0.6 and 6.8% and approximately 1%, respectively, of Y chromosome-containing tubular cells in kidneys of male patients, who received a renal transplant from a female patient.[54,55] Nishida and colleagues[56] have also reported the contribution of BM cells to renal regeneration in a 7-year-old female patient who received a male BM transplant, suggesting a clinical application for BM cells.

Sex-mismatched transplantation of whole BM, predominantly in mice, has generated a lot of controversy over BM plasticity for the kidney. In female recipients of wild-type whole BM, Y chromosome-positive tubular cells expressing epithelial markers have been reported without induction of renal injury.[55] Further evidence for

BM contribution to tubular cells has been provided by Fang and co-workers,[57] who showed that about 10% of regenerating tubular cells come from the BM and are capable of DNA synthesis after folic acid-induced injury and treatment with granulocyte-colony stimulating factor (G-CSF). On the contrary, Szczypka and colleagues[58] have demonstrated that BM-derived cells rarely contribute to repair of renal tubules in uninjured or folic acid-treated mouse kidneys. In addition, inducing renal ischemia reperfusion injury (IRI) in chimeric mice did not result in tubular regeneration by BM cells, as examined by three separate detection approaches.[59,60]

Morigi and colleagues[61] have found that the MSC population has the primary capacity to participate in renal tubule repair after toxic injury, whereas the HSC mediate a lesser protective effect. Similar findings have been reported by Herrera and his group[62] following transplantation of GFP-expressing MSC into mice that were subjected to glycerol-induced tubular injury. However, others have found that purified MSC did not incorporate into tubules of ischemic mice, although renal function was improved, probably due to immunomodulatory mechanisms rather than renewal of tubular cells.[59,60,63,64] The role of HSC in renal repair has also been debated, with some groups reporting no evidence for HSC repopulating the kidney using GFP as a marker, but without inducing any specific renal damage.[65,66] Conversely, following HSC transplantation from β-gal transgenic ROSA26 mice into wild-type recipients, two studies described the presence of X-gal positive cells in cortex and medulla that stained positive for epithelial markers after renal IRI.[67,68] In one of these studies, it was also shown that sorted HSC have a functional role in the repair of the kidney as they could partially reverse blood urea in injured chimeric mice.[67] By changing the donor mouse strain from ROSA26 to eGFP transgenic mice, Lin et al.[52] later suggested that tubular regeneration after IRI is predominantly due to indigenous proliferating renal cells with HSC making only a small contribution.

Glomeruli

Glomerular mesangial cells provide structural support in the glomerular capillary tufts. The mesangial cells are modified smooth muscle cells and regulate blood flow through the glomerular capillaries by their contractile activity. Mesangial cells may be injured by immunological insults and play a key role in the development of scarring in many progressive glomerular diseases, including glomerulonephritis and diabetic nephropathy. Mesangial cell injury manifested as mesangiolysis, proteinuria, proliferation, and hypercellularity, if sustained, may lead to impaired renal function. Therefore, the repair process following glomerular injury needs a well-balanced recruitment of glomerular endothelial and mesangial cells.

In recent years, the role of BM as a reservoir for mesangial cells during kidney repair has been well investigated. Mesangial progenitor cells have been shown to derive from the BM of GFP transgenic donor rats in vivo, and they stain for desmin and respond to angiotensin II stimulation in vitro.[43,44] In addition, BM-derived cells have been shown to incorporate into glomeruli as specialized glomerular mesangial cells after folic acid injury in mice.[58] However, in these studies the exact stem cell population in the BM which provides these progenitor cells has not been elucidated. Later studies sought to define the exact origin of the engrafting cells in the BM and showed that cloned progeny of a single HSC can transdifferentiate into glomerular mesangial cells, which respond to angiotensin II.[69] In contrast, other groups using a slightly different method of HSC purification failed to detect donor-derived glomerular mesangial cells in mice transplanted with single HSC.[66]

In the disease setting, contribution of BM to development and progression of glomerulosclerosis has been very elegantly shown in two studies. Cornacchia and colleagues[41] have demonstrated that mouse mesangial cell progenitors originate from the BM and transmit both the sclerotic lesions and the glomerular hypertrophy of donor kidneys to normal glomeruli. In diabetic nephropathy, where mesangial cell proliferation and mesangial sclerosis are pathologic hallmarks, Zheng et al.[70] have shown that BM-derived mesangial cell progenitors from type II diabetic mice may also transfer the disease genotype and phenotype into normal recipients, which develop albuminuria and severe glomerular lesions.

Recently, several groups have provided evidence for a functional role of BM-derived mesangial cell progenitors in improvement of renal disease. Guo et al.[71] showed that transplantation of wild-type BM prevents or attenuates progression of mesangial sclerosis in the Wt1+/− mouse model of renal disease, most probably by replacement of mesangial cells with BM cells.[71] BM transplantation has been shown to attenuate mesangial cell activation in Thy 1.1 nephritic rats[45] and reduce mortality and pathological findings in fatal progressive glomerulosclerosis.[47] However, whether these cells originated from resident BM cells, and/or injected BM cells was not determined in these studies.

The origin of glomerular epithelium and especially podocytes has been less well studied compared to other parts of the nephron. Podocytes form part of the glomerular filtration barrier and support the capillary tuft and regulate glomerular filtration. Podocytes also have phagocyte-like functions, as they remove any large molecules trapped in the outer layers of the filter. They are predominantly terminally differentiated cells with little or no capacity of renewal.

Poulsom and colleagues[55] were the first to observe that cells located in the periphery of a glomerulus resembled podocytes and stained with vimentin and could be BM-derived. However, other specific phenotypic markers were not used to identify them unequivocally. Since then, a few groups supported a small contribution of BM cells to podocyte regeneration in mice by staining them with antibodies to a specific podocyte marker, WT-1 protein.[71] An alternative and possibly efficient way to use cell therapy in renal disease may be to condition or otherwise manipulate stem cells before their delivery in vivo.

A recent study showed that culturing canine BM-derived cells on plastic, type IV collagen substrate, which resembles matrix ordinarily seen by podocytes in vivo, promotes their partial differentiation in vitro into a podocyte-like phenotype.[72] Whether these cultured cells could ever become functional podocytes in vivo is unknown, but this in vitro conditioning strategy with stem cells clearly underscores the importance of cell–matrix interrelationships in achieving appropriate phenotypes.

Recent studies have also reported that whole BM transplantation has a functional effect in a mouse model for Alport's syndrome. Alport's syndrome is a progressive disease that ultimately leads to renal failure. There is no specific therapy and it is fatal, if renal replacement therapy is not provided once kidneys fail to function.

In the murine model, mice that lack the $\alpha 3$ chain of collagen IV ($Col4\alpha 3^{-/-}$) develop progressive glomerular damage leading to renal failure. The proposed mechanism is that podocytes fail to synthesize normal GBM, so the collagen IV network is unstable and easily degraded. Two recent studies have shown for the first time that BM cells replace defective podocytes and produce Col4α3, thereby improving functional and structural parameters of renal disease in Alport mice.[73,74] Although, the lineage of BM-derived cells that were recruited to the damaged glomeruli was not clearly established in these studies, preliminary data suggest that BM-derived MSC fail to reverse disease in this model,[73,75] suggesting that the HSC compartment might be exerting the beneficial effects observed. Although more experimental data are needed before BM transplantation can be applied to patients, these observations provide new hope for treating Alport's disease by stem cell therapy.

These data demonstrate that BM proves a highly promising, ethically accepted, and readily accessible source of adult stem/progenitor cells for the remodeling of injured kidney.

De Novo Kidney Creation

Growing new organs in situ by implanting developing animal organ anlagen/primordia represents a novel solution to the problem of the limited supply of human donor organs that offers advantages relative to transplanting ES cells or xenotransplantation of developed organs. Renal primordia (metanephroi) transplanted into animal hosts undergo organogenesis in situ, become vascularized by blood vessels of host origin, and exhibit excretory function.[76] Metanephric mesenchymal tissue harvested from donors at an early stage in development (E13-E15) was transplanted into neonatal mouse kidney and was shown to create functioning nephrons.[77,78] Transplantation of developing metanephroi into adult rats has resulted in functional chimeric kidneys vascularized by the host and producing urine after anastomosis to the host's ureter.[79] Metanephroi can be also preserved prior to transplantation and differentiate in situ before being introduced into animal hosts to develop into functional kidneys.[80,81] In addition, human metanephroi can be induced in vivo to grow and develop into mature nephrons following transplantation into mice.[82] Moreover, xenotransplanted early kidney embryonic precursor cells, of both human and pig origin, can form functional miniature kidneys in mice, although it was not shown whether the urine they produced had been concentrated by the structures formed.[83] These studies demonstrate the possibility of integrating new filtering nephrons into kidneys. Critical to providing organ function replacement through cell therapy is the need for the isolation and growth in vitro of specific cells, such as kidney progenitors, that could potentially create new kidney segments or entire nephrons appropriate for transplantation. A very promising study recently showed that human MSC injected into in vitro cultured developing rodent embryos and subjected to further organ culture could be reprogrammed to contribute to kidney cell lineages, such as podocytes and tubular epithelial cells.[84]

Artificial Kidney (See Chapter 3)

Hemodialysis replaces some of the filtration functions of the kidney but does not recapitulate the endocrine/metabolic activities of renal cells. To address this deficiency, a bioartificial tubule, which uses cultured epithelial progenitor cells on appropriate membranes and biomatrices that confer immunoprotection and long-term functional performance, has been developed. Humes et al.[85] have created a synthetic hemofiltration cartridge and a renal tubule assist device (RAD) containing human or porcine cells in an extracorporeal circuit. Cells are grown as confluent monolayers along the inner surface of hollow fibers within a standard hemofiltration cartridge.[86,87] The RAD has been used for the treatment of acutely uremic dogs and increases excretion of ammonia and enhances glutathione metabolism and $1,25(OH)_2D_3$ production during 24 h of treatment.

A Phase I/II trial in 10 humans with ARF and multi-organ failure has been safely conducted and RAD treatment resulted in declines in pro-inflammatory cytokines (G-CSF, IL-10, and IL-6/IL-10 ratios).[88] A controlled, randomized Phase III trial is currently underway. The RAD was recently shown to modify sepsis to improve survival in ARF.[89] However, existing bioartificial kidneys are large and they use intensive labor, making the miniaturization of the bioartificial kidney a prerequisite before applying this novel technology. The differentiated growth of human tubular epithelial cells on thin-film and nanostructured materials strongly suggests that this miniaturization will be soon feasible.[90,91]

Diabetes

Diabetes mellitus affects over 6% of the population worldwide and the World Health Organization expects that the number of diabetic patients will increase to 300 million by 2025 (57). Type I diabetes is a chronic disease and results from autoimmune-mediated destruction of insulin-secreting β-cells in the islets of Langerhans of the pancreas. Once activated the continued destruction of β-cells leads to a progressive loss of insulin, then to clinical diabetes, and finally in almost all affected to a state of absolute insulin deficiency.[92] Type II diabetes is due to systemic insulin resistance and reduced insulin secretion by pancreatic β-cells. Although the etiology of type II diabetes remains obscure, obesity and a sedentary lifestyle are the most common epidemiologic factors associated with development of the disease. The absence of insulin is life-threatening, thus requiring diabetic patients to take daily hormone injections. However, insulin injections do not adequately mimic beta cell function, which results in the development of diabetic complications such as neuropathy, nephropathy, retinopathy, and diverse cardiovascular disorders. Long-term normalization of glucose metabolism is a prerequisite for prevention of secondary complications and to date has only been achieved with transplantation of the whole organ or with a reasonable number of islets. However, the chief limitation to transplantation, either whole gland or islets, is the paucity of donors. Islet transplantation is mainly limited because of the difficulty in obtaining sufficiently large numbers of purified islets from cadaveric donors and treatment can be offered to only an estimated 0.5% of needy recipients.[93] Additionally, differentiated β-cells cannot be expanded efficiently in vitro and senesce rapidly.[94] Several approaches are now being investigated to generate insulin-producing cells either by genetic engineering of β-cells or by utilizing various β-cell precursor cells, and stem/progenitor cells. Insulin-secreting cells could be transplanted into patients to help maintain blood glucose homeostasis, reduce the burden of diabetes-related complications, and overcome the limitation of donor organs.

Stem Cell Therapy for Diabetes

ES cells have been proposed as a potential source for cell replacement therapy in the treatment of diabetes. Several studies have demonstrated that by manipulating culture conditions and using growth and transcription factors of the β-cell lineage (in particular *Pdx-1* and *Pax4*), ES cells can differentiate in vitro into insulin-producing cells.[10,95,96] Soria et al.[97] transplanted an insulin-secreting cell clone from undifferentiated ES into the spleen of streptozotocin-induced diabetic animals. Although transplanted animals corrected hyperglycemias within 1 week, an intraperitoneal glucose tolerance test showed a slower recovery in transplanted versus control mice. Fujikawa et al.[98] cultured and differentiated embryonic cells into insulin and c-peptide positive cells. When the cultured cells were transplanted into diabetic mice, they reversed the hyperglycemic state for approximately 3 weeks, but the rescue failed due to immature teratoma formation. An encapsulated solid tumor was found at each transplanted site in 6 of 10 transplanted mice.

The risk of teratoma formation would need to be eliminated before ES cell-based therapies for the treatment of diabetes are considered. Promising data regarding the potential of BM stem cells to reconstitute the β-cell endocrine portion of the pancreas has been produced by Ianus and co-workers.[99] Irradiated female wild-type mice were injected with BM stem cells expressing enhanced green fluorescent protein (EGFP) under the control of the murine insulin promoter. Up to 3% of total cells per islet were found to express EGFP at 4–6 weeks post-transplantation. Further RT-PCR analysis of sorted cells showed the expression of β-cell markers including insulin I, insulin II, GLUT2, IPF-1, HNF1α, HNF1β, HNF3β, and Pax-6. Finally, demonstration of glucose-dependent and incretin-enhanced insulin secretion was reported as proof of functionality. However, another group using a similar strategy failed to show any GFP positive cells within the pancreatic parenchyma of transplanted animals.[100] As this was not informative per se of pancreatic engraftment, another series of experiments was conducted using BMDS cells expressing GFP under the control β-actin promoter. Despite the large degree of engraftment none of the GFP positive cells co-expressed insulin or the β-cell transcription factors Pdx-1 or Nkx6.1, while >99.9% expressed the pan-hematopoietic marker CD45 as well as myeloid antigens. The authors concluded that although BM stem cells demonstrated efficient pancreatic engraftment, a hematopoietic cell fate was almost exclusively retained. Hess et al.[101] used murine model of streptozotocin-induced pancreatic damage to induce hyperglycemia and transplanted the mice with BM-derived stem cells expressing GFP. They observed that pancreatic injury was a prerequisite for BM stem cells taking on an insulin-producing phenotype within the pancreatic parenchyma, an observation also made by other researchers.[102] They have detected only up to 2.5% donor-derived insulin positive cells. Moreover there was no expression of Pdx-1 in these cells. Also, a large proportion of donor cells documented in ductal or islet regions were of endothelial lineage, thus associating the regenerative process with various endothelial interactions. Similarly, Lechner et al.[103] failed to detect donor-derived cells in animals with induced pancreatic damage and treated with BM stem cells. Kang et al.[104] showed that HSC transplantation prevents diabetes in NOD mice but does not contribute to significant islet cell regeneration once disease was established. Successful BM engraftment before diabetes onset prevented disease in all mice for 1 year after transplantation. However, despite obtaining full hematopoietic engraftment in over 50 transplanted mice, only one mouse became insulin independent. However, BM stem cells transplanted into the renal capsule and the distal tip of the spleen of streptozotocin-diabetic mice reversed the existing hyperglycemia and the animals' ability to respond to in vivo glucose challenges. Furthermore, Banerjee et al.[105] showed that multiple injections of BM stem cells improved glycemic control in streptozotocin-treated mice. Ende et al.[106] transplanted human umbilical cord blood mononuclear cells into non-obese diabetic mice with autoimmune type I diabetes were able to reduce blood glucose levels and improve survival compared to untreated animals.

Tang et al.[107] pre-differentiated BM stem cells into insulin-producing cells, transplanted them in streptozotocin-induced diabetic mice, and achieved reversal of hyperglycemia and improved metabolic profiles in response to intraperitoneal glucose tolerance testing. Oh et al.[107,108] transplanted BM stem cells transdifferentiated into insulin-producing cell aggregates and showed lowered circulating blood glucose levels and maintained comparatively normal glucose levels in mice for up to 90 days post-transplantation. These studies indicated that pre-transplantation in vitro cell manipulation may provide a useful tool for delivering large numbers of predefined cells, thus avoiding complications such as suboptimal delivery rates and cell differentiation down non-pancreatic pathways.

Clinical Studies

The first reported data on cellular therapy for type I and II diabetes were presented by Fernandez Vina et al.[109,110]. They have treated 23 patients with type I diabetes with $CD34^+CD38^-$ cells isolated from BM and followed them up for 90 days. After 90 days from cell transplantation, the blood sugar decreased by 9.7% and c-peptide significantly increased by 55%. It was also observed that the requirement for exogenous insulin, taken daily by the patients, decreased by 17% suggesting that autologous BM stem cells could improve pancreatic function. Similar results were obtained for type II diabetes patients where autologous $CD34^+CD38^-$ cells were transplanted via spleen artery into 16 patients. Ninety days post-transplantation the blood sugar significantly decreased by 27%, while c-peptide and insulin increased by 26 and 19%, respectively. Even more impressive is the fact that 90 days post-transplantation, 84% of treated patients did not need any more anti diabetic drugs or insulin.

Liver Diseases

Liver diseases impose a heavy burden on society and affect approximately 17% of the population.[111] The main causes of cirrhosis, the end result of long-term liver damage, are hepatitis B and C and alcohol abuse. At the cirrhotic stage, liver disease is considered irreversible and the only solution is orthotopic liver transplantation (OLT). However, the increasing incidence of liver disease, the widening donor–recipient gap, and the poor outcome in patients not supported by liver transplantation mean that there is obviously a demand for new strategies to supplement OLT.

New strategies such as cell therapy are under investigation. Potential sources include the expansion of existing hepatocytes, ES cells, progenitor/stem cells in the liver, and BM stem cells. Hepatocyte transplantation has been accomplished in small number of patients with metabolic deficiencies and acquired liver disease.[112-114] The major limiting factor is the inability to produce large quantity of hepatocytes and to keep them ready for use on demand, short duration of the functioning replacement cells, and the need for immunosuppression.[115,116] These limitations generated the interest in stem cells as a stable and expandable source, expected to provide large numbers of cells for hepatic disorders.

Stem Cell Therapy for Liver Diseases

Several studies have shown in vitro hepatic differentiation of ES cells, showing expression of alpha-feto protein (AFP), albumin, alpha-1-antitrypsin, and transthyretin.[117,118] Co-culture with Thy1-positive cells in vitro induced the maturation of AFP-producing cells isolated from ES cell cultures into hepatocytes.[119] Moreover, AFP-positive cells isolated from cultured ES cells differentiated into hepatocytes when transplanted into livers of apolipoprotein-E- (ApoE) or haptoglobin-deficient mice.[120] Yamada et al.[121] and Chinzei et al.[122] demonstrated that ES cells growing in embryoid bodies express mRNAs for albumin, AFP, and other mature hepatocyte markers. They also incorporate into hepatic plates, produce albumin, and morphologically resemble adjacent hepatocytes when transplanted into mice.

More work has been done on adult extrahepatic stem cells such as HSC. Petersen et al.[123] transplanted male BM stem cells into injured livers of female mice. They demonstrated that regenerated hepatic cells were of BM origin by using Y chromosome, dipeptidyl peptidase IV enzyme, and L21-6 antigen as markers to identify donor-derived cells. Grompe et al.[124] used $FAH^{(-/-)}$ mice, an inducible animal model of tyrosinemia type I, a lethal hereditary liver disease and showed repopulation of injured liver by donor-derived BM cells. Twenty-two weeks after transplantation one-third of the liver comprised BM-derived cells, suggesting that BM stem cells contribute to hepatocyte generation, when regenerative potential of hepatocytes is impaired. Sakaida et al.[125] showed that BM stem cells can reduce liver fibrosis, probably by expressing matrix metalloproteases, which enable degradation of hepatic scars. Mallet et al.[126] induced hepatic apoptosis in mice by JO$_2$ antibody, the murine anti-Fas agonist and transplanted unfractionated BM cells expressing Bcl-2 under the control of a liver-specific promoter. BM-derived hepatocytes expressing Bcl-2 were only seen in the liver of the mice, which received JO$_2$ antibody injections. Moreover, in mice with induced liver cirrhosis, 25% of the recipient liver was repopulated in 4 weeks by BM-derived hepatocytes.[127] Similarly, murine HSC converted into viable hepatocytes with increasing liver injury and restored liver function 2–7 days after transplantation, suggesting that HSC contribute to liver regeneration by differentiating into functional hepatocytes.[128]. However, some studies have shown that BM stem cells can repopulate liver even in the absence of liver injury. Theise et al.[129] identified up to 2.2% donor-derived hepatocytes when they transplanted BM or CD34$^+$lin$^-$ cells into irradiated mice without acute liver injury. HSC transplanted into irradiated mice engrafted in several organs, including liver, gastrointestinal tract, bronchus and skin of recipient animals, and generated albumin-expressing hepatocyte-like cells.[130]

In contrast, several other studies failed to show the contribution of BM stem cells to liver regeneration. HSC reconstituted blood leukocytes of irradiated mice, but did not contribute to non-hematopoietic tissues, including liver, brain, kidney, gut, and muscle.[66] Several groups failed to show a significant contribution of BM stem cells to liver regeneration using various liver injury models.[131] Although the contribution of HSC to hepatocyte lineages in vivo still remains divisive, the differences between the studies may in part reflect the types of cells used, different injury models used and the method used to detect engrafted stem cells.

Several studies have also shown the presence of cells of BM origin in the human liver. Alison et al.[132] examined livers from female patients that received BM transplantation and found donor-derived hepatocytes, suggesting that extrahepatic stem cells can colonize the liver. Theise et al.[133] identified hepatocytes and cholangiocytes of BM origin in archival autopsy and biopsy liver specimens. Using double-staining analysis, they found a large number of engrafted hepatocytes (4–43%) and cholangiocytes (4–38%), derived from extrahepatic circulating stem cells, suggesting BM stem cells can replenish large numbers of hepatic parenchymal cells. However, in a similar study, Korbling et al.[134] found only 4–7% BM-derived hepatocytes. Ng et al.[135] identified only small proportion of donor-derived hepatocytes (1.6%) in liver allografts, most donor-derived cells were macrophages/Kupffer cells. Two other studies did not detect any BM-derived hepatocytes at all.[136,137] The differences in the published studies could be due to use of different techniques to identify recipient derived hepatocytes in transplanted patients. Also, various markers can be used for hepatocyte identification and the accuracy of the methods used for identification is variable.

Clinical Studies

Recent success in a few studies using stem cell treatment for liver diseases has raised hopes for the patients that cell therapy may be feasible treatment for their disease. Only three clinical studies using BM stem cells for liver disease have been published so far. In the first study, three patients with large central hepatobiliary malignancies were treated with autologous CD133$^+$ cells.[138] CD133$^+$ cells highly enriched from autologous BM were selectively implanted to the left-lateral portal branches subsequent to selective portal vein embolization of right liver segments. Mean daily hepatic growth determined by CT scan volumetry rates was 2.5-fold higher compared to the patients that had been subjected to portal vein embolization without CD133$^+$ application. These data suggested that stem cell therapy enhances and accelerates liver regeneration and may bear the potential for augmentation of liver regeneration before extensive hepatectomy. The second study using adult HSC in treatment of liver diseases was performed by our group.[139] We treated five patients with liver insufficiency and mobilized their stem cells by G-CSF. Between 1×10^6 and 2×10^8 CD34$^+$ cells were injected into the either portal vein or hepatic artery. Three of the five patients showed improvement in serum bilirubin and four of five in serum albumin. Clinically, the procedure was well tolerated with no observed procedure-related complications. The data suggested that stem cells contributed to the regeneration of liver damage and are encouraging for the future development of stem cell therapy for liver diseases. In the third study, nine liver cirrhosis patients were treated with autologous BM.[140] Mononuclear cells (CD34+, CD45+, c-kit+) were infused via the peripheral vein the total number of the infused cells was 5.20+/−0.63 × 10⁹. They reported of significant improvement in serum albumin levels, total protein, and improved Child–Pugh score.

Myocardial Infarction/Heart Disease

Coronary artery disease with its clinical sequelae continues to be one of the leading causes of congestive heart failure. Following myocardial infarction, cardiomyocyte death and segmental scarring eventually contribute to the development of replacement fibrosis. The impact of myocardial fibrosis on the remaining healthy myocardium may range from subclinical to detrimental. The remodeling process initiated will eventually lead to impairment of left ventricular function. In an attempt to reverse the natural progress of the disease, several alternative novel approaches are being considered. These include cellular transplantation in which de novo introduced cells are expected to regenerate/repair areas of diseased myocardium.

Stem Cell Therapy for Ischemic Heart Diseases

The main types of stem cells currently being investigated include embryonic, umbilical cord blood, and adult stem cells. Undebatable proof for the ability of ES cells to differentiate into cardiomyocytes cannot be other than the spontaneous contraction observed in embryoid bodies.[8] Besides spontaneous "beating", cells from these areas exhibit typical immunophenotypical, molecular, and electrophysiological properties of cardiomyocytes.[8,141] Following intramyocardial transplantation into rodent models of myocardial infarction, engraftment with subsequent cardiac-lineage differentiation has been reported by many groups; and sustained improvement in cardiac function was also noted.[142,143] Recent data also suggest that ES cells are capable of homing to myocardial injury following peripheral delivery by being chemoattracted to locally released cytokines.[144] Although a high degree of in vitro electromechanical coupling has been documented for ES cells and cardiomyocytes,[145] there are still concerns regarding underlying arrhythmogenic potential.[146]

Although the totipotent/pluripotent ES cells may seem to be the ideal candidate, their clinical application is not foreseeable in the near future. Serious ethical considerations remain the main drawback; other issues complicating clinical adaptation include insufficient availability, associated disadvantages of allograft transplantation, and unpredictable electrical behavior as well as the risk of tumor formation. The lack of these side effects probably with the exception of arrhythmogenicity has allowed the majority of available adult stem cell types to enter the clinical trial setting.

Extensive preclinical work in small and large animal infarction models preceded the introduction of adult stem cell therapy in the experimental clinical setting. This ongoing body of research established feasibility and provided the necessary support via demonstration of myocardial regeneration/repair and functional improvement.[147,148] The use of crude BM versus pre-selected stem cell populations remains contentious, the main argument being synergy versus specification, respectively. By definition crude preparations are less concentrated in potent stem cells and encompass a variety of different cell types. This in turn may expose subjects to unjustifiable procedure-associated risks with potentially unwanted side effects.[149,150] On the other hand, pre-selected populations may require to undergo multiple population doublings in vitro prior to delivery in order to achieve sufficient cell counts.[151] Prolonged passaging in culture is not without risk since replicative senescence,[152] changes in multipotentiality,[153] and spontaneous transformation[154] have all been associated with long-term in vitro culture. Finally, data concerning the arrythmogenic potential of transplanted MSC has emerged from in vitro experimental work.[155]

The sole assay available at present for identification of HSC remains the reconstitution of the hemopoietic system of a myeloablated host. Surface markers such as CD34 or the more primitive CD133 help in distinguishing subpopulations enriched in HSC in humans; these include the CD34+CD38− cell population as well as the side population. The latter cell type may reside in various organs besides the BM and there is conflicting data as to the origin of these cells with some evidence supporting the fact of them actually being BM-derived HSC rather than tissue specific.[156,157] As murine progenitor cells do not express the same surface markers, lineage depletion (Lin⁻) is the main criterion to identify enriched populations.[158] In Orlic's landmark paper,[21] transplanted Lin⁻c-kit⁺ were demonstrated to form new myocytes, endothelial cells, and smooth muscle cells, leading thus to de novo myocardial regeneration. Similar data have also been produced with human peripheral blood CD34⁺ cells.[159] Nonetheless, controversy remains as to whether HSC are capable of transdifferentiation into cardiomyocytes[160,161] or even confer any functional improvement whatsoever.[162]

Endothelial progenitor cells (EPC) or angioblasts and HSC are thought to share a common precursor, the hemangioblast.[163] Studies have shown the connection between angioblasts residing within the BM and neovascularization.[164,165] EPC are recruited to sites of ischemic injury and promote angiogenesis. Fazel and colleagues[166] suggested that this is achieved via regulation of the myocardial levels of various angiogenic cytokines such as the angiopoietins 1 and 2 and vascular endothelial growth factor (VEGF). Absolute numbers and functional activity of EPC appear to be inversely correlated with risk factors for coronary artery disease;[167,168] an issue to consider for the design of clinical studies if one bears in mind target population characteristics.

MSC have two main characteristics: the ability to adhere to culture dishes as well as to differentiate into a variety of tissues under the appropriate conditioning. In addition, they appear uniformly negative for typical "hematopoietic" surface markers. Apart from innate plasticity, MSC may exhibit immunomodulatory effects[169] that may allow for allogeneic in vivo transplantation with minimal risk of immune rejection.[170] Possible co-delivery of MSC with BM-derived mononuclear cells in order to maximize clinical effect has also been proposed.[148]

A very appealing adult BM-derived population of high plasticity was reported by the Minnesota group.[171] These cells which are known as multipotent adult progenitor cells (MAPCs) were isolated from MSC cultures and maintain the ability to differentiate in vitro in cells of the three germ layers. Only recently another group has reported the identification of a similar subpopulation from adult human BM.[151] Intramyocardial transplantation of these cells in a rodent myocardial infarction model lead to in vivo differentiation into multiple lineages including cardiac, endothelial, and smooth muscle cell phenotypes.

Clinical Studies

From the clinical standpoint, a plethora of studies have been published incorporating BM – and blood-derived stem cells. Design heterogeneity (cell type, number of delivered cells, etc.) along with the fact that majority of studies consist of small cohorts with short follow-up warrant cautious interpretation of the results. The route of administration may also vary depending mostly on the underlying disease. Techniques involving transepicardial, intravascular (both intracoronary and intravenous), and transendocardial delivery have been developed and are in clinical use. Although the majority of large randomized studies demonstrate improvement in left ventricular ejection fraction, one must notice that two of these show minimal to no clinical benefit.

Mechanisms of Action

The exact mechanisms that govern the functional improvement observed in animal and human studies remain a highly debatable issue. The inability for routine pathological examination of specimens in the clinical trial setting necessitates data collection from experimental models to investigate this. The initial – and to a certain extent simplistic– consensus was to attribute all benefit to the innate plasticity of transplanted stem cells. Cells committed to cardiomyogenic lineages have been considered to be produced from delivered cells via transdifferentiation,[21,172] fusion with resident end-differentiated cells,[173] or even a combination of both mechanisms.[174] Although both transdifferentiation and fusion provide an acceptable theoretical platform at the cellular level for the documented functional recovery, it is by now widely accepted that their collective clinical effect is probably negligible due to their diminutive frequency of occurrence.

A very interesting notion is that transplanted cells may promote restoration of resident cardiac stem cell niches. This falls under the wider suggestion that stem cells exert their beneficial effect via paracrine pathways. In a rat model of myocardial infarction, transplantation of MSC induced greater expression of proangiogenic and homing cytokines while reducing the expression of the proapoptotic protein Bax compared with medium-treated control hearts.[175] Stem cell recruitment in a murine model of myocardial infarction was also shown to establish a proangiogenic milieu in the infarct border zone leading neoangiogenesis and the formation of an extensive myofibroblast-rich repair tissue.[166] By providing improvement in local blood supply,[176] in addition to further recruitment of resident and peripheral stem cells to the site of injury via paracrine factor secretion, recovery of the local microenvironment is supported. An interaction also exists with the ECM leading to the induction of reverse remodeling.

Stem Cells and Cardiac-Related Bioengineering

Steady advancements in the field of pediatric cardiac surgery have increased the demand for exogenous myocardial "building blocks", mainly in the form of right ventricular outflow tract conduits as well as transannular patches. Synthetic biomaterials, heterologous glutaraldehyde-preserved bovine pericardium/jugular vein, and glutaraldehyde-preserved homografts currently represent the mainstay of options available to surgeons. Several limitations render these implants far from ideal; inability to follow the recipients' growth may limit considerably conduit life span and make repeated surgery necessary. From a physiological point of view, failure of electromechanical integration deprives the pulmonary arterial circulation of pulsatile blood flow. Similarly, both mechanical and available biological valves (xenografts or allografts) are linked with a need for life-long anticoagulation associated morbidity and limited durability respectively.

While production of a total bioengineered heart remains wishful thinking, many research groups are addressing the construction of viable myocardial patches. The aim remains a viable autologous construct that may contract, achieve electromechanical coupling, and integrate within the native vascular network. Although encouraging data utilizing fetal or neonatal cardiomyocytes[177–179] are being gradually produced, the nature of these cells probably precludes their transition to the clinical level. Cardiomyocytes are difficult to obtain and have limited capacity for proliferation, with such constructs not reflecting the actual cellular organization of the myocardial wall. On the other hand stem cells are easily obtained and expanded as well as having by definition the capacity to differentiate into a variety of tissue types including endothelial, smooth muscle, and nerve cells. After seeding BrdU-labeled MSC into porous acellular bovine pericardium, Wei et al.[180] proceeded to repair a surgically created right ventricular myocardial defect in a rat model. Both epicardial and endocardial surfaces were neo-mesothelialized and neo-endothelialized, respectively, avoiding thus the formation of adhesions and thrombi. Evidence of tissue regeneration (neo-muscle fibers, neo-capillaries, and smooth muscle cells) within the MSC patch was documented with many of these cells staining positive for BrdU. Unfortunately, the MSC patch appeared akinetic via echocardiography, possibly due to an inadequate number of cardiomyocytes present within the patch.

Heart valve tissue engineering incorporates (autologous) cell seeding onto biodegradable scaffolds, anticipating gradual replacement of the scaffold by cells and matrix produced by the implanted cells. Proof of principal was first published more than a decade ago by seeding a polyglycolic acid scaffold with a mixed population of autologous endothelial cells and fibroblasts; this was subsequently transplanted as an orthotopic single pulmonary valve leaflet in an ovine model.[181] Hoerstrup et al. showed that MSC were a reliable cell source for heart valve tissue engineering.[182] The created trileaflet valve demonstrated morphological features and mechanical properties similar to those of native valves, while MSC differentiation into cells of myofibroblast phenotype was reported. Based on previous in vitro work,[183] Sutherland and colleagues demonstrated prolonged (>4 months) in vivo function of a stem cell-engineered valve constructed from MSC and a biodegradable heart valve scaffold.[184] Even more interestingly, the sequential seeding of biodegradable leaflet scaffolds with human fetal mesenchymal progenitors and umbilical cord blood-derived endothelial progenitor cells lead to constructs comparable with native heart valve leaflets.[185] Growing out of this important contribution, prenatal chorionic villus sampling may allow surgeons to perform autologous valve replacements immediately after birth.

Stem Cells and Pulmonary Regeneration

Lung parenchyma is organized around a complex 3-D array of proximal and distal airways lined with numerous types of distinct epithelia. Architectural complexity alongside multiple in situ cell lineages is the main limitations to reconstruct pulmonary units via tissue engineering. Resident stem cell populations have been described to exist within the proximal airways,[186,187] distal airways,[188,189] and the alveoli.[190,191] The actual stemness of these populations remains at issue, as the term "reparative cells" has been recently proposed to indicate cell populations involved in lung remodeling following injury.[192] BM-derived stem cells have been described to populate the pulmonary parenchyma,[193,194] while recruitment of non-resident stem cells appears to be associated with injury.[195–197] Interestingly, cells recruited to injury do not always participate in tissue repair; circulating fibrocytes have the opposite effect, as these cells are known to contribute to the pathogenesis of pulmonary fibrosis.[198] Distal lung epithelial cell progenitors have been generated from ES cells[199] but small cell yields along with ethical considerations of ES cell research. Probably make this approach very remote at present to clinical transition. Mondrinos and co-workers[200] recently demonstrated in vitro generation of branching sacculated 3-D pulmonary tissue constructs with mixed populations of murine fetal pulmonary isolates, cultured in 3-D hydrogels in the presence of tissue-specific growth factors. Seeding of ovine somatic lung progenitor cells onto polyglycolic acid or Pluronic F-127 scaffolds leads to production of identifiable pulmonary structures;[201] although polymers performed likewise in vitro, Pluronic F-127 scaffolds generated less tissue inflammation in vivo resulting in tissue organization comparable to normal pulmonary parenchyma.

From the clinical front, stem cell therapy is about to make its debut in pulmonary disease.[202] Peripheral mobilized autologous mononuclear cells engineered with human nitric oxide synthase will be directly infused within the pulmonary arterial tree of patients with idiopathic pulmonary arterial hypertension. Extensive preclinical work has shown restoration of the integrity of the pulmonary microcirculation as well as reversal of established pulmonary hypertension in relevant animal models. Of all developments, this trial from Toronto is probably the most anticipated in the field of pulmonary stem cell therapy.

Central Nervous System Diseases

Replacement cell therapy in the central nervous system (CNS) is arguably the most complex topic in regenerative medicine. Lessons learned from countless studies have begun to outline what is required of the transplanted cells in order to be successful. Within the CNS, cells must migrate to the site of injury, and differentiate into the appropriate cell type according to disease. Differentiated cells must integrate with existing neural cells, create functional synapse formations with existing circuitry, and restore saltatory conductivity when appropriate. Neurotransmitter release and uptake must have a regulatory mechanism. In most degenerative diseases of the CNS, a concerted regeneration of multiple types of neural cells must occur for functional recovery. In vitro investigation has demonstrated that ES cells, fetal derived stem, and progenitor cells, as well as cells from non-neural sources are capable of exhibiting phenotypic, genetic, and electrophysiological characteristics of neural cells. Animal models of CNS diseases are proof positive that stem cells are capable of restoring appropriate motor function. However, the molecular mechanisms of repair remain unknown making long-term effects of transplantation uncertain. Here, we discuss the feasibility of stem cell therapy in CNS regeneration in the most likely candidates for clinical use, Parkinson's disease (PD), and stroke.

Parkinson's Disease

Parkinson's disease (PD) is a neurodegenerative disease characterized by a progressive loss of mesencephalic dopaminergic neurons. Symptoms include tremor, rigidity, and hypokinesia.[203] The pathology of PD becomes more complicated as there are thought to be symptoms which are due to subsequent degeneration of other neuronal systems. Current treatments include administration of L-DOPA, deep brain stimulation, dopamine (DA) agonists, and inhibitors of DA breakdown.[204,205] Current treatments temporarily alleviate physical symptoms of Parkinson's, but do not impede progression of the disease. In addition, there are drawbacks to available therapy which include dyskinesia and the loss of the efficacy with disease progression. Ideally, clinical cell-based therapy should provide long-lasting major improvements of mobility, suppression of dyskinesias, and improvement of symptoms that are resistant to other treatments such as balance problems.

Cell transplantation therapy would be ideal in diseases like PD where the pathology is restricted to only one part of the brain, the A9 region of the striatum, and the damage is to a specific subset of dopaminergic neurons. Transplantation experiments of fetal neural tissue in animals and humans have enabled researchers to identify the requirements that need to be satisfied by stem cells in order to achieve clinical recovery in PD. First, the cells must have the capacity for regulated dopamine synthesis and release while showing phenotypic, morphological, and electrophysical properties of dopaminergic neurons of the substantia pars compacta. Second, in animal models of PD, these cells must be able to ameliorate motor symptoms while surviving over long-term periods. A third and important requirement is that grafted dopaminergic neurons must demonstrate functionality, integrating into the hosts' terminal network of nerve cells.[204,205]

Stem Cell Therapy in Parkinson's Disease

Neurons exhibiting a dopaminergic phenotype reportedly have been generated from mouse, monkey, and human ES cells as well as from fetal rodent and human neural stem cells (NSC) and non-neural tissue. Strategies for efficient induction of dopamine neurons from ES cells have been developed using forced gene expression, growth factor cocktails, retinoic acid, and co-culture experiments. For example, nuclear receptor related-1 (Nurr-1) is a transcription factor which plays a role in the differentiation of dopaminergic neurons; driving Nurr-1 expression in ES cells successfully induces the dopaminergic phenotype in vitro.[206] In rat models of PD, transplants of ES cells over-expressing Nurr-1 successfully integrated into the site of lesion and expressed tyrosine hydroxylase (TH), the enzyme involved in dopamine synthesis.[206] Another example of inducing dopaminergic differentiation of ES cells is by stromal cell-derived inducing activity (SDIA).[207] Co-culture of ES cells with PA6 stromal cell line yields dopamine secreting TH+ neurons, which upon transplantation into 6-OHDA PD animal models, graft into the striatum and continue to express TH.[207,208] Although hopeful results have been demonstrated using mouse ES cells, issues surrounding the genetic stability of ES cells need to be addressed before ES cells can be used in human trials. Long-term culture of mouse ES cells can lead to chromosomal aberrations which have also been observed in mid-term cultured human ES cell lines, implying potential detrimental long-term effects associated with ES cell transplantation.[209,210]

Stem cells derived from tissues other than the brain are also currently being explored as a possible source for autologous transplant. Increasing numbers of investigations are exploring the possibility of generating dopaminergic neurons from post-natal stem cells derived from other tissues such as BM, peripheral blood, and umbilical cord.[204,211,212] The transdifferentiation of HSC and MSC into neural cells is very controversial, the differentiation of cells from one-germ lineage to another still raises doubts despite growing evidence of alternative sources of tissue committed neural cells such as in BM.[212] In vitro, multipotent BM-derived stem cells are capable of exhibiting neuron-like morphology and phenotype and expressing several neuronal-specific markers including TH.[204,211,213] Transplantation experiments using GFP-labeled BM-derived stem cells demonstrate migration, differentiation, and long-term survival of these cells in rodent models of PD.[204,211,212] Umbilical cord stem cells have also been successfully induced to differentiate into TH+ neurons, using neuron-conditioned media supplemented with FGF-8 and sonic hedgehog.[214]

Clinical Studies

During development, fetal ventral mesencephalic tissue contains a mixture of two subtypes of dopaminergic neurons, making it an ideal candidate for transplantation therapy. Difficulties in identifying surface markers which are differentially expressed between neuronal subtypes, creates a problem in trying to purify a population of dopaminergic neurons specific to the substantia nigra pars compacta. Using transgenic mice and retrograde axonal tracing, Thompson et al.[215] has demonstrated that dopaminergic neurons which innervate the substantia nigra pars compacta (SNpc) almost exclusively express the transcription factor Girk2. The SNpc is the A9 region of the brain which is affected during Parkinson's disease. These results imply axonal guidance mechanisms take place in the CNS, suggesting that cell transplantation therapies for PD may only be efficient if transplanted fetal cells are capable of differentiating into the correct DA phenotype specific to the SNpc. Researchers in the clinical setting do not yet have an accurate measure of the neuronal cell type which engrafts in transplantation. As a marker of graft viability, clinical studies measure fluorodopa (^{18}F-dopa) uptake on positron emission (PET). However, this measures total F-dopa uptake and cannot distinguish between the uptake from endogenous neurons and the grafted neurons.[216] Results from clinical trials remain unclear because of contrasting results from different groups.

In open-label clinical trials, human fetal ventral mesencephalic tissue transplants have shown long-term survival and restoration of dopaminergic networks in the striatum.[216–220] However, it is not entirely clear if transplanted cells are able to synthesize and secrete dopamine in a regulated manner. Grafts contained a mixed population of neural cells, 5–10% of which were dopaminergic neurons[205] thus, it is unclear whether the success of engraftment was due specifically to transplanted dopaminergic neurons, or possibly due to a role of accompanying glial cells. Increasing evidence points to an important role of astrocytes during neuronal fate specification of neural stem and precursor cells.[221] Initial transplantations of fetal brain tissue were promising, and in the best case, a patient showed marked symptomatic relief for up to 10 years post-transplant, without the need for additional anti-Parkinsonian medication such as L-dopa.[218] In a 59-year-old patient who received two transplants from seven donors, post-mortem histopathological investigation of the grafted area showed TH immunoreactive cells and dopaminergic fibers proximal to the grafted area and extended to host tissue indicating that dopaminergic processes crossed the graft–host interface and innervated the Parkinsonian striatum.[216] Despite graft survival and integration, some patients have developed post-transplant dyskinesia even in the absence of anti-Parkinsonian medication.[218] It has been speculated that this may be due to uneven innervation of grafted cells, inflammation, different populations of DA neurons, or inappropriate synaptic graft–host connections.[218,219,222] This alludes to a lack of proper regulatory mechanisms of DA synthesis and release.

Although open-label clinical trials have demonstrated the viability and innervations of fetal transplants, results from more recent double-blind trials showed contrasting evidence, stating that no significant alleviation of motor symptoms of PD were found after fetal mesencephalic tissue transplantation. Two recent double-blind placebo-controlled clinical trials both reported that the grafts failed to improve primary endpoints in PD patients.[218–220] Between the two trials, 73 patients in total were divided into two groups, one of which received fetal nigral transplantation, and the other a sham surgery, in both studies, only the neurosurgeon was aware of the type of surgery conducted on each patient. There were no significant differences in the overall treatment effect between the transplantation group and the sham surgery group in either study, as both failed to meet the primary end point. The primary outcome was the difference in the UPDRS (Unified Parkinson's Disease Rating Scale) motor score between the baseline reading prior to surgery and final physician visits post-operatively.

A big problem with transplantation of fetal mesencephalic tissue is that 15% of patients develop dyskinesia.[219,220,223] It was thought that overgrowth of grafted cells may lead to excess DA release subsequently causing dyskinesias. However, no correlation has been found between graft-induced dyskinesia and high levels of F-dopa post-operatively.[223] Dyskinesia may have also resulted from abnormal regulatory mechanisms of DA synthesis and release from transplanted cells.[223] There are conflicting reports which compare putaminal F-dopa uptake in grafted patients with and without dyskinesias. Ma et al.[224] reported that in dyskinetic patients, there is an imbalance between dopaminergic innervation in the ventral and dorsal putamen. In contrast, Olanow et al.[220] reported no such regional differences of F-dopa levels between patients with and without graft-induced dyskinesia. Differences in outcome between the open-label trials and the double-blind trials have not been explained as there are many differences among the studies such as patient selection criteria, immunosuppression regimes, and donor tissue preparation. Although it is promising that fetal nigral transplants survive, integrate with host tissue, and express TH, fetal cell transplantation cannot be recommended at this time as it has not shown long-term symptomatic relief nor has it been shown to stop progression of the disease.

Although results of cell transplantation studies seem hopeful and cell integration can be seen, there is no proof of dopamine secretion by the exogenous cells. In addition, there has not been a clear demonstration that DA neurons generated *in vitro* can efficiently reinnervate the striatum, release dopamine in a regulated manner, and provide functional recovery from PD once transplanted into animal models. The optimal number of grafted cells required remains unknown, and efforts to standardize fetal tissue transplantations have failed to pin point the number of donor required for human transplant.[218] Although functional recovery is temporarily observed after transplantation, perhaps further investigations should focus on the mechanisms of symptomatic relief and exploiting endogenous means of dopaminergic neuronal repair. Investigators have observed an increase in neurogenesis after delivery of lesion to the dopaminergic system, while other studies find that lesion to the DA system stimulates a glial response rather than an increase in neuronal generation.[205,225]

Stroke

In stroke, a cerebral artery is blocked, causing a focal ischemia and loss of neurons and glia. Subsequently, multifactorial motor, sensory, and cognitive capacities are impaired, and there is neither a cure nor an effective means of promoting recovery. Thus, therapy which has potential of neuron regeneration is attractive. There are two main arms of investigation in the search for stem cell therapy in stroke: (i) directly transplanting stem and progenitor cells and (ii) stimulating the proliferation of endogenous neural stem cells which would ideally migrate to the penumbra region and replace degenerated neurons and glia.

Stem Cell Therapy in Stroke

ES cells have been successfully transplanted in models of PD, before their therapeutic potential in cerebral ischemia was explored. The challenge here is that unlike PD, where damage is specific to dopaminergic neurons in a defined region of the brain SNpc, stroke affects glia and varying types of neurons, leaving the brain susceptible to damage followed by the possibility of inflammation and glial scar. Thus, specifically defining which neural cell type to transplant remains challenging.

Neural precursor cells (NPC) can be derived from ES cells, expanded as neurospheres and, upon attachment to a substrate, can be differentiated into mixed cultures of glia and mature neurons. ES cell-derived NPC transplanted into a rodent stroke model survive and differentiate into glia and electrophysiologically mature neurons of different neurotransmitter subtypes.[226,227] Tracking NPC using a GFP tag showed that after transplantation, these cells survived and matured into glutaminergic, gabaergic, dopaminergic, serotonergic, and cholinergic neurons.[226,227] In stroke models, ES cells genetically modified to over-express the anti-apoptotic gene *bcl-2* have increased survival relative to normal ES cells. Also, there is an increase in the ES cell-derived neuronal fraction of the transplanted cells. After focal ischemia, animals that received Bcl-2 over-expressing ES cells demonstrated significant functional recovery relative to animals that received non-genetically modified ES cells and control animals that received culture medium.[228] There are two controversial findings with regard to neural differentiation from cells originating in non-neural tissue. First, several groups have independently identified stem and progenitor cells which express neural lineage markers circulating in the peripheral blood and residing in the BM.[211,212,229,230] Second, cells derived from non-neural tissues such as cord blood, umbilical cord, peripheral blood, and BM have been induced to have neural phenotypes in vitro.[213,231–234] Are there stem cells in non-neural tissue that are truly plastic? Or are investigators differentiating pre-determined neural committed progenitor cells?

In rat stroke models, intravenous administration of CD34+ hUCBCs within 1 day of ischemic induction, lead to significant improvement of functional recovery. CD34+ hUCBCs selectively migrated to the injured tissue, survived, and differentiated in the brain but there was no significant reduction in the lesion volume. The majority of cells were found at the ischemic boundary,[235] perhaps due to the lack of blood supply in the lesion itself. In lieu of replacing damaged cells and integrating into host circuitry, the administration of hUCBCs and their migration to injury may instead stimulate trophic factors, endogenous neuroprotection, and brain recovery mechanisms.[235] The same group has shown that after stroke, intravenous administration of BM stromal cells enhances angiogenesis at the ischemic boundary of the host brain, which is important in promoting repair and restoration of blood flow to the ischemic area. The administration of BM stromal cells promotes endogenous secretion of VEGF and the upregulation of VEGF receptor 2 (VEGFR2), which mediate angiogenesis.[236] Animal transplantation studies have shown that MSC transplantation into ischemic brain models leads to functional recovery, providing relief in sensory-motor symptoms caused by stroke.[225,237] However, close immunohistological examination of post-mortem tissue shows evidence that functional recovery may have been mediated by molecular signals secreted by the transplanted MSC.[225] Although MSC provide a therapeutic effect, genetically modified MSC programmed to hypersecrete trophic factors such as brain-derived neurotrophic factor (BDNF) and glial cell line-derived neurotrophic factor (GDNF) have a greater therapeutic effect relative to non-genetically altered MSC.[237,238] Cerebral ischemia induces the release of several neurotrophic factors in the brain including GDNF and BDNF which are thought to have neuroprotective properties.[238] Treatment with intravenous BDNF after stroke improves functional motor recovery in animal models.[239] BDNF rescues motoneurons, hippocampal neurons, and dopaminergic neurons from brain injury, and its upregulation after focal cerebral ischemia suggests that BDNF may have a neuroprotective role in stroke.[240] Topical treatment of focal ischemia with GDNF significantly reduces infarct volume.[241] Investigators have thus explored the potential of transfecting MSC with vectors containing BDNF and GDNF.[237,242] BDNF gene-modified human MSC (BDNF-MSC) intravenously administered to rats with cerebral occlusion reduced lesion volume and increased functional improvement compared to animals that received MSC alone.[242] In addition, intravenous administration of MSC transfected with GDNF (GDNF-MSC) also showed a greater reduction in the lesion volume, increase in GDNF in the penumbra region, and improvement in behavioral defects.[237,242] Although these results show promise in gene-modified MSC transplantation therapy for stroke, the long-term effects of receiving gene-modified cells remain uncertain.

Clinical Study

There has been one safety and feasibility trial for cell transplantation in stroke. This open-label trail consisted of 12 patients with at least a basal ganglionic infarct. Patients received LBS-Neurons (from Layton Bio-Science) which are produced from the NT2/D1 human precursor cell line and induced to differentiate into neurons. Two million cells per injection were administered stereotactically, and patients received between 1 and 3 injections ($2–6 \times 10^6$ cells). Six out of 12 patients showed an improved functional outcome, but three patients deteriorated, exhibiting decreased motor performance relative to baseline performance prior to surgery. Although this trial may have proved that transplantation is safe, its efficacy is poor and there were no consistent signs of improvement in patients.[243]

Conclusions

Despite a great amount of interest and development in stem cell biology and therapy in the past few years, many questions are yet to be answered before stem cell therapy can be applied to its fullest potential in the clinic. Which cells should be used in order to maximize potential benefits and what is the best method of their delivery? The ideal route for administering stem cells has still yet to be determined, but it is important to take certain factors into consideration. The strength of homing signals may vary in different clinical scenarios. In more acutely ischemic scenarios, the stem cells may be administered either peripherally or locally through the circulatory system. When the homing signals may be less intense, injection of the cells directly into the damage tissue may produce a more favorable outcome. It also remains to be determined how cell survival can be optimized and how cells can be tracked once delivered to ensure that they reach the right location. An important issue concerning the therapeutic use of stem cells is the quantity of cells necessary to achieve an optimal effect. Ideally, cells should expand extensively in vitro have minimal immunogenicity and be able to reconstitute tissue when transplanted into damaged tissue. It must also be defined which patients are suitable for this therapy and which stem cell types are the most effective given the underlying pathology. Currently, it is not possible to fully anticipate long-term side effects, since most of the trials are very recent. In addition, there is growing evidence that transplanted cells not just simply replace missing tissue but also trigger local mechanisms to initiate a repair response and secret factors useful for tissue protection or neovascularization.

Ultimately, large clinical trials will have to be conducted and at the same time, we need to continue the basic research to elucidate the underlying mechanism of stem cell therapy.

References

1. Assmus B, Schachinger V, Teupe C, Britten M, Lehmann R, Dobert N, et al. Transplantation of Progenitor Cells and Regeneration Enhancement in Acute Myocardial Infarction (TOPCARE-AMI). *Circulation*. December 10, 2002;106(24):3009–17.
2. Wollert KC, Meyer GP, Lotz J, Ringes-Lichtenberg S, Lippolt P, Breidenbach C, et al. Intracoronary autologous bone-marrow cell transfer after myocardial infarction: the BOOST randomised controlled clinical trial. *Lancet*. July 10–16, 2004;364(9429):141–8.
3. Thomson JA, Itskovitz-Eldor J, Shapiro SS, Waknitz MA, Swiergiel JJ, Marshall VS, et al. Embryonic stem cell lines derived from human blastocysts. *Science*. November 6, 1998;282(5391):1145–7.
4. Brivanlou AH, Gage FH, Jaenisch R, Jessell T, Melton D, Rossant J. Stem cells. Setting standards for human embryonic stem cells. *Science*. May 9, 2003;300(5621):913–6.
5. Reubinoff BE, Pera MF, Fong CY, Trounson A, Bongso A. Embryonic stem cell lines from human blastocysts: somatic differentiation in vitro. *Nat Biotechnol*. April 2000;18(4):399–404.
6. Schuldiner M, Yanuka O, Itskovitz-Eldor J, Melton DA, Benvenisty N. Effects of eight growth factors on the differentiation of cells derived from human embryonic stem cells. *Proc Natl Acad Sci USA*. October 10, 2000;97(21):11307–12.
7. Kaufman DS, Hanson ET, Lewis RL, Auerbach R, Thomson JA. Hematopoietic colony-forming cells derived from human embryonic stem cells. *Proc Natl Acad Sci USA*. September 11, 2001;98(19):10716–21.
8. Kehat I, Kenyagin-Karsenti D, Snir M, Segev H, Amit M, Gepstein A, et al. Human embryonic stem cells can differentiate into myocytes with structural and functional properties of cardiomyocytes. *J Clin Invest*. August 2001;108(3):407–14.
9. Levenberg S, Golub JS, Amit M, Itskovitz-Eldor J, Langer R. Endothelial cells derived from human embryonic stem cells. *Proc Natl Acad Sci USA*. April 2, 2002;99(7):4391–6.
10. Assady S, Maor G, Amit M, Itskovitz-Eldor J, Skorecki KL, Tzukerman M. Insulin production by human embryonic stem cells. *Diabetes*. August 2001;50(8):1691–7.
11. Gearhart J. New human embryonic stem-cell lines–more is better. *N Engl J Med*. March 25, 2004;350(13):1275–6.
12. Robertson JA. Human embryonic stem cell research: ethical and legal issues. *Nat Rev Genet*. January 2001;2(1):74–8.
13. Weissman IL. Stem cells: units of development, units of regeneration, and units in evolution. *Cell*. January 7, 2000;100(1):157–68.
14. Fuchs E, Tumbar T, Guasch G. Socializing with the neighbors: stem cells and their niche. *Cell*. March 19, 2004;116(6):769–78.
15. Slack JM. Stem cells in epithelial tissues. *Science*. February 25, 2000;287(5457):1431–3.
16. Kucia M, Ratajczak J, Reca R, Janowska-Wieczorek A, Ratajczak MZ. Tissue-specific muscle, neural and liver stem/progenitor cells reside in the bone marrow, respond to an SDF-1 gradient and are mobilized into peripheral blood during stress and tissue injury. *Blood Cells Mol Dis*. January–February 2004;32(1):52–7.
17. Kucia M, Ratajczak J, Ratajczak MZ. Bone marrow as a source of circulating CXCR4+ tissue-committed stem cells. *Biol Cell*. February 2005;97(2):133–46.
18. Till JE, McCulloch E. A direct measurement of the radiation sensitivity of normal mouse bone marrow cells. *Radiat Res*. February 1961;14:213–22.
19. Bianco P, Riminucci M, Gronthos S, Robey PG. Bone marrow stromal stem cells: nature, biology, and potential applications. *Stem Cells*. 2001;19(3):180–92.
20. Pittenger MF, Mackay AM, Beck SC, Jaiswal RK, Douglas R, Mosca JD, et al. Multilineage potential of adult human mesenchymal stem cells. *Science*. April 2, 1999;284(5411):143–7.
21. Orlic D, Kajstura J, Chimenti S, Jakoniuk I, Anderson SM, Li B, et al. Bone marrow cells regenerate infarcted myocardium. *Nature*. April 5, 2001;410(6829):701–5.
22. Gussoni E, Soneoka Y, Strickland CD, Buzney EA, Khan MK, Flint AF, et al. Dystrophin expression in the mdx mouse restored by stem cell transplantation. *Nature*. September 23, 1999;401(6751):390–4.
23. Mezey E, Chandross KJ, Harta G, Maki RA, McKercher SR. Turning blood into brain: cells bearing neuronal

24. Nash K, Hafeez A, Hou S. Hospital-acquired renal insufficiency. *Am J Kidney Dis*. May 2002;39(5):930–6.
25. Yamamoto M, Cui L, Johkura K, Asanuma K, Okouchi Y, Ogiwara N, et al. Branching ducts similar to mesonephric ducts or ureteric buds in teratomas originating from mouse embryonic stem cells. *Am J Physiol Renal Physiol*. January 2006;290(1):F52–60.
26. Steenhard BM, Isom KS, Cazcarro P, Dunmore JH, Godwin AR, St John PL, et al. Integration of embryonic stem cells in metanephric kidney organ culture. *J Am Soc Nephrol*. June 2005;16(6):1623–31.
27. Kobayashi T, Tanaka H, Kuwana H, Inoshita S, Teraoka H, Sasaki S, et al. Wnt4-transformed mouse embryonic stem cells differentiate into renal tubular cells. *Biochem Biophys Res Commun*. October 21 2005;336(2):585–95.
28. Kramer J, Steinhoff J, Klinger M, Fricke L, Rohwedel J. Cells differentiated from mouse embryonic stem cells via embryoid bodies express renal marker molecules. *Differentiation*. March 2006;74(2–3):91–104.
29. Vigneau C, Zheng F, Polgar K, Wilson PD, Striker G. Stem cells and kidney injury. *Curr Opin Nephrol Hypertens*. May 2006;15(3):238–44.
30. Kim D, Dressler GR. Nephrogenic factors promote differentiation of mouse embryonic stem cells into renal epithelia. *J Am Soc Nephrol*. December 2005;16(12):3527–34.
31. Lanza RP, Chung HY, Yoo JJ, Wettstein PJ, Blackwell C, Borson N, et al. Generation of histocompatible tissues using nuclear transplantation. *Nat Biotechnol*. July 2002;20(7):689–96.
32. Poulsom R, Prodromidi EI, Pusey CD, Cook HT. Cell therapy for renal regeneration – time for some joined-up thinking? *Nephrol Dial Transplant*. December 2006;21(12):3349–53.
33. Reinders ME, Rabelink TJ, Briscoe DM. Angiogenesis and endothelial cell repair in renal disease and allograft rejection. *J Am Soc Nephrol*. April 2006;17(4):932–42.
34. Williams GM, Alvarez CA. Host repopulation of the endothelium in allografts of kidneys and aorta. *Surg Forum*. 1969;20:293–4.
35. Sinclair RA. Origin of endothelium in human renal allografts. *Br Med J*. October 7, 1972;4(831):15–6.
36. Lagaaij EL, Cramer-Knijnenburg GF, van Kemenade FJ, van Es LA, Bruijn JA, van Krieken JH. Endothelial cell chimerism after renal transplantation and vascular rejection. *Lancet*. January 6, 2001;357(9249):33–7.
37. Xu W, Baelde HJ, Lagaaij EL, De Heer E, Paul LC, Bruijn JA. Endothelial cell chimerism after renal transplantation in a rat model. *Transplantation*. November 15, 2002;74(9):1316–20.
38. Kerjaschki D, Huttary N, Raab I, Regele H, Bojarski-Nagy K, Bartel G, et al. Lymphatic endothelial progenitor cells contribute to de novo lymphangiogenesis in human renal transplants. *Nat Med*. February 2006;12(2):230–4.
39. Rookmaaker MB, Tolboom H, Goldschmeding R, Zwaginga JJ, Rabelink TJ, Verhaar MC. Bone-marrow-derived cells contribute to endothelial repair after thrombotic microangiopathy. *Blood*. February 1, 2002;99(3):1095.
40. Dekel B, Shezen E, Even-Tov-Friedman S, Katchman H, Margalit R, Nagler A, et al. Transplantation of human hematopoietic stem cells into ischemic and growing kidneys suggests a role in vasculogenesis but not tubulogenesis. *Stem Cells*. May 2006;24(5):1185–93.
41. Cornacchia F, Fornoni A, Plati AR, Thomas A, Wang Y, Inverardi L, et al. Glomerulosclerosis is transmitted by bone marrow-derived mesangial cell progenitors. *J Clin Invest*. December 2001;108(11):1649–56.
42. Rookmaaker MB, Smits AM, Tolboom H, Van 't Wout K, Martens AC, Goldschmeding R, et al. Bone-marrow-derived cells contribute to glomerular endothelial repair in experimental glomerulonephritis. *Am J Pathol*. August 2003;163(2):553–62.
43. Imasawa T, Utsunomiya Y, Kawamura T, Zhong Y, Nagasawa R, Okabe M, et al. The potential of bone marrow-derived cells to differentiate to glomerular mesangial cells. *J Am Soc Nephrol*. July 2001;12(7):1401–9.
44. Ito T, Suzuki A, Imai E, Okabe M, Hori M. Bone marrow is a reservoir of repopulating mesangial cells during glomerular remodeling. *J Am Soc Nephrol*. December 2001;12(12):2625–35.
45. Uchimura H, Marumo T, Takase O, Kawachi H, Shimizu F, Hayashi M, et al. Intrarenal injection of bone marrow-derived angiogenic cells reduces endothelial injury and mesangial cell activation in experimental glomerulonephritis. *J Am Soc Nephrol*. April 2005;16(4):997–1004.
46. Ikarashi K, Li B, Suwa M, Kawamura K, Morioka T, Yao J, et al. Bone marrow cells contribute to regeneration of damaged glomerular endothelial cells. *Kidney Int*. May 2005;67(5):1925–33.
47. Li B, Morioka T, Uchiyama M, Oite T. Bone marrow cell infusion ameliorates progressive glomerulosclerosis in an experimental rat model. *Kidney Int*. February 2006;69(2):323–30.
48. Hayakawa M, Ishizaki M, Hayakawa J, Migita M, Murakami M, Shimada T, et al. Role of bone marrow cells in the healing process of mouse experimental glomerulonephritis. *Pediatr Res*. August 2005;58(2):323–8.
49. Grimm PC, Nickerson P, Jeffery J, Savani RC, Gough J, McKenna RM, et al. Neointimal and tubulointerstitial infiltration by recipient mesenchymal cells in chronic renal-allograft rejection. *N Engl J Med*. July 12, 2001;345(2):93–7.
50. Sun DF, Fujigaki Y, Fujimoto T, Yonemura K, Hishida A. Possible involvement of myofibroblasts in cellular recovery of uranyl acetate-induced acute renal failure in rats. *Am J Pathol*. October 2000;157(4):1321–35.
51. Direkze NC, Forbes SJ, Brittan M, Hunt T, Jeffery R, Preston SL, et al. Multiple organ engraftment by bone-marrow-derived myofibroblasts and fibroblasts in bone-marrow-transplanted mice. *Stem Cells*. 2003;21(5):514–20.
52. Lin F, Moran A, Igarashi P. Intrarenal cells, not bone marrow-derived cells, are the major source for regeneration in postischemic kidney. *J Clin Invest*. July 2005;115(7):1756–64.
53. Roufosse C, Bou-Gharios G, Prodromidi E, Alexakis C, Jeffery R, Khan S, et al. Bone marrow-derived cells do not contribute significantly to collagen I synthesis in a murine model of renal fibrosis. *J Am Soc Nephrol*. March 2006;17(3):775–82.
54. Gupta S, Verfaillie C, Chmielewski D, Kim Y, Rosenberg ME. A role for extrarenal cells in the regeneration following acute renal failure. *Kidney Int*. October 2002;62(4):1285–90.
55. Poulsom R, Forbes SJ, Hodivala-Dilke K, Ryan E, Wyles S, Navaratnarasah S, et al. Bone marrow contributes to renal parenchymal turnover and regeneration. *J Pathol*. September 2001;195(2):229–35.

56. Nishida M, Kawakatsu H, Shiraishi I, Fujimoto S, Gotoh T, Urata Y, et al. Renal tubular regeneration by bone marrow-derived cells in a girl after bone marrow transplantation. *Am J Kidney Dis*. November 2003;42(5): E10–2.
57. Fang TC, Alison MR, Cook HT, Jeffery R, Wright NA, Poulsom R. Proliferation of bone marrow-derived cells contributes to regeneration after folic acid-induced acute tubular injury. *J Am Soc Nephrol*. June 2005;16(6):1723–32.
58. Szczypka MS, Westover AJ, Clouthier SG, Ferrara JL, Humes HD. Rare incorporation of bone marrow-derived cells into kidney after folic acid-induced injury. *Stem Cells*. 2005;23(1):44–54.
59. Duffield JS, Bonventre JV. Kidney tubular epithelium is restored without replacement with bone marrow-derived cells during repair after ischemic injury. *Kidney Int*. November 2005;68(5):1956–61.
60. Duffield JS, Park KM, Hsiao LL, Kelley VR, Scadden DT, Ichimura T, et al. Restoration of tubular epithelial cells during repair of the postischemic kidney occurs independently of bone marrow-derived stem cells. *J Clin Invest*. July 2005;115(7):1743–55.
61. Morigi M, Imberti B, Zoja C, Corna D, Tomasoni S, Abbate M, et al. Mesenchymal stem cells are renotropic, helping to repair the kidney and improve function in acute renal failure. *J Am Soc Nephrol*. July 2004;15(7):1794–804.
62. Herrera MB, Bussolati B, Bruno S, Fonsato V, Romanazzi GM, Camussi G. Mesenchymal stem cells contribute to the renal repair of acute tubular epithelial injury. *Int J Mol Med*. December 2004;14(6):1035–41.
63. Lange C, Togel F, Ittrich H, Clayton F, Nolte-Ernsting C, Zander AR, et al. Administered mesenchymal stem cells enhance recovery from ischemia/reperfusion-induced acute renal failure in rats. *Kidney Int*. October 2005;68(4):1613–7.
64. Togel F, Hu Z, Weiss K, Isaac J, Lange C, Westenfelder C. Administered mesenchymal stem cells protect against ischemic acute renal failure through differentiation-independent mechanisms. *Am J Physiol Renal Physiol*. July 2005;289(1):F31–42.
65. Krause DS, Theise ND, Collector MI, Henegariu O, Hwang S, Gardner R, et al. Multi-organ, multi-lineage engraftment by a single bone marrow-derived stem cell. *Cell*. May 4, 2001;105(3):369–77.
66. Wagers AJ, Sherwood RI, Christensen JL, Weissman IL. Little evidence for developmental plasticity of adult hematopoietic stem cells. *Science*. Sep 27, 2002;297(5590):2256–9.
67. Kale S, Karihaloo A, Clark PR, Kashgarian M, Krause DS, Cantley LG. Bone marrow stem cells contribute to repair of the ischemically injured renal tubule. *J Clin Invest*. July 2003;112(1):42–9.
68. Lin F, Cordes K, Li L, Hood L, Couser WG, Shankland SJ, et al. Hematopoietic stem cells contribute to the regeneration of renal tubules after renal ischemia-reperfusion injury in mice. *J Am Soc Nephrol*. May 2003;14(5):1188–99.
69. Masuya M, Drake CJ, Fleming PA, Reilly CM, Zeng H, Hill WD, et al. Hematopoietic origin of glomerular mesangial cells. *Blood*. March 15, 2003;101(6):2215–8.
70. Zheng F, Cornacchia F, Schulman I, Banerjee A, Cheng QL, Potier M, et al. Development of albuminuria and glomerular lesions in normoglycemic B6 recipients of db/db mice bone marrow: the role of mesangial cell progenitors. *Diabetes*. September 2004;53(9):2420–7.
71. Guo JK, Ardito TA, Kashgarian M, Krause DS. Prevention of mesangial sclerosis by bone marrow transplantation. *Kidney Int*. September 2006;70(5):910–3.
72. Perry J, Tam S, Zheng K, Sado Y, Dobson H, Jefferson B, et al. Type IV Collagen Induces Podocytic Features in Bone Marrow Stromal Stem Cells In Vitro. *J Am Soc Nephrol*. January 2006;17(1):66–76.
73. Prodromidi EI, Poulsom R, Jeffery R, Roufosse CA, Pollard PJ, Pusey CD, et al. Bone Marrow Derived-Cells Contribute to Podocyte Regeneration and Amelioration of Renal Disease in a Mouse Model of Alport Syndrome. *Stem Cells*. November 2006; 24(11):2448–55.
74. Sugimoto H, Mundel TM, Sund M, Xie L, Cosgrove D, Kalluri R. Bone-marrow-derived stem cells repair basement membrane collagen defects and reverse genetic kidney disease. *Proc Natl Acad Sci USA*. 2006 May 9, 2006;103(19):7321–6.
75. Ninichuk V, Gross O, Segerer S, Hoffmann R, Radomska E, Buchstaller A, et al. Multipotent mesenchymal stem cells reduce interstitial fibrosis but do not delay progression of chronic kidney disease in collagen4A3-deficient mice. *Kidney Int*. July 2006;70(1):121–9.
76. Hammerman MR. Renal organogenesis from transplanted metanephric primordia. *J Am Soc Nephrol*. May 2004;15(5):1126–32.
77. Woolf AS, Palmer SJ, Snow ML, Fine LG. Creation of a functioning chimeric mammalian kidney. *Kidney Int*. November 1990;38(5):991–7.
78. Woolf AS, Hornbruch A, Fine LG. Integration of new embryonic nephrons into the kidney. *Am J Kidney Dis*. June 1991;17(6):611–4.
79. Rogers SA, Lowell JA, Hammerman NA, Hammerman MR. Transplantation of developing metanephroi into adult rats. *Kidney Int*. July 1998;54(1):27–37.
80. Hammerman MR. Growing new kidneys in situ. *Clin Exp Nephrol*. September 2004;8(3):169–77.
81. Rogers SA, Hammerman MR. Transplantation of metanephroi after preservation in vitro. *Am J Physiol Regul Integr Comp Physiol*. August 2001;281(2):R661–5.
82. Dekel B, Amariglio N, Kaminski N, Schwartz A, Goshen E, Arditti FD, et al. Engraftment and differentiation of human metanephroi into functional mature nephrons after transplantation into mice is accompanied by a profile of gene expression similar to normal human kidney development. *J Am Soc Nephrol*. April 2002;13(4):977–90.
83. Dekel B, Burakova T, Arditti FD, Reich-Zeliger S, Milstein O, Aviel-Ronen S, et al. Human and porcine early kidney precursors as a new source for transplantation. *Nat Med*. January 2003;9(1):53–60.
84. Yokoo T, Ohashi T, Shen JS, Sakurai K, Miyazaki Y, Utsunomiya Y, et al. Human mesenchymal stem cells in rodent whole-embryo culture are reprogrammed to contribute to kidney tissues. *Proc Natl Acad Sci USA*. March 1 2005;102(9):3296–300.
85. Humes HD, Fissell WH, Weitzel WF, Buffington DA, Westover AJ, MacKay SM, et al. Metabolic replacement of kidney function in uremic animals with a bioartificial kidney containing human cells. *Am J Kidney Dis*. May 2002;39(5):1078–87.
86. Humes HD, MacKay SM, Funke AJ, Buffington DA. Tissue engineering of a bioartificial renal tubule assist

device: in vitro transport and metabolic characteristics. *Kidney Int.* June 1999;55(6):2502–14.
87. Nikolovski J, Gulari E, Humes HD. Design engineering of a bioartificial renal tubule cell therapy device. *Cell Transplant.* July–August 1999;8(4):351–64.
88. Humes HD, Weitzel WF, Bartlett RH, Swaniker FC, Paganini EP, Luderer JR, et al. Initial clinical results of the bioartificial kidney containing human cells in ICU patients with acute renal failure. *Kidney Int.* October 2004;66(4):1578–88.
89. Tiranathanagul K, Brodie J, Humes HD. Bioartificial kidney in the treatment of acute renal failure associated with sepsis. Nephrology (Carlton). August 2006;11(4):285–91.
90. Fissell WH. Developments towards an artificial kidney. *Expert Rev Med Devices.* March 2006;3(2):155–65.
91. Fissell WH, Manley S, Westover A, Humes HD, Fleischman AJ, Roy S. Differentiated growth of human renal tubule cells on thin-film and nanostructured materials. *Asaio J.* May–June 2006;52(3):221–7.
92. Devendra D, Liu E, Eisenbarth GS. Type 1 diabetes: recent developments. *Bmj.* March 27, 2004;328(7442):750–4.
93. Lechner A, Habener JF. Stem/progenitor cells derived from adult tissues: potential for the treatment of diabetes mellitus. *Am J Physiol Endocrinol Metab.* Feb 2003;284(2):E259–66.
94. Halvorsen TL, Beattie GM, Lopez AD, Hayek A, Levine F. Accelerated telomere shortening and senescence in human pancreatic islet cells stimulated to divide in vitro. *J Endocrinol.* July 2000;166(1):103–9.
95. Hori Y, Rulifson IC, Tsai BC, Heit JJ, Cahoy JD, Kim SK. Growth inhibitors promote differentiation of insulin-producing tissue from embryonic stem cells. *Proc Natl Acad Sci USA.* December 10, 2002;99(25):16105–10.
96. Miyazaki S, Yamato E, Miyazaki J. Regulated expression of pdx-1 promotes in vitro differentiation of insulin-producing cells from embryonic stem cells. *Diabetes.* April 2004;53(4):1030–7.
97. Soria B, Roche E, Berna G, Leon-Quinto T, Reig JA, Martin F. Insulin-secreting cells derived from embryonic stem cells normalize glycemia in streptozotocin-induced diabetic mice. *Diabetes.* February 2000;49(2):157–62.
98. Fujikawa T, Oh SH, Pi L, Hatch HM, Shupe T, Petersen BE. Teratoma formation leads to failure of treatment for type I diabetes using embryonic stem cell-derived insulin-producing cells. *Am J Pathol.* June 2005;166(6):1781–91.
99. Ianus A, Holz GG, Theise ND, Hussain MA. In vivo derivation of glucose-competent pancreatic endocrine cells from bone marrow without evidence of cell fusion. *J Clin Invest.* March 2003;111(6):843–50.
100. Taneera J, Rosengren A, Renstrom E, Nygren JM, Serup P, Rorsman P, et al. Failure of transplanted bone marrow cells to adopt a pancreatic beta-cell fate. *Diabetes.* February 2006;55(2):290–6.
101. Hess D, Li L, Martin M, Sakano S, Hill D, Strutt B, et al. Bone marrow-derived stem cells initiate pancreatic regeneration. *Nat Biotechnol.* July 2003;21(7):763–70.
102. Mathews V, Hanson PT, Ford E, Fujita J, Polonsky KS, Graubert TA. Recruitment of bone marrow-derived endothelial cells to sites of pancreatic beta-cell injury. *Diabetes.* January 2004;53(1):91–8.
103. Lechner A, Yang YG, Blacken RA, Wang L, Nolan AL, Habener JF. No evidence for significant transdifferentiation of bone marrow into pancreatic beta-cells in vivo. *Diabetes.* March 2004;53(3):616–23.
104. Kang EM, Zickler PP, Burns S, Langemeijer SM, Brenner S, Phang OA, et al. Hematopoietic stem cell transplantation prevents diabetes in NOD mice but does not contribute to significant islet cell regeneration once disease is established. *Exp Hematol.* June 2005;33(6):699–705.
105. Banerjee M, Kumar A, Bhonde RR. Reversal of experimental diabetes by multiple bone marrow transplantation. *Biochem Biophys Res Commun.* March 4, 2005;328(1):318–25.
106. Ende N, Chen R, Reddi AS. Effect of human umbilical cord blood cells on glycemia and insulitis in type 1 diabetic mice. *Biochem Biophys Res Commun.* December 17, 2004;325(3):665–9.
107. Tang DQ, Cao LZ, Burkhardt BR, Xia CQ, Litherland SA, Atkinson MA, et al. In vivo and in vitro characterization of insulin-producing cells obtained from murine bone marrow. *Diabetes.* July 2004;53(7):1721–32.
108. Oh SH, Muzzonigro TM, Bae SH, LaPlante JM, Hatch HM, Petersen BE. Adult bone marrow-derived cells trans-differentiating into insulin-producing cells for the treatment of type I diabetes. *Lab Invest.* May 2004;84(5):607–17.
109. Fernandez Vina R, Saslavsky J, Andrin O, Vrsalovick F, Ferreyra de Silva J, Ferreyra O, et al. First word reported datas from Argentina of implant and cellular therapy with autologous adult stem cells in type 2 diabetic patients (Teceldiar study 1). 4th ISSCR Annual Meeting, Toronto; 2006.
110. Fernandez Vina R, Andrin O, Saslavsky J, Ferreyra de Silva J, Vrsalovick F, Camozzi L, et al. Increase of 'c' peptide level in type 1 diabetics patients after direct pancreas implant by endovascular way of autologous adult mononuclears CD34+CD38 (–) cells (Teceldiab 2 study). 4th ISSCR Annual Meeting, Toronto; 2006.
111. Health Mo. Annual Report of the Chief Medical Officer. London: Ministry of Health, UK; 2001.
112. Fox IJ, Chowdhury JR, Kaufman SS, Goertzen TC, Chowdhury NR, Warkentin PI, et al. Treatment of the Crigler-Najjar syndrome type I with hepatocyte transplantation. *N Engl J Med.* May 14, 1998;338(20):1422–6.
113. Strom SC, Fisher RA, Thompson MT, Sanyal AJ, Cole PE, Ham JM, et al. Hepatocyte transplantation as a bridge to orthotopic liver transplantation in terminal liver failure. *Transplantation.* February 27 1997;63(4):559–69.
114. Bilir BM, Guinette D, Karrer F, Kumpe DA, Krysl J, Stephens J, et al. Hepatocyte transplantation in acute liver failure. *Liver Transpl.* January 2000;6(1):32–40.
115. Ohashi K, Park F, Kay MA. Hepatocyte transplantation: clinical and experimental application. *J Mol Med.* November 2001;79(11):617–30.
116. Najimi M, Sokal E. Liver cell transplantation. *Minerva Pediatr.* October 2005;57(5):243–57.
117. Hamazaki T, Iiboshi Y, Oka M, Papst PJ, Meacham AM, Zon LI, et al. Hepatic maturation in differentiating embryonic stem cells in vitro. *FEBS Lett.* May 18, 2001;497(1):15–9.
118. Jones EA, Tosh D, Wilson DI, Lindsay S, Forrester LM. Hepatic differentiation of murine embryonic stem cells. *Exp Cell Res.* January 1, 2002;272(1):15–22.

119. Ishii T, Yasuchika K, Fujii H, Hoppo T, Baba S, Naito M, et al. In vitro differentiation and maturation of mouse embryonic stem cells into hepatocytes. *Exp Cell Res.* September 10 2005;309(1):68–77.
120. Yin Y, Lim YK, Salto-Tellez M, Ng SC, Lin CS, Lim SK. AFP(+), ESC-derived cells engraft and differentiate into hepatocytes in vivo. *Stem Cells.* 2002;20(4):338–46.
121. Yamada T, Yoshikawa M, Kanda S, Kato Y, Nakajima Y, Ishizaka S, et al. In vitro differentiation of embryonic stem cells into hepatocyte-like cells identified by cellular uptake of indocyanine green. *Stem Cells.* 2002;20(2):146–54.
122. Chinzei R, Tanaka Y, Shimizu-Saito K, Hara Y, Kakinuma S, Watanabe M, et al. Embryoid-body cells derived from a mouse embryonic stem cell line show differentiation into functional hepatocytes. *Hepatology.* July 2002;36(1):22–9.
123. Petersen BE, Bowen WC, Patrene KD, Mars WM, Sullivan AK, Murase N, et al. Bone marrow as a potential source of hepatic oval cells. *Science.* May 14, 1999;284(5417):1168–70.
124. Grompe M, Lindstedt S, al-Dhalimy M, Kennaway NG, Papaconstantinou J, Torres-Ramos CA, et al. Pharmacological correction of neonatal lethal hepatic dysfunction in a murine model of hereditary tyrosinaemia type I. *Nat Genet.* August 1995;10(4):453–60.
125. Sakaida I, Terai S, Yamamoto N, Aoyama K, Ishikawa T, Nishina H, et al. Transplantation of bone marrow cells reduces CCl4-induced liver fibrosis in mice. *Hepatology.* December 2004;40(6):1304–11.
126. Mallet VO, Mitchell C, Mezey E, Fabre M, Guidotti JE, Renia L, et al. Bone marrow transplantation in mice leads to a minor population of hepatocytes that can be selectively amplified in vivo. *Hepatology.* April 2002;35(4):799–804.
127. Terai S, Sakaida I, Yamamoto N, Omori K, Watanabe T, Ohata S, et al. An in vivo model for monitoring transdifferentiation of bone marrow cells into functional hepatocytes. *J Biochem (Tokyo).* October 2003;134(4):551–8.
128. Jang YY, Collector MI, Baylin SB, Diehl AM, Sharkis SJ. Hematopoietic stem cells convert into liver cells within days without fusion. *Nat Cell Biol.* June 2004;6(6):532–9.
129. Theise ND, Badve S, Saxena R, Henegariu O, Sell S, Crawford JM, et al. Derivation of hepatocytes from bone marrow cells in mice after radiation-induced myeloablation. *Hepatology.* January 2000;31(1):235–40.
130. Wang X, Ge S, McNamara G, Hao QL, Crooks GM, Nolta JA. Albumin-expressing hepatocyte-like cells develop in the livers of immune-deficient mice that received transplants of highly purified human hematopoietic stem cells. *Blood.* May 15, 2003;101(10):4201–8.
131. Kanazawa Y, Verma IM. Little evidence of bone marrow-derived hepatocytes in the replacement of injured liver. *Proc Natl Acad Sci USA.* September 30, 2003;100(Suppl 1):11850–3.
132. Alison MR, Poulsom R, Jeffery R, Dhillon AP, Quaglia A, Jacob J, et al. Hepatocytes from non-hepatic adult stem cells. *Nature.* July 20, 2000;406(6793):257.
133. Theise ND, Nimmakayalu M, Gardner R, Illei PB, Morgan G, Teperman L, et al. Liver from bone marrow in humans. *Hepatology.* July 2000;32(1):11–6.
134. Korbling M, Katz RL, Khanna A, Ruifrok AC, Rondon G, Albitar M, et al. Hepatocytes and epithelial cells of donor origin in recipients of peripheral-blood stem cells. *N Engl J Med.* Mar 7, 2002;346(10):738–46.
135. Ng IO, Chan KL, Shek WH, Lee JM, Fong DY, Lo CM, et al. High frequency of chimerism in transplanted livers. *Hepatology.* October 2003;38(4):989–98.
136. Fogt F, Beyser KH, Poremba C, Zimmerman RL, Khettry U, Ruschoff J. Recipient-derived hepatocytes in liver transplants: a rare event in sex-mismatched transplants. *Hepatology.* July 2002;36(1):173–6.
137. Wu T, Cieply K, Nalesnik MA, Randhawa PS, Sonzogni A, Bellamy C, et al. Minimal evidence of transdifferentiation from recipient bone marrow to parenchymal cells in regenerating and long-surviving human allografts. *Am J Transplant.* September 2003;3(9):1173–81.
138. am Esch JS, 2nd, Knoefel WT, Klein M, Ghodsizad A, Fuerst G, Poll LW, et al. Portal application of autologous CD133+ bone marrow cells to the liver: a novel concept to support hepatic regeneration. *Stem Cells.* April 2005;23(4):463–70.
139. Gordon MY, Levicar N, Pai M, Bachellier P, Dimarakis I, Al-Allaf F, et al. Characterisation and Clinical Application of Human Cd34+ Stem/Progenitor Cell Populations Mobilised into the Blood by G-Csf. *Stem Cells.* July 2006;24(7):1822–30.
140. Terai S, Ishikawa T, Omori K, Aoyama K, Marumoto Y, Urata Y, et al. Improved liver function in liver cirrhosis patients after autologous bone marrow cell infusion therapy. *Stem Cells.* October 2006;24(10):2292–8.
141. Wei H, Juhasz O, Li J, Tarasova YS, Boheler KR. Embryonic stem cells and cardiomyocyte differentiation: phenotypic and molecular analyses. *J Cell Mol Med.* October–December 2005;9(4):804–17.
142. Min JY, Yang Y, Sullivan MF, Ke Q, Converso KL, Chen Y, et al. Long-term improvement of cardiac function in rats after infarction by transplantation of embryonic stem cells. *J Thorac Cardiovasc Surg.* February 2003;125(2):361–9.
143. Hodgson DM, Behfar A, Zingman LV, Kane GC, Perez-Terzic C, Alekseev AE, et al. Stable benefit of embryonic stem cell therapy in myocardial infarction. *Am J Physiol Heart Circ Physiol.* September 2004;287(2):H471–9.
144. Min JY, Huang X, Xiang M, Meissner A, Chen Y, Ke Q, et al. Homing of intravenously infused embryonic stem cell-derived cells to injured hearts after myocardial infarction. *J Thorac Cardiovasc Surg.* April 2006;131(4):889–97.
145. Kehat I, Khimovich L, Caspi O, Gepstein A, Shofti R, Arbel G, et al. Electromechanical integration of cardiomyocytes derived from human embryonic stem cells. *Nat Biotechnol.* November 2004;22(10):1282–9.
146. Zhang YM, Hartzell C, Narlow M, Dudley SC, Jr. Stem cell-derived cardiomyocytes demonstrate arrhythmic potential. *Circulation.* September 3, 2002;106(10):1294–9.
147. Ye L, Haider H, Sim EK. Adult stem cells for cardiac repair: a choice between skeletal myoblasts and bone marrow stem cells. *Exp Biol Med (Maywood).* January 2006;231(1):8–19.
148. Minguell JJ, Erices A. Mesenchymal stem cells and the treatment of cardiac disease. *Exp Biol Med (Maywood).* January 2006;231(1):39–49.
149. Yoon YS, Park JS, Tkebuchava T, Luedeman C, Losordo DW. Unexpected severe calcification after transplantation of bone marrow cells in acute myocardial infarction. *Circulation.* June 29 2004;109(25):3154–7.
150. Kang HJ, Kim HS, Zhang SY, Park KW, Cho HJ, Koo BK, et al. Effects of intracoronary infusion of peripheral

blood stem-cells mobilised with granulocyte-colony stimulating factor on left ventricular systolic function and restenosis after coronary stenting in myocardial infarction: the MAGIC cell randomised clinical trial. *Lancet.* March 6, 2004;363(9411):751–6.
151. Yoon YS, Wecker A, Heyd L, Park JS, Tkebuchava T, Kusano K, et al. Clonally expanded novel multipotent stem cells from human bone marrow regenerate myocardium after myocardial infarction. *J Clin Invest.* February 2005;115(2):326–38.
152. Stenderup K, Justesen J, Clausen C, Kassem M. Aging is associated with decreased maximal life span and accelerated senescence of bone marrow stromal cells. *Bone.* December 2003;33(6):919–26.
153. Vacanti V, Kong E, Suzuki G, Sato K, Canty JM, Lee T. Phenotypic changes of adult porcine mesenchymal stem cells induced by prolonged passaging in culture. *J Cell Physiol.* November 2005;205(2):194–201.
154. Rubio D, Garcia-Castro J, Martin MC, de la Fuente R, Cigudosa JC, Lloyd AC, et al. Spontaneous human adult stem cell transformation. *Cancer Res.* April 15, 2005;65(8):3035–9.
155. Chang MG, Tung L, Sekar RB, Chang CY, Cysyk J, Dong P, et al. Proarrhythmic potential of mesenchymal stem cell transplantation revealed in an in vitro coculture model. *Circulation.* April 18 2006;113(15):1832–41.
156. Majka SM, Jackson KA, Kienstra KA, Majesky MW, Goodell MA, Hirschi KK. Distinct progenitor populations in skeletal muscle are bone marrow derived and exhibit different cell fates during vascular regeneration. *J Clin Invest.* February 2003;111(1):71–9.
157. Summer R, Kotton DN, Sun X, Fitzsimmons K, Fine A. Translational physiology: origin and phenotype of lung side population cells. *Am J Physiol Lung Cell Mol Physiol.* September 2004;287(3):L477–83.
158. Osawa M, Hanada K, Hamada H, Nakauchi H. Long-term lymphohematopoietic reconstitution by a single CD34-low/negative hematopoietic stem cell. *Science.* July 12, 1996;273(5272):242–5.
159. Yeh ET, Zhang S, Wu HD, Korbling M, Willerson JT, Estrov Z. Transdifferentiation of human peripheral blood CD34+-enriched cell population into cardiomyocytes, endothelial cells, and smooth muscle cells in vivo. *Circulation.* October 28, 2003;108(17):2070–3.
160. Murry CE, Soonpaa MH, Reinecke H, Nakajima H, Nakajima HO, Rubart M, et al. Haematopoietic stem cells do not transdifferentiate into cardiac myocytes in myocardial infarcts. *Nature.* April 8, 2004;428(6983): 664–8.
161. Balsam LB, Wagers AJ, Christensen JL, Kofidis T, Weissman IL, Robbins RC. Haematopoietic stem cells adopt mature haematopoietic fates in ischaemic myocardium. *Nature.* April 8, 2004;428(6983):668–73.
162. Deten A, Volz HC, Clamors S, Leiblein S, Briest W, Marx G, et al. Hematopoietic stem cells do not repair the infarcted mouse heart. *Cardiovasc Res.* January 1, 2005;65(1):52–63.
163. Choi K, Kennedy M, Kazarov A, Papadimitriou JC, Keller G. A common precursor for hematopoietic and endothelial cells. *Development.* February 1998;125(4): 725–32.
164. Asahara T, Masuda H, Takahashi T, Kalka C, Pastore C, Silver M, et al. Bone marrow origin of endothelial progenitor cells responsible for postnatal vasculogenesis in physiological and pathological neovascularization. *Circ Res.* August 6, 1999;85(3):221–8.
165. Kalka C, Masuda H, Takahashi T, Kalka-Moll WM, Silver M, Kearney M, et al. Transplantation of ex vivo expanded endothelial progenitor cells for therapeutic neovascularization. *Proc Natl Acad Sci USA.* March 28, 2000;97(7):3422–7.
166. Fazel S, Cimini M, Chen L, Li S, Angoulvant D, Fedak P, et al. Cardioprotective c-kit+ cells are from the bone marrow and regulate the myocardial balance of angiogenic cytokines. *J Clin Invest.* July 2006;116(7):1865–77.
167. Vasa M, Fichtlscherer S, Aicher A, Adler K, Urbich C, Martin H, et al. Number and migratory activity of circulating endothelial progenitor cells inversely correlate with risk factors for coronary artery disease. *Circ Res.* July 6, 2001;89(1):E1–7.
168. Hill JM, Zalos G, Halcox JP, Schenke WH, Waclawiw MA, Quyyumi AA, et al. Circulating endothelial progenitor cells, vascular function, and cardiovascular risk. *N Engl J Med.* February 13, 2003;348(7):593–600.
169. Jiang XX, Zhang Y, Liu B, Zhang SX, Wu Y, Yu XD, et al. Human mesenchymal stem cells inhibit differentiation and function of monocyte-derived dendritic cells. *Blood.* May 15, 2005;105(10):4120–6.
170. Amado LC, Saliaris AP, Schuleri KH, St John M, Xie JS, Cattaneo S, et al. Cardiac repair with intramyocardial injection of allogeneic mesenchymal stem cells after myocardial infarction. *Proc Natl Acad Sci USA.* August 9, 2005;102(32):11474–9.
171. Jiang Y, Jahagirdar BN, Reinhardt RL, Schwartz RE, Keene CD, Ortiz-Gonzalez XR, et al. Pluripotency of mesenchymal stem cells derived from adult marrow. *Nature.* July 4, 2002;418(6893):41–9.
172. Kajstura J, Rota M, Whang B, Cascapera S, Hosoda T, Bearzi C, et al. Bone marrow cells differentiate in cardiac cell lineages after infarction independently of cell fusion. *Circ Res.* January 7, 2005;96(1):127–37.
173. Nygren JM, Jovinge S, Breitbach M, Sawen P, Roll W, Hescheler J, et al. Bone marrow-derived hematopoietic cells generate cardiomyocytes at a low frequency through cell fusion, but not transdifferentiation. *Nat Med.* May 2004;10(5):494–501.
174. Zhang S, Wang D, Estrov Z, Raj S, Willerson JT, Yeh ET. Both cell fusion and transdifferentiation account for the transformation of human peripheral blood CD34-positive cells into cardiomyocytes in vivo. *Circulation.* December 21, 2004;110(25):3803–7.
175. Tang YL, Zhao Q, Qin X, Shen L, Cheng L, Ge J, et al. Paracrine action enhances the effects of autologous mesenchymal stem cell transplantation on vascular regeneration in rat model of myocardial infarction. *Ann Thorac Surg.* July 2005;80(1):229–36; discussion 36–7.
176. Kamihata H, Matsubara H, Nishiue T, Fujiyama S, Tsutsumi Y, Ozono R, et al. Implantation of bone marrow mononuclear cells into ischemic myocardium enhances collateral perfusion and regional function via side supply of angioblasts, angiogenic ligands, and cytokines. *Circulation.* August 28, 2001;104(9): 1046–52.
177. Zhao YS, Wang CY, Li DX, Zhang XZ, Qiao Y, Guo XM, et al. Construction of a unidirectionally beating 3-dimensional cardiac muscle construct. *J Heart Lung Transplant.* August 2005;24(8):1091–7.

178. Furuta A, Miyoshi S, Itabashi Y, Shimizu T, Kira S, Hayakawa K, et al. Pulsatile cardiac tissue grafts using a novel three-dimensional cell sheet manipulation technique functionally integrates with the host heart, in vivo. *Circ Res.* March 17, 2006;98(5):705–12.
179. Baar K, Birla R, Boluyt MO, Borschel GH, Arruda EM, Dennis RG. Self-organization of rat cardiac cells into contractile 3-D cardiac tissue. *Faseb J.* February 2005;19(2):275–7.
180. Wei HJ, Chen SC, Chang Y, Hwang SM, Lin WW, Lai PH, et al. Porous acellular bovine pericardia seeded with mesenchymal stem cells as a patch to repair a myocardial defect in a syngeneic rat model. *Biomaterials.* November 2006;27(31):5409–19.
181. Shinoka T, Breuer CK, Tanel RE, Zund G, Miura T, Ma PX, et al. Tissue engineering heart valves: valve leaflet replacement study in a lamb model. *Ann Thorac Surg.* December 1995;60(6 Suppl):S513–6.
182. Hoerstrup SP, Kadner A, Melnitchouk S, Trojan A, Eid K, Tracy J, et al. Tissue engineering of functional trileaflet heart valves from human marrow stromal cells. *Circulation.* September 24, 2002;106(12 Suppl 1):I143–50.
183. Perry TE, Kaushal S, Sutherland FW, Guleserian KJ, Bischoff J, Sacks M, et al. Thoracic Surgery Directors Association Award. Bone marrow as a cell source for tissue engineering heart valves. *Ann Thorac Surg.* March 2003;75(3):761–7; discussion 7.
184. Sutherland FW, Perry TE, Yu Y, Sherwood MC, Rabkin E, Masuda Y, et al. From stem cells to viable autologous semilunar heart valve. *Circulation.* May 31, 2005;111(21):2783–91.
185. Schmidt D, Mol A, Breymann C, Achermann J, Odermatt B, Gossi M, et al. Living autologous heart valves engineered from human prenatally harvested progenitors. *Circulation.* July 4, 2006;114(1 Suppl):I125–31.
186. Hong KU, Reynolds SD, Watkins S, Fuchs E, Stripp BR. In vivo differentiation potential of tracheal basal cells: evidence for multipotent and unipotent subpopulations. *Am J Physiol Lung Cell Mol Physiol.* April 2004;286(4):L643–9.
187. Hong KU, Reynolds SD, Watkins S, Fuchs E, Stripp BR. Basal cells are a multipotent progenitor capable of renewing the bronchial epithelium. *Am J Pathol.* February 2004;164(2):577–88.
188. Reynolds SD, Hong KU, Giangreco A, Mango GW, Guron C, Morimoto Y, et al. Conditional clara cell ablation reveals a self-renewing progenitor function of pulmonary neuroendocrine cells. *Am J Physiol Lung Cell Mol Physiol.* June 2000;278(6):L1256–63.
189. Boers JE, Ambergen AW, Thunnissen FB. Number and proliferation of clara cells in normal human airway epithelium. *Am J Respir Crit Care Med.* May 1999;159(5 Pt 1):1585–91.
190. Adamson IY, Bowden DH. The type 2 cell as progenitor of alveolar epithelial regeneration. A cytodynamic study in mice after exposure to oxygen. *Lab Invest.* January 1974;30(1):35–42.
191. Evans MJ, Cabral LJ, Stephens RJ, Freeman G. Transformation of alveolar type 2 cells to type 1 cells following exposure to NO2. *Exp Mol Pathol.* February 1975;22(1):142–50.
192. Weiss DJ, Berberich MA, Borok Z, Gail DB, Kolls JK, Penland C, et al. Adult stem cells, lung biology, and lung disease. NHLBI/Cystic Fibrosis Foundation Workshop. *Proc Am Thorac Soc.* May 2006;3(3):193–207.
193. Pereira RF, Halford KW, O'Hara MD, Leeper DB, Sokolov BP, Pollard MD, et al. Cultured adherent cells from marrow can serve as long-lasting precursor cells for bone, cartilage, and lung in irradiated mice. *Proc Natl Acad Sci USA.* May 23, 1995;92(11):4857–61.
194. Pereira RF, O'Hara MD, Laptev AV, Halford KW, Pollard MD, Class R, et al. Marrow stromal cells as a source of progenitor cells for nonhematopoietic tissues in transgenic mice with a phenotype of osteogenesis imperfecta. *Proc Natl Acad Sci USA.* February 3, 1998;95(3):1142–7.
195. Abe S, Boyer C, Liu X, Wen FQ, Kobayashi T, Fang Q, et al. Cells derived from the circulation contribute to the repair of lung injury. *Am J Respir Crit Care Med.* December 1, 2004;170(11):1158–63.
196. Rojas M, Xu J, Woods CR, Mora AL, Spears W, Roman J, et al. Bone marrow-derived mesenchymal stem cells in repair of the injured lung. *Am J Respir Cell Mol Biol.* August 2005;33(2):145–52.
197. Macpherson H, Keir P, Webb S, Samuel K, Boyle S, Bickmore W, et al. Bone marrow-derived SP cells can contribute to the respiratory tract of mice in vivo. *J Cell Sci.* June 1, 2005;118(Pt 11):2441–50.
198. Phillips RJ, Burdick MD, Hong K, Lutz MA, Murray LA, Xue YY, et al. Circulating fibrocytes traffic to the lungs in response to CXCL12 and mediate fibrosis. *J Clin Invest.* August 2004;114(3):438–46.
199. Rippon HJ, Polak JM, Qin M, Bishop AE. Derivation of distal lung epithelial progenitors from murine embryonic stem cells using a novel three-step differentiation protocol. *Stem Cells.* May 2006;24(5):1389–98.
200. Mondrinos MJ, Koutzaki S, Jiwanmall E, Li M, Dechadarevian JP, Lelkes PI, et al. Engineering three-dimensional pulmonary tissue constructs. *Tissue Eng.* April 2006;12(4):717–28.
201. Cortiella J, Nichols JE, Kojima K, Bonassar LJ, Dargon P, Roy AK, et al. Tissue-engineered lung: an in vivo and in vitro comparison of polyglycolic acid and pluronic F-127 hydrogel/somatic lung progenitor cell constructs to support tissue growth. *Tissue Eng.* May 2006;12(5):1213–25.
202. http://controlled-trials.com/ISRCTN14519481/ ISRCTN14519481 (accessed 8 October 2006).
203. Arenas E. Stem cells in the treatment of Parkinson's disease. *Brain Res Bull.* April 2002;57(6):795–808.
204. Hellmann MA, Djaldetti R, Israel Z, Melamed E. Effect of deep brain subthalamic stimulation on camptocormia and postural abnormalities in idiopathic Parkinson's disease. *Mov Disord.* September 13, 2006.
205. Lindvall O, Kokaia Z, Martinez-Serrano A. Stem cell therapy for human neurodegenerative disorders-how to make it work. *Nature Medicine.* July 2004;10(Suppl:):S42–50.
206. Kim J-H, Auerbach JM, Rodriguez-Gomez JA, Velasco I, Gavin D, Lumelsky N, et al. Dopamine neurons derived from embryonic stem cells function in an animal model of Parkinson's disease. *Nature.* 2002;418(6893):50–6.
207. Kawasaki H, Mizuseki K, Nishikawa S, Kaneko S, Kuwana Y, Nakanishi S, et al. Induction of midbrain dopaminergic neurons from ES cells by stromal cell-derived inducing activity. *Neuron.* October 2000;28:31–40.
208. Morizane A, Takahashi J, Takagi Y, Sasai Y, Hashimoto N. Optimal conditions for in vivo induction of dopaminergic neurons from embryonic stem cells through

stromal cell-inducing activity. *J Neurosci Res.* September 15, 2002;69(6):934–9.
209. Draper JS, Smith K, Gokhale P, Moore HD, Maltby E, Johnson J, et al. Recurrent gain of chromosomes 17q and 12 in cultured human embryonic stem cells. *Nat Biotechnology.* 2004;22(1):53–4.
210. Longo L, Bygrave A, Grosveld F, Pandolfi PP. The chromosome make-up of mouse embryonic stem cells is predictive of somatic and germ cell chimaerism. *Transgenic Res.* September 1997;6(5):321–8.
211. Blondheim N, Levy Y, Ben-Zur T, Burshtein A, Cherlow T, Kan I, et al. Human mesenchymal stem cells express neural genes, suggesting a neural predisposition. *Stem Cells Dev.* April 2006;15(2):141–64.
212. Kucia M, Zhang YP, Reca R, Wysoczynski M, Machalinski B, Majka M, et al. Cells enriched in markers of neural tissue-committed stem cells reside in the bone marrow and are mobilized into the peripheral blood following stroke. *Leukemia.* 2005;20(1):18–28.
213. Jiang Y, Henderson D, Blackstad M, Chen A, Miller RF, Verfaillie CM. Neuroectodermal differentiation from mouse multipotent adult progenitor cells. *Proc Natl Acad Sci USA.* September 302003;100 Suppl 1:11854–60.
214. Fu YS, Cheng YC, Lin MY, Cheng H, Chu PM, Chou SC, et al. Conversion of human umbilical cord mesenchymal stem cells in Wharton's jelly to dopaminergic neurons in vitro: potential therapeutic application for Parkinsonism. *Stem Cells.* January 2006;24(1):115–24.
215. Thompson L, Barraud P, Andersson E, Kirik D, Bjorklund A. Identification of dopaminergic neurons of nigral and ventral tegmental area subtypes in grafts of fetal ventral mesencephalon based on cell morphology, protein expression, and efferent projections. *J Neurosci.* July 6, 2005;25(27):6467–77.
216. Kordower JH, Freeman TB, Snow BJ, Vingerhoets FJ, Mufson EJ, Sanberg PR, et al. Neuropathological evidence of graft survival and striatal reinnervation after the transplantation of fetal mesencephalic tissue in a patient with Parkinson's disease. *N Engl J Med.* April 27, 1995;332(17):1118–24.
217. Clarkson ED, Freed CR. Development of fetal neural transplantation as a treatment for Parkinson's disease. *Life Sci.* October 29, 1999;65(23):2427–37.
218. Correia AS, Anisimov SV, Li JY, Brundin P. Stem cell-based therapy for Parkinson's disease. *Ann Med.* 2005;37(7):487–98.
219. Freed CR, Greene PE, Breeze RE, Tsai WY, DuMouchel W, Kao R, et al. Transplantation of embryonic dopamine neurons for severe Parkinson's disease. *N Engl J Med.* March 8, 2001;344(10):710–9.
220. Olanow CW, Goetz C, Kordower JH, Stoessl AJ, Sossi V, Brin M, et al. A double-blind controlled trail of bilateral fetal nigral transplantation in Parkinson's disease. *Ann Neurol.* August 2003;54(3):403–14.
221. Song Z-M, Undie AS, Koh PO, Fang YY, Zhang L, Dracheva S, et al. D1 dopamine receptor regulation of microtubule-associated protein-2 phosphorylation in developing cerebral cortical neurons. *J Neurosci.* July 15, 2002;22(14):6092–105.
222. Hagell P, Piccini P, Bjorklund A, Brundin P, Rehncrona S, Widner H, et al. Dyskinesias following neural transplantation in Parkinson's disease. *Nat Neurosci.* July 2002;5(7):627–8.
223. Piccini P, Pavese N, Hagell P, Reimer J, Bjorklund A, Oertel WH, et al. Factors affecting the clinical outcome after neural transplantation in Parkinson's disease. *Brain.* December 2005;128(Pt 12):2977–86.
224. Ma N, Stamm C, Kaminski A, Li W, Kleine HD, Muller-Hilke B, et al. Human cord blood cells induce angiogenesis following myocardial infarction in NOD/scid-mice. *Cardiovasc Res.* April 1, 2005;66(1):45–54.
225. Zhao LR, Duan WM, Reyes M, Verfaillie CM, Low WC. Immunohistochemical identification of multipotent adult progenitor cells from human bone marrow after transplantation into the rat brain. *Brain Res Brain Res Protoc.* March 2003;11(1):38–45.
226. Buhnemann C, Scholz A, Bernreuther C, Malik CY, Braun H, Schachner M, et al. Neuronal differentiation of transplanted embryonic stem cell-derived precursors in stroke lesions of adult rats. *Brain.* December 2006;129(pt12):3238–48.
227. Takagi Y, Nishimura M, Morizane A, Takahashi J, Nozaki K, Hayashi J, et al. Survival and differentiation of neural progenitor cells derived from embryonic stem cells and transplanted into ischemic brain. *J Neurosurg.* August 2005;103(2):304–10.
228. Wei L, Cui L, Snider BJ, Rivkin M, Yu SS, Lee CS, et al. Transplantation of embryonic stem cells overexpressing Bcl-2 promotes functional recovery after transient cerebral ischemia. *Neurobiol Dis.* June–July 2005;19(1–2):183–93.
229. Goolsby J, Marty MC, Heletz D, Chiappelli J, Tashko G, Yarnell D, et al. Hematopoietic progenitors express neural genes. *Proc Natl Acad Sci USA.* December 9, 2003;100(25):14926–31.
230. Habich A, Jurga M, Markiewicz I, Lukomska B, Bany-Laszewicz U, Domanska-Janik K. Early appearance of stem/progenitor cells with neural-like characteristics in human cord blood mononuclear fraction cultured in vitro. *Exp Hematol.* July 2006;34(7):914–25.
231. Munoz-Elias G, Woodbury D, Black IB. Marrow stromal cells, mitosis, and neuronal differentiation: stem cell and precursor functions. *Stem Cells.* 2003;21(4):437–48.
232. Ortiz-Gonzalez XR, Keene CD, Verfaillie CM, Low WC. Neural induction of adult bone marrow and umbilical cord stem cells. *Curr Neurovasc res.* July 2004;1(3):207–13.
233. Padovan CS, Jahn K, Birnbaum T, Reich P, Sostak P, Strupp M, et al. Expression of neuronal markers in differentiated marrow stromal cells and CD133+ stem-like cells. *Cell Transplant.* 2003;12(8):839–48.
234. Woodbury D, Schwarz EJ, Prockop DJ, Black IB. Adult rat and human bone marrow stromal cells differentiate into neurons. *J Neurosci Res.* August 15, 2000;61(4): 364–70.
235. Chen J, Sanberg PR, Li Y, Wang L, Lu M, Willing AE, et al. Intravenous administration of human umbilical cord blood reduces behavioral deficits after stroke in rats. *Stroke.* November 2001;32(11):2682–8.
236. Chen SL, Fang WW, Ye F, Liu YH, Qian J, Shan SJ, et al. Effect on left ventricular function of intracoronary transplantation of autologous bone marrow mesenchymal stem cell in patients with acute myocardial infarction. *Am J Cardiol.* July 1, 2004;94(1):92–5.
237. Horita Y, Honmou O, Harada K, Houkin K, Hamada H, Kocsis JD. Intravenous administration of glial cell line-derived neurotrophic factor gene-modified human mesenchymal stem cells protects against injury in a

cerebral ischemia model in the adult rat. *J Neurosci Res.* September 22 2006;84(7):1495–504.
238. Kurozumi K, Nakamura K, Tamiya T, Kawano Y, Ishii K, Kobune M, et al. Mesenchymal stem cells that produce neurotrophic factors reduce ischemic damage in the rat middle cerebral artery occlusion model. *Mol Ther.* January 2005;11(1):96–104.
239. Schabitz WR, Berger C, Kollmar R, Seitz M, Tanay E, Kiessling M, et al. Effect of brain-derived neurotrophic factor treatment and forced arm use on functional motor recovery after small cortical ischemia. *Stroke.* April 2004;35(4):992–7.
240. Schabitz WR, Schwab S, Spranger M, Hacke W. Intraventricular brain-derived neurotrophic factor reduces infarct size after focal cerebral ischemia in rats. *J Cereb Blood Flow Metab.* May 1997;17(5):500–6.
241. Zhang WR, Hayashi T, Iwai M, Nagano I, Sato K, Manabe Y, et al. Time dependent amelioration against ischemic brain damage by glial cell line-derived neurotrophic factor after transient middle cerebral artery occlusion in rat. *Brain Res.* June 8, 2001;903(1–2):253–6.
242. Nomura T, Honmou O, Harada K, Houkin K, Hamada H, Kocsis JD. I.V. infusion of brain-derived neurotrophic factor gene-modified human mesenchymal stem cells protects against injury in a cerebral ischemia model in adult rat. *Neuroscience.* 2005;136(1):161–9.
243. Kondziolka D, Wechsler L, Goldstein S, Meltzer C, Thulborn KR, Gebel J, et al. Transplantation of cultured human neuronal cells for patients with stroke. *Neurology.* August 22, 2000;55(4):565–9.

10

Composite Tissue Transplantation: A Stage Between Surgical Reconstruction and Cloning

Earl R. Owen and Nadey S. Hakim

There is no doubt the entire brief and brilliant history of transplantation is about a temporary, far from ideal, and only partially successful solution to the desperate attempt of our profession to keep people alive and functioning. With the present advances in nanosurgery, miniscopes, cloning, stem cell culturing and placement, laser solder bonding, ultrasonics, chemogenomics, and microrobotics involving physical and chemical manipulations of even single cell components, seasoned transplantation researchers in the most advanced laboratories are looking for better therapy than transplants to replace worn out, diseased, or failing tissues. These new methods, now being developed, will take over from surgeons having to perform allografts, which still require immunosuppression of the body's incredibly evolved, individually personalized immunological recognition system.

The first Composite Tissue Allograft (CTA) was magnificently unsuccessful! It is, however, suitably emblazoned into the "literature", particularly as a color feature and transplantation icon as there are approximately 29 beautiful paintings since the 1600s, several of which are in the Vatican, of the event that made Saints out of Doctor's Damian and Cosmos. In the 4th century AD, they are reported to have transplanted the leg of a dead black man to replace that of a white amputee, despite the obvious lack of immunosuppressives at the time. For such an outrageous attempt, even by a surgeon, to "play God", these worthy experimental surgeons were, of course, tried, condemned, and crucified by their conservative colleagues at that time.

The second lower limb CTA was also a magnificent failure. Alexis Carrel from Lyon, France,[1] received the Nobel Prize for Medicine in 1912. Carrel used his earlier researched vessel anastomotic technique,[2] together with Dr Guthrie from USA to actually "swap" (or double allograft) the left hind legs of a black and white pair of greyhound dogs in an initially surgically successful experiment.[3] In the limited time they survived, these canine CTAs were sketched and the illustration of the standing dogs appeared in the New York newspapers at the time.

The first modern attempt at a genuinely specific human limb or hand allograft[4] was an inevitable failure. In Ecuador in 1964, ignoring any need for early immunosuppression and based on a mistake of family relationship between the dead donor and live hand amputee, this allograft failed after the surgery despite the recipient being later airlifted to a Florida hospital for Imuran and steroid therapy too late to be useful.

The frontier of CTA was considered to have been crossed, in a blaze of publicity, on September 23, 1998, in Lyon, France, when our team of international surgeons and specialists performed a terminal forearm and hand allograft.[5] The donor was a French road traffic accident victim and the recipient a New Zealand-born man who had lost his dominant right hand in an accident while he was in jail some 14 years previously. It had been an objective of at least two of the surgeons to aim their lifetime research toward CTAs. For the past 31 years, they had been accumulating microsurgical and immunological drug expertise and techniques with their unit's laboratory research programs as well as their department's clinical experiences during the development of both transplantation and microsurgery.

It is pertinent to consider how many scientific innovations had to merge in order that the daunting Frontier of Composite Tissue Allografts (CTAs) be crossed.

Medical innovation tends to occur almost simultaneously in different parts of the world. Thus, it was in the 1950s that alert surgical minds became enthralled with the idea of operating on smaller and smaller parts of the body, which led to microsurgery. Simultaneously intelligent surgeons with increasing research opportunities started to attempt to reconstruct or replace parts of the body beginning with organs that were in terminal failure. The surgical world from then on saw the fields of microsurgery and transplantation merge. It was on the east coast of America that Julius Jacobson and Anasto Suarez defined the word and performed the earliest practice of microvascular surgery by consistently anastomosing arteries of 1 mm diameter.[6] At the same time, Dr Sun Lee of Korea was experimenting on the west coast with similar microvascular techniques not only to join small vessels but also to perform organ transplants in rodents using his amazing surgical skills in research, although his medical degrees never allowed him to practice in the United States.[7] Sun Lee advanced the knowledge and scope of transplantation and immunology by technically describing and carrying out transplantations of the kidney, liver, spleen, stomach, heart, heart and lung, uterus, ovary, intestines, and even the pancreas in his years of surgical rodent research.[8] He proved this could be done cheaper and faster and with more certainty across larger series than those experiments which were also being attempted all around the world in larger animals such as rabbits, dogs, and pigs.

The early history of successful kidney transplantation occurred during this 1950s intellectual awakening of medicos and Murray's outstandingly successful kidney transplantations[9] using identical twins as donors from 1954 onwards in itself spurred the already exciting development of immunology.

A definition for CTA is simply the simultaneous allotransplantation of multiple heterogeneous livable nonorgan bodily tissues. It must, by definition, include the supplying of a functioning blood supply, and preferably a nerve supply, but skin does not necessarily need to be included in the CTA to have the composite tissues satisfy the definition.

The First Successful Hand Transplant (CTA)

The recipient of the first successful human hand CTA had sought a possible hand transplant in several countries and joined a group of similar one- and two-handed amputees in Australia hoping for transplants who were otherwise fit and healthy throughout 1997. Up until September 1998, they had been tutored by one of us in Sydney, Australia, on all elements of the possible approaching procedure.

Their extremities were color photographed, measured, X-rayed, angiograms were taken and their forearm muscles, tendons, and nerves carefully examined, tested, and well mapped. They were commenced on forearm muscle strengthening exercises and their motives, states of mind, determination, flexibility, personality strength, sanguinity, and absence of family psychiatric history evaluated by psychiatric and psychological specialists.

Their complete medical history and routine pre-transplantation blood and serum biology were assessed. Apart from the lecture discussions these potential recipients were given homework of all the relevant review articles and books on transplantation to enlighten them thoroughly on the "pros and cons" of what they were about to undertake.[10] Their legal position as regards to possible complications, and their legal agreements to actually give their full permission and co-operation to follow the proposed protocols were drawn up and they gave their signed agreements. This included that they set up a system for the early months of post-operation care, when they would need to be able to contact their treating doctors in any emergency.

The teams so far performing hand and face CTAs have had healthy recipients, who are fit and disease free, highly motivated, and co-operative. Being quite healthy, they differ from the usual debilitated and infirm allograft organ recipient. They have agreed that they will fully co-operate with their physicians and therapists to give themselves and their team the best chance for the allograft to succeed. They realize how important it is to stay closely in touch with their treating team members with regular follow-ups.

By June 1998, the five most appropriate amputees, four men and one woman, were adjudged ready to not only be knowledgeable and eager candidates for this possibly physically and personality disturbing ordeal, but also be ready-to-board an aircraft to fly to Europe at the receipt of a phone call signifying that a suitably compatible donor was available.

The international team, four already in France, two in Australia, and one each from Italy and England met by arrangement in Lyon and awaited an appropriate donor. While waiting they rehearsed the operation procedures with the various already organ allograft-experienced physicians, nurses, therapists, operating room staff, and administrators. Prior to this alignment of experienced expert talent, the permissions required to actually plan and carry out this procedure had been sought, explained, and eventually approved by all the authorities involved. This actually involved people from the highest authorities in the French Parliament through National, Civil, State, local Government, University, and Hospital managements and even including the obtaining of the approval of the French Patient's Protection Association.

We were privileged to have had the cooperation of the France-wide organization of the French Ministry of Health's Etablissement Frances des Greffes, wherein the well-trained and smoothly functioning seven sectional teams of doctors and nurses are alerted to all France's possible organ/tissue donors. This network (which also connects to the Eurotransplant system) keeps the thorough computerized details of the potential donors online and matches them with appropriate recipient waiting lists. It not only swiftly and efficiently notifies the awaiting transplant teams who harvest the donor materials, but also delicately and compassionately approaches and comforts and supports the donor's relatives at the point of donation.

Previously in Australia, discussions for a hand transplantation from a dead man to a living man had been arranged, debated, and approved by the most senior Australian representatives of all the world's major religions.

Over the past few years, in individual countries as well as international gatherings of transplantation experts, the feelings invoked by the concept of hand and other CTAs had swung around to show less opposition and finally definite statements that the "time was now ripe".[11] Most of the debates were over the obvious fact that a hand or face transplant was not a life-saving one but rather a "quality of life" enabling and effecting procedure. The other contentious hurdle was the argument that the powerful drugs to prevent rejection had very serious side effects such as diabetes induction, or the increased susceptibility to infection and cancer, and even perhaps other life-threatening conditions, and would possibly need to be taken for the rest of the recipient's life.

It is often thought that there must be a big difference between CTAs and the now more familiar and regular "solid" organ allografts. But, are the solid organ allografts actually basically only the one tissue? With very few exceptions all the cells of all tissues have both a blood supply and have or are within close range of a nerve supply. A "solid" organ such as a liver has kilometers of its three main tubular structures, arteries, veins, and ducts, as well as nerves and connective tissues and a remarkable variety of differing sheets of specialized liver cells carrying out unique manufacturing, reprocessing, and excretory functions. The exploration of the microanatomy, physiology, and biochemistry of the amazing variety of liver cells is far from complete, as is the knowledge of its recuperative powers, yet the success of liver allografts with all its many tissues was the basis for our drug regime for our CTAs.

Before we decided on the actual date to carry out the preparations for this, our first single-hand allograft, we were encouraged that a CTA's rejection of the hand with its basically untried human-skin-grafted component could be controlled by our selected cocktail of immunosuppressive drugs by several earlier groups' successes. Giumberteau and Baudet's team had successfully allografted a digital muscle flexion system for the hand in 1989,[12] and Hoffman and Kirschner had successfully begun allografting knee joints[13] and the femoral diaphysis[14] following the lead of Chiron's adventurous operative technique.[15]

Early attempts to transplant skin across even minor histocompatibility barriers, first, within the same animal species by Medawar, had proven how difficult it could be.[16] In the following 50 years of immunology research when skin transplants and allografts had been attempted, it was proven that skin tissue rejection was the most difficult rejection to control. We knew that this could be our major hurdle. The team leader had to deal with the other members of the international team who were keen to start our CTA series (we had permission in mid-1998 to go ahead with the first five cases in France), with a bilateral amputee, to refute the possible objections that to do just a one-handed allograft might be considered an unnecessary procedure and that a single-handed man could still carry out a productive and worthwhile occupation. The team leader argued that the area of skin on two hands might prove to be too much skin area for the chosen drugs regime to protect, and so there was a much greater chance for success if only one hand with its already considerable surface area of skin was attempted. As we had in our overall team a leading French dermatologist with transplantation experience and the use of an antirejection drug ointment available to bolster skin rejection suppression if necessary, we felt confident to progress to obtain an appropriate donor. This took longer to arrange than we had anticipated despite the fact that in France, all citizens who die are eligible in French law to be donors of organs or tissues unless they have specifically written in to the Department of Health to refuse such permission.

Whereas an organ allograft is not seen by the recipient, a hand or face allograft is seen as soon as the patient awakens from the operation's anesthetic. So not only the donor's blood type and, preferentially, tissue types should match, but so should the skin color, texture, and hair distribution as well as the actual size and shape of the donor parts.

Surgical Technique

Human ingenuity encompassed the trephining of skulls to release cerebral hematomas some 5000 years ago in Egypt, as testified by the specimens viewable in Medical Museums today. The late 1950s, the 1960s, and early 1970s were exciting times for experimental surgeons worldwide and the early enthusiasts from all over the world corresponded and formed meetings to start the International Microsurgical Society and the Transplantation Society, both in 1967, which saw the coming together of extraordinary medical and scientific minds. So in the past 50 years skillful surgeons have replanted, reconstructed, and repositioned completely severed human bones, tendons, nerves, muscles, intestines, skin, tongue, limbs, joints, hands, digits, scalps, ears, larynxes, and penises, requiring delicate anastomozing techniques.

CTA recipients are subjected to all routine pre-transplant investigations with the addition of the suitable special tests to specifically define the available functional anatomy and physiology and thus the perceived capacity to activate the allograft post-operatively. The detailed surgery of those first successful single and double forearm and hand allografts has been well described by the members of the French/Australian and the Austrian, American, and Chinese teams.[17]

The actual surgical procedure in the September 1998 operation was to first carefully dissect and mark the donor's end tissues, whose blood vessels had previously been perfused with cold University of Wisconsin's solution at harvesting. The lower forearm donor bones were osteotomized at the chosen lengths to match the lengths to the recipient's desired both arms of equal natural length. After application of a tourniquet, the donor's and recipient's bones were fixed together with metal plates and 4.5 mm screws to stabilize all further surgery. The radial and ulnar arteries and then the cephalic and the largest veins were available and were carefully anastomosed with 8/0 microsutures. The previously applied tourniquet was released and the graft reperfused with recipient's blood. This took slightly longer than we expected, as the donor tissues had been cold preserved for 12 h, so we warm wet wrapped the area once it was in normal color and left it to warm up while we took a 20-min break. After a celebratory hot drink, we rescrubbed and gowned and returned to carefully suture the tendons and muscles in layers and microsurgically the ulnar and median nerves. This was done 20 and 21 cm, respectively, proximal to the wrist skin crease, to take advantage of the shorter healthy remaining recipient's and the freely excessive amount of donor's nerves. To encourage strong bone union, we harvested iliac crest autologous cancellous bone chips and spread them around the osteosynthesis sites. The recipient's skin was sutured to the generously shaped donor skin, even including a wedge of split skin graft from the recipient's right thigh, as we had learned from 28 years of arm replantations around the distal forearm to allow space for possible initial swelling or compartment syndrome. We left two Penrose drains in site, the wrist slightly extended, the elbow flexed 45°, and the distal limb gently bandaged, splint supported, and elevated.

Obviously more donor tissue than would be required was harvested in each case as the actual condition of the available viable and actionable tissue in the recipient's limb stumps was never precisely known until seen at operative dissection. In over 28 cases of the so-called "hand allografts" now surviving it would appear that longer lengths of donor nerve tissue than were originally planned in these cases was routinely used and we believe this does give a better eventual functional result, as recipient's nerve tissue has usually suffered functionally regressive partial degradement.

When the patient awoke and immediately saw his hand he exclaimed, "I have my hand back!", but it was not until the local anesthetic to his right axilla had worn off and he tried out gentle flexion of the fingers that he was convinced. Physiotherapy for two sessions a day started only 10 h after the surgery and rehabilitation by controlled motion passive- and active-supervised exercises were continued for 3 months. Psychological support daily was less intensive after 3 weeks had passed. Skin biopsies were taken once a week together with a program of close observation in case it might be needed more frequently, should commencement of rejection be suspected. No surgical complications occurred in this case, who was correctly supervised in Lyon for the first 3 post-operative months. He then went off, by himself, quite contrarily to the pre-operatively psychological assessments by experts both in Australia and in France and went his own way. He would not keep regular follow-up sessions, could only be contacted by mobile phone, and that too occasionally. He learned about the onset of mild rejection by observing his mild pink skin rash and treated himself by increasing his daily dose of prednisone for 1 or 2 days until the rash subsided. At the occasional times when one of us could examine him, we were surprised how rapidly the patient's nails and his ulnar and median nerves grew. These were checked first by Tinel's sign, and then with delicate nerve conduction studies as the feeling grew down to his fingertips in the first 12 months. At 2 years post-operation he was found touring the United States where he deliberately then ceased his immunosuppressives, and then demanded that the team amputate the slowly rejecting part. When this was carried out 5 months later on the still very healthy patient some 28 months post-operation, and the transplanted tissues were then examined, only the skin was actually proved to be rejecting. All this team's later double hand allographs were far more co-operative and have done very well.[18] They use their hands and fingers well at daily tasks and at work and report that their lives have been transformed back to being normal.

One of the most intriguing understandings that has come out of the hand transplantation program is the insight science that has gained into the way the brain can adapt to changing circumstances. That there really is brain area plasticity was shown in progressive fMRIs from pre-operative to post-operative observations that peripheral input can modify cortical hand representational organization in both sensory and motor regions. Relatively blank areas of cortex in the previously amputated patient's brain regained activity as the allografted hands regained activity when seen as early as 6 months post-operatively and continued to be more activated as the movements and feelings matured.[19]

Immunology

The choice of immunosuppression in our hand allograft program was not an easy one. The team discussed many possibilities and rejected pre-operative complete irradiation of the recipients bone marrow, but settled for commencing on antilymphocyte antibody just prior to the attachment of the CTA and then utilizing what we called a "cocktail" of well-proven drugs that sustained liver allografts. Several following CTAs in the United States, Austria, and China also adopted this "starting with a clean plate" (having cleared out the recipient's lymphocytes) approach which had been well tried in many organ allograft programs worldwide.

That and the current immunosuppressive protocol includes loading doses of Thymoglobulin® (polyclonal antibodies) 1.25 mg/kg/d for the first 10 days, and then three main drugs after loading doses were continued with

- Tacrolimus (FK506)0.2 mg/kg/day keeping blood levels between 15 and 20 μgm/kg/day in the first month;
- Mycophenolate mofetil 2/g/day;
- Prednisone 250 mg on day 1, 1 mg/kg for 10 days, then tapered down to 20 mg daily, reduced to 15 mg/day at 6 months; and
- wide-spectrum antibiotics for the first 10 days.

Should early serum sickness occur, monoclonal antibodies can be administered in short courses. In some patients transient hyperglycemia occurred which was treated initially with insulin I.V.I. for a short time.

We somewhat suspect that a mechanism that protects these allografts from chimerism and graft versus host disease and perhaps even chronic rejection is involved. To that end current papers accepted for publications of our own and others' research works with co-allografting vascularized lengths of donor femurs with rat lower limb allografts is encouraging as we have found that larger amounts of transplanted donor bone marrow lessen the need in the rat model for immunosuppressants. Bone marrow transplantation in order to create a chimerism has been a feature of our more recent allografts and those of other authors.

Although it is well known that major histocompatibility (MHA) antigens should ideally be matched in any allograft donor/recipient pair our first four hand allografts cases, one single, and three double hand cases (totaling seven allografted hands) did not have even the luxury of one of the major MHA matches. Both serologic and molecular genetic testing of matching MHAs is available and so the CTA teams are hopeful of the sort of help with allograft outcome that has been shown to occur when there is matching for HLA-A, for -B and for -DR in kidney organ allografts will occur in future CTAs. We recognize that 1% of the general population, without having had a blood transfusion, can have preformed antibodies that could react to alloantigens,[20] and of course check both ABO compatibility and check for any history of prior immunological stimulation, but neither have nor had expected any hyperacute rejection episodes on our regime.

We recognize that a chronic rejection process may develop as it can in nearly all solid organ allografts, with the usual vasculopathy described early on as a transplant arteriosclerosis.[21]

We have not yet had biopsy evidence of any such chronic rejection so far but as we necessarily allograft active blood-generating donor bone marrow in these cases we are aware it has been shown to continue producing blood cells.[22]

The best descriptions so far in the literature on the normal, the allografted, and the allograft-rejecting skin's three cellular layers have been clearly outlined in detail and illustrated by our Dermatologist Jean Kanitakis in Lyon.[23] There are no really detailed reports available on other CTAs such as the larynx and the knee joint; however, biopsies when they are reported show the same open-vascular infiltrate of mostly T-cell lymphocytes that we have all been familiar with since the earliest skin allografts in mice more than 50 years ago.

In some hand-allografted patients early skin rejection occurs, seen as a distinct maculo-papular rash of pink lesions. They have a mild, nonitchy inflammatory response, and biopsies show a peri-vascular and dermal mononuclear heavily staining recipient cell infiltration. This rash is easily reversed by increasing the oral steroids and applying topical immunosuppressive ointment. Maintenance doses were given to keep tacrolimus blood levels between 5 and 10 μg/ml, with Solupred® at 5 mgm/d and mycopherolate mofetil at 2 g/d.

The phenomenon of the pink rash acts as a warning system that the immunosuppression regime is not optimum. It was first noted by the first single-hand allograft recipient, who began to use the appearance of pink spots as a means to judge his own treatment. He was able to conserve his drug supply by voluntarily lessening his doses in the second year post-operation, until the rash appeared. He would then adjust the doses upward and again stabilize before gradually dropping the dosages again. This, of course, was at the stage where he was staying away from his medical team for long periods, as he was by no means an ideal patient. It may be recalled that after 16 months with his allograft, one of us had to appear on worldwide television to appeal to him, wherever he was, to come back to any one of us in any of our countries for his delayed follow up and to obtain more drugs. Owing to his nonconformity, this patient allowed skin rejection to progress so that one of us had no choice but to amputate at 28 months. The histopathological examination of the allografted terminal forearm and hand was remarkable as the only microscopic signs of rejection were those of the skin.[24] The patient had no other body signs or symptoms and was otherwise fit after this amputation.

The Face Allograft

The 2006 face allograft in Amiens, France, involved full thickness facial soft tissue fine reconstruction of a woman's face over dry bone in a large oval defect measuring 16 × 15 cm^2 from just beneath her orbicularis oculus muscles and above the nose to below the chin and jaw. This flap of tissue between skin and mouth mucosa consisted of tendons, muscles, fat, motor and sensory nerves, and vessels. The deceased donor tissue including the nose of similar skin color and shape to that of the recipient provided a fully functioning face and also return to a normal life for the delighted recipient.

Some years ago a Hollywood film called *Face Off* brought to the general public a "hot" controversy that had been previously challenging Transplantation Units worldwide. In the film the faces of a "bad guy" and a "good guy" who was chasing him were first cross-allografted ("swapped"), and then "swapped" back again at the film's end. This would have given the public the idea that such operations were quite feasible and technically easy, with no mention of immunosuppression, but such intricate surgery is far from simple.

The deformed or damaged face has been the subject of many clever techniques of repair, and plastic surgery history abounds with complex-staged procedures to reconstruct parts of faces. The success of the first 28 hand allografts showed that large areas of skin could be allografted possibly allowing a CTA for those whose facial damage could not be functionally corrected by even the most experienced Reconstructive Plastic Surgery teams.

Our international team considered in 1999 that, following our and the world's experience with CTAs, we would consider a face allograft if a suitable case occurred and came to our attention, and such a case fell within the group of tissues we already had obtained permission to reconstruct by CTAs. The history of reconstructions of small parts of the face goes back thousands of years and includes the use of tube pedicle skin transfer almost 500 years ago by the Italian Gasparo Dagliacozzi (1557–1599). We remember the heroic efforts of plastic surgeons to restore skin cover and shape to the severely burned and hideously disfigured faces of those pilots in World War II, who survived their cabin fires, as the work of Sir Archibald McIndoe at East Grinstead Hospital, West Sussex in England, was detailed in films and reports.[25]

We considered the 37 published cases of replantation of the scalp that we found in the literature of our Microsurgical colleagues since the first report of successful replacement of an avulsed scalp.[26] This had been followed by increasing numbers of reports of scalp replants, which included as well as scalp such differing tissues as with a complete ear cartilage in 1978,[27] and other "skin plus" tissues in 1983 such as the penis, nose, ear, and scalp.[28]

Applications to actually perform clinical face transplants had been submitted to two other French (2004) and US (2006) authorities and had received approval before the case of the 38-year-old woman with severe facial tissue ablation was referred to the Facio-Maxillary Surgery Department in Amiens, France, in May, 2005.

The controversies about a possible "Facial Transplant" had been extensively discussed by transplantation units for years and had led to ethical committees of some countries and long-established surgical colleges investigating and issuing informed reports on the subject in the early 2000s.[29,30]

In this case, a large family dog had found his mistress in a deep sleep and savaged her face. The almost oval bite, measuring 15 × 16 cm^2 from just below the lower eyelids to below the jaw encompassing all tissue, including the nose, down to bone and teeth, was totally unsuitable for replantation when discovered. The horrific gap, unequally present on both sides of the midline, would, untreated, inevitably fibrose and retract and was treated with wet dressings. After confirming the French authorities' agreement to go ahead, the search for a suitable donor was notified to the Etablissement Frances des Greffes and the Lyon and Amiens surgeons began detailing and practicing the procedures necessary to provide a sustainable and acceptable CTA. The search for the right donor was agonizingly long for both the patient and the readied operative teams, as the retraction of the oval-shaped defect's edges constricted to such an extent that the apparent gap lessened considerably as the upper and lower teeth became almost tightly pressed together, when feeding by mouth and talking became a great difficulty.

It took almost 7 months for a suitably compatible donor to be discovered and the operation commenced on November 27, 2005, in Professor Bernard Devauchelle's Maxillo Facial Surgery Department by the team jointly led by him and Professor Jean-Michel Dubernard. The intricate surgery required motor facial and sensory trigeminal nerve branch anastomoses and muscle and tendon and nasal reconstruction, well-practiced facial vascular anastomoses, and gentle plastic surgical skin alignment together with the bold immunosuppressive regime. The outstanding result is now apparent in the almost completely functioning and esthetically delightful result 2 years later.

The immunosuppressive drug combination, now well tried in hand CTAs was followed but in the 10 days after the operation two separate injections of donor bone marrow hemopoietic cells were administered, even though this bold attempt to invoke a micro-chimerism had only been tried experimentally. This triumph of surgical and immunosuppressive virtuosity demonstrates how co-operation among experienced specialists can achieve what may have seemed impossible only a short time before.

Laryngeal Transplantation

The human larynx has evolved as an extraordinarily complex of cartilages, mostly covered with mucosa, joints, muscles, and ligaments and an efficient large nerve and vascular supply. Everyone can remember at least one episode of laryngeal discomfort, such as when coughing, or a feeling of choking, or of having a sore throat and not speaking with one's normal voice. Just understanding how the anatomy and physiology of the larynx work is extremely difficult even for those who have studied medicine. The internal muscles shorten, lengthen, or relax the vocal cords, so we can speak and sing, whereas the upper muscles can raise and lower the Epiglottis and direct food posteriorly to the esophagus to allow the beginning of swallowing, or else allow air from both the mouth and the nasal passages into the trachea and on into the lungs, usually without mixing up these two essential functions.

Such a complex dual purpose essential mechanical instrument mostly works automatically, so when it misfires from just one sectional defect the physician is usually quickly consulted. If a disease such as a laryngeal cancer has progressed so that laryngeal excision is required, it is comforting to know that extensive research on laryngeal allografting has occurred since 1966,[31,32,33] and a partial CTA was surgically performed in 1969,[34] and a successful complete laryngeal CTA in 1970.[35] As the first was mainly an attempt to remove cancerous mucosa and graft in some vascularized mucosal tissue, it was at first seen to have survived on the immunosuppressive regime. Unfortunately cancerous tissue, presumably from the cartilaginous bed, did overwhelm the mucosa and the patient died 8 months later. It is presumed that the higher dosed, less-sophisticated immunosuppression then used might have encouraged the conditions to allow freer tumor cell multiplication in the drugs causing an absence of any body cell defense mechanism. The disappointment of this case dampened down enthusiasm for such allografts. There is no man-made substitute yet for the quite bewilderingly intricate complex that is the human larynx, capable of such extraordinary control of the vocal cords, swallowing, and diameter of the shared passages for air and food, but research continued.

The first successful laryngeal CTA occurred 30 years later when in 1998 a very dedicated group of Cleveland Clinic throat specialists performed a CTA with a large fully matched complex of the larynx and its pharynx as well as the thyroid and parathyroid glands, and upper five tracheal rings. This also required anastomosis of the upper laryngeal nerves and one recurrent laryngeal nerve with its complex's complete extensive blood supply. A 40-month follow-up biopsy of the trachea was normal. That such a surgical triumph worked and to date is still functioning is most encouraging.

The immunosuppressive regime was similar for that used in the other CTAs, except that cyclosporine rather than tacrolimus was initially used in the basic three drug-sustaining cocktail. Tacrolimus was introduced after a rejection episode began at 15 months post-operation and since then the drugs have been steadily reduced.

This recipient, a no skin, but otherwise very varied composite tissue transplantation, supposedly used his "new" voice 3 days post-operatively, and is now, over 8 years later successfully talking, eating, and breathing within normal limits, within a one octave but quite serviceable vocal range. This operation is, like those hands and face transplantations, excellent examples of CTAs providing near normal quality of life outcomes, which would not have been otherwise conventionally surgically possible.

The success of this extraordinary CTA has been repeated 16 times since. These highly technical procedures require in the one institution a functioning, multidisciplinary, and co-operative team led by strong, confident, and excellent specialist surgeons, immunologists, physicians, and paramedics, all prepared to provide prolonged obsessive care at every step of the lifelong journey of the patient. The way forward in this field was best presented by a review in 2006 by the US group.[36]

Uterine CTAs

In April 2007, the First International Symposium on this subject was held in Gothenburg, Sweden. Since the first technically successful attempt at Uterine CTA was performed[37] in Saudi Arabia in April 2000, much further research has occurred, yet a fully successful human uterine transplantation has not been reported.

That first case proved that a uterus from a living donor, together with its fallopian tubes, could be technically implanted in the recipient after a hysterectomy, and actually later respond to combined estrogen–progesterone hormone treatment causing thickening of the endometrial uterine tissue bed and withdrawal bleeding. The attempt was abandoned requiring a further hysterectomy after 99 days due to massive necrosis of the uterus due, no doubt, to vascular occlusion. The original surgical approach from a living donor precluded the use of its similar length uterine vascular supply, so saphenous vein grafts were employed to the uterine arteries and veins on both sides and the blood shunted to and from the internal iliac arteries of the recipient. The absence of adequate structural support fixing the donor uterus and tubes in place may also have contributed to the vascular occlusion. The immunosuppressive protocol, similar to our CTAs, was quite successful as there was no evidence of rejection in the harvested necrosed uterus.

In the time since then a great deal of subsequent research has rationalized and optimized the donor organ harvesting, from either a living altruistic woman (a technically difficult vascular approach), or a fresh cadaver where a large dissection is required to obtain sufficient length of large blood vessels might prove more appropriate.

The uterine transplantation program must be all inclusive as regards medical ethics, national, and international laws be able to be fully evaluated as regards both donor and recipient selection and follow the proper assessment of the efficiency of the differing drug regimes on these tissues. Then, there are the problems of the effect of immunosuppressive drugs on the development of the offspring-embryo, fetus, and baby, even including the effect of drug dose by breast feeding. The problem of detailing early rejection in the pregnant uterus and some of the drug-related uncertainties has been studied in women who became pregnant while on immunosuppressives for other organ transplants.

As it is such a tragedy when a woman's ability and desire to conceive children is prevented by various uterine abnormalities, the ingenious research protocols in the literature, with those voiced at recent symposiums make it seem inevitable that fully successful uterine/fallopian tubes CTA will soon be performed. There are hundreds of research articles carefully debating the controversies involved in this field, of which several seem the most pertinent and discuss the pressing issues such as operative techniques and dangers to both the women and their offspring due to immunosuppressives, as well as the alternatives to transplantation.[38]

Pregnancy outcomes after immunosuppressive therapy during pregnancy[39] suggested more pre-term deliveries and congenital deformities than the norm, but other studies in experimented animals,[40,41] do not reinforce this conclusion even though some work suggests teratogenic effects on animal offspring due to prednisolone.

Alternatives to CTAs for female sterility of uterine origin now include many cases of successful surrogacy. Researchers have grown uterine and other specialized tissue in rabbits, and using embryonic human stem cells and tissue engineering can now grow most human-specialized organs and other tissues,[42] including uterine endometria.[43]

The moral, ethical, religious, medical, legal, individual country, as well as the administrative, technical, child, and gender issues in this absorbing field all come together as the uterus, so far in human evolution, has been mandatory to civilization. We will hear far more about this highly debatable and essential topic in the future.

Peripheral Nerve Transplantation

Peripheral nerve defects are and have been restored as whole, cable, or fascicular replantations, usually utilizing one or even both sural nerves since 1970s.[44] In 1976, the first vascularized nerve graft was performed by Taylor and Ham in Australia.[45] This early attempt was not immediately repeated until greater numbers of trained microsurgeons came on the scene to perfect fascicular and small vessel anastomoses under the operating microscope. It was found that increasing lengths of gently harvested, nontraumatized sural nerve alone could provide the pathway for the regrowth of a patient's own long peripheral nerves, such as, the median, ulnar, and sciatic where no immunosuppression was required. This was more successful in children where one of us (E.R.O.) used lengths of sural nerve to bridge a 12-cm gap using nerve anastomoses between the sciatic nerve and the main trunks of the lateral popliteal and posterior tibial nerves, with such function that the child's only defect several years later was the feeling to his big and second toe, and he grew up to walk and run normally.

Nonetheless, extensive peripheral nerve defects where using the patient's own nerves is impossible or impractical can require a donor-vascularized nerve.[46] A 10-year study of the results of allotransplants for both upper and lower limb traumas have been studied, primarily in the McKinnen team from St Louis and by our Hand Transplantation Team (pp. 29, 24, 25, 31). Patients can indeed regain almost full sensitivity and function with donor nerves also anastmotized with their supplying arteries up to lengths of 19 cm on the routine three main immunosuppressive drug regime. Positive Tinel's tests are used to plot the down growth of viable nerve tissue and on an average the drugs can be tailed right off in 18 months. That way iatrogenic complications can be avoided.

We have described in our hand CTAs, as has Dr S. McKinnen's work shown for many years, that with some immunosuppressive drugs, particularly Tacrolimus, the advance of nerve tissue and its activity down the grafted nerves occurs faster with the drugs than it does with or without an accompanying blood supply.[47,48,49,50]

The presence of a sustaining blood supply for a nerve graft to survive and duly function is essential. The longer the nerve length required the less likely it is to pick up lengthy and adequate blood supply from the surrounding tissue alone, hence the need for concomitant vascular supply. There are, of course, other factors in peripheral nerve transplantation. Some of the grafts are interpositional rather than terminal, and so the graft's rates of growth may be adequate, but when they reach the distally severed nerve end that tissue will have had no recent nerve stimulation and may have fibrosed and become more difficult to re-innovate.

The preservation of nerves prior to transplantation and the effects of the drugs on the nerve tissue and Schwann cells are becoming increasingly important.[51] While most CTAs and organ transplants require relatively large blood vessels, needed to supply to large amounts of tissues, nerve grafts and transplants use much smaller blood vessels, yet the tissues making up a peripheral nerve are small and tightly packed with their essential capillary blood supply which is so easily obstructed by even slight pressure from surrounding tissue pressures.

It must therefore be emphasized that in any CTA requiring an essential nerve component transplantation, the normal surgical principles of any delicate surgery, particularly those concerning the absence of pressure and the use of gravity drainage (if at all possible), must be even more rigorously observed than is usual.

Tongue Transplantation

Dr Rolf Evers, speaking for the Vienna General Hospital team led by Dr Christian Kermer and Dr Franz Watzinger that carried out the first successful total tongue transplant was happy with the initial result. He was quoted worldwide on television stating that "other organs such as liver and kidneys are complicated, but the tongue is just muscle"; however, we believe it to be a CTA. For it to function as a tongue it must have significant vascular and nerve tissues transplanted with it. The transplant, done in July 2003 following removal of a large carcinoma of the tongue and jaw of a 42-year-old man, showed it to be technically possible. We believe that this brave attempt to assist a stricken patient was not fully successful and have not as yet seen any pathological studies. We respect the deliberations of the Royal College of Surgeons of England who in 2003 issued a Working Party Report suggesting much more research into many issues should go into tongue and face and other potential CTAs, and to date no more tongue transplants have been reported.[52] It would seem that in general terms it would be perhaps counter-productive to contemplate a CTA in a patient with an advancing tumor, as the necessary immunosuppression drugs would only accelerate the growth of secondary tumors.

Penis Transplantation

The technicality of transplanting a donor penis has been well proved by the many penis replantations carried out since the 1970s. One of us (E.R.O.) replanted the completely amputated penis of a nine-year-old boy at the Royal Alexandra Hospital for Children in 1970, which was not published and only briefly mentioned in that Hospital's Annual General Hospital Report in the Research section, at the request of the child's parents. He had been masturbating with a relatively narrow necked milk bottle in the bathroom and slipped and fell, leaving only a 1-cm stump. Brought to the hospital within an hour, and with the experience of having successfully already replanted a 2-year-old boy's completely amputated index finger months before, the operation proceeded as a succession of anastomoses. These were the urethra first and the deep fascia about it of the corpora spongiosa, both deep penile arteries, the two corporal cavernosa's penile tunica fascia, the deep dorsal vein, and the fine dorsal nerves on either side, and the very small dorsal arteries beside, then the large dorsal vein of the penis. Some deep fascia was next and then the skin was joined with interrupted buried sutures of fine microsurgery nylon with ends cut very short, which was left inside. The boy was sedated and gently cool packed for over a week and developed into a very well-behaved boy and man, capable of having quite normal erections. One of us, Jean Michel Dubernard combined with Dr Gelet at The Edouard Herriot Hospital complex in Lyon, France, performed another functioning and normally sensitized replantation, also joining the dorsal nerve of the penis. These replants were not publicized, and were done, as were some other successful replants in China and Taiwan, long before a highly publicized penile replant was completed in the United States.

The recent first penis transplant, a Chinese case,[53] had specialized microsurgery, some immunological support, but had to be reamputated after 3 days. It seems, because it is technically possible and because the CTAs so far have shown that allograft skin can be defended against rejection, that it is only a matter of time before other cases of penile allografts will be completed and announced.

Conclusion

The second successful single-hand CTA is now 8 years on, and our first three double hands allografts at seven, three, and almost 1 year post-operation are functioning very well indeed. Over 28 hand allografts and many other CTAs have now been performed in many countries.

The initial hand CTAs achieved the goals of motor and sensory function equal to or approaching those of properly replanted traumatically injured hands, and certainly superior to that of myoelectrical prostheses. Patient satisfaction and personal delight in having working esthetically normal limbs again with good social integration and work potential justifies the costly labor-intensive procedure. The drug doses, although potentially having debilitating side effects, can be greatly reduced over time and can be well controlled by the astute patient under supervision. When rejection episodes occur, the skin of the donor is the "early warning system" that let the patient know to report back for simple known reversal measures to resume their balanced state. The face CTA in France is presently 26 months post-allograft, with an expressive face, going about her daily life pleased to be a normal woman. The scars are not visible with light make up, and the patient's drugs are already greatly reduced. The first laryngeal CTA is into his 8th year being very satisfied with his extraordinary allograft which functions virtually normally. A partial Hand CTA consisting of half the palmar tissues and all four fingers still in its first post-operative year has been seen to be doing well in China, The Chinese penis allograft is reported to be well satisfied with "his" restored manhood. Unfortunately we believe that all the attempted knee joint CTAs have not survived.

That donated human organs and other body structures, such as tendons, muscles, nerves, and intestine can also join skin in being able to be guarded from rejection is heartening and useful as there is no other way for certain tissue loss replacements to be replaced at this time. There is thus a present need for some well-prepared patients to have CTAs to enable them to have a life worth living. All the arguments against the considerable risks entailed in CTAs have been talked out and written about, and those frontiers have been crossed without loss of life, or worsening of the situations. Experience with years of careful following up of CTAs shows just how useful they are and how grateful are the individual recipients when the protocols are scrupulously carried out.

We do believe that in the most deserving of select cases in a well balanced, otherwise healthy body, the potential benefits of hand and certain other CTAs outweigh the risks of early infection and late possible malignancy, or early onset of diabetes. We have found out that technically and theoretically the donor-to-recipient operation should be, but not always is, easier than the replacement of severed parts to the same body. This is due to the form of injury and the response of peripheral nerves to severance and trauma, which cause a "die back" phenomenon with shrinkage and also tissue swelling that hampers normal nerve conduction on the recipient side.

We believe that face CTAs are the correct form of treatment for a small select group of patients that cannot be otherwise adequately reconstructed by even brilliant conventional plastic surgical departments.

The more we know about cell metabolism, the more we realize how much we do not know. Yet how each cell functions is the key to its health and survival, and therefore our survival. CTAs provide huge collections of living cells to replace dead, diseased, cancerous, or amputated parts of our bodies. Surgery, from the point of view of the single cell, has always been a gross and clumsy procedure. The more we can actually see when we operate, the more precise can be our application of our surgical principles. The Monocular Operating Microscope, originally used by Nylen and Holingren in Sweden[54] in 1921, allowed surgery nearly 90 years ago on the ossicles and the labyrinth of the ear. Later developments led to binocular-operating microscopes with foot, mouth, and other remote controls with brilliant lighting allowing for smaller and smaller precise microsurgery techniques. The advances since in microscopy allow scanning of single living cells and even manipulation within those cells. Science now discovers particles that are smaller than the essential parts of a single atom and is also researching the genetic composition as well as the actual structure of the plethora of human cell components. Biochemists are engineering ways of influencing (turning on or off) the activities of molecules within a cell component and that could be the "surgery" of the future.

Perhaps surgeons will eventually be needed only to repair gross injuries, such as happen in accidents, wars, and catastrophic natural disasters. As the population of this globe increases, those with the available medical facilities and necessary food and water live longer lives than the previous generations.

As future genetic engineered babies grow up without congenital diseases or proclivities, and automatically diagnosed ailing cells are replaced with technologically manufactured individual stem cell derivatives by minimally invasive new methods by remote control, the readers of this book may wonder how long such a cellularly engineered human being's life span might turn out to be.

References

1. Carrel A. La technique operatoire des anastomoses vasculaires et al. transplantation des visceres. *Lyon Med.* 1902;98:859.
2. Carrel A. Results of the Transplantation of blood vessels, organs and limbs. *JAMA.* 1908;51:1662.
3. Carrel A, Guthrie CC. Uniterminal and biterminal venous transplantations. *Surg Gynae and Obst.* 1906;2:266.
4. Gilbert R. Transplant is successful with a cadaver forearm. *Med Trib News.* 1964;5:20.
5. Dubernard JM, Owen E, Herzberg G, Lanzetta M, Martin X, Kapila H, Davahra M, Hakim N. Human hand allograft: report on first six months. *Lancet.* 1999;353: 1315–1320.
6. Jacobson JH 2nd, Suarez E. Microsurgery in anastomoses of small vessels. *Surg Forum; Clin Congr,* Vol. II. American College of Surgeons, Chicago, 1960:243.
7. Fisher B, Lee SH. Microvascular surgical techniques in research with special reference to renal transplantation on the rat. *Surg.* 1965;58:904.
8. Lee SH. Experiences with organ transplantation in the rat (series begun in 1961) IX. Implantation vs Transplantation of the Ovary. *J Res Inst Med Sci, Korea.* 1974;6:112.
9. Murray JE, Merrill JP, Harrison JH. Kidney Transplantation between seven pairs of identical twins. *Ann Surg.* 1958;148:343.
10. Hakim NS. Introduction to Organ Transplantation. Imperial College Press, London; 1997. ISMB 1_ 86094-025-0.
11. Seigler M. Ethical issues in innovative surgery: should we attempt a cadaveric hand transplant in a human. *Transplant Proc.* 1998;30 (6):2779–1782.
12. Guimberteau JC, Baudet J, Panconi B, Boileau L. Human allotransplant of a digital flexion system vascularised on the ulnar pedicle: a preliminary report and one year follow-up of two cases. *Plast Reconstr Surg.* 1992;89: 1135–1147.
13. Hofmann GO, Kirschner MH, Wagner FD, Land W, Bukren V. Allogeneic vascularised grafting of a human knee joint with post-operative immunosuppression. *Arch Orthop Trauma Surg.* 1997;116:125–128.
14. Hoffman GO, Kirschner MH, Wagner FD, Brauns L, Gonschorek O, Buhran V. Allogeneic vascularised transplantation of human femoral diaphyses and total knee joints – first clinical experiences. *Transp Proc.* 1998;30:2754–2761.

15. Chiron P, Columbier JA, Tricoire JL, Puget J, Utheza G, Glock Y, Puel P. A large vascularised allograft of the Femoral Diaphysis in man. *Int Orthop.* 1990;14:26–272.
16. Medawar PB. The Behaviour of skin autografts and skin homografts in rabbits. *J. Anat.* 1944;78:176.
17. Francois CG, Breidenbach WC, Maldonado C, Kaloulidis TP, Hodges A, Dubernard JM, Owen ER, Pei G, Ren X, Barker JH. Hand Transplantation: comparisons and observations on the first four clinical cases. *Microsurgery.* 2000;20:360–371.
18. Petruzzo P, Revillard JP, Kanitakis J, Lanzetta M, Hakim NS, Lefrancol SN, Owen ER, Dubernard JM. First Human Double Hand transplantation: efficacy of a conventional immunosuppressive protocol. *Clin Transplant.* 2003;17:1–6.
19. Giraux P, Sirigu A, Schneider F, Dubernard JM. Functional cortical reorganisation after transplantation of both hands as revealed by fMRI. *Nat Neurosci.* 2001;4:691–692.
20. Scorpik JC, Saloman DR, Howard RJ, Pfaff WW. Evaluation of Antibody Synthesis in Broadly Sensitised Patients. *Transplantation.* 1988; 45:95–100.
21. Billingham ME. Cardiac Transplant Arteriosclerosis. *Transplant Proc.* 1987;19:19–25.
22. Granger DK, Briedenback WC, Pidwell DJ, Jones JW, Baxter-Lowe LA, Kauffman CL. Lack of Donor Hyporesponiveness and Donor Chimerism After Clinical Transplantation of the Hand. *Transplantation.* 2002; 74: 1624–1630.
23. Kanitakis J. Histopathology of Human Composite Tissue Allografts. *Composite Tissue Allografts* Hakim NS, Owen ER, Dubernard JM (eds.). Imperial College Press; 2006.
24. Kanitakis J, Jullien D, Petruzzo P, et al. Clinicopathologic features of graft rejection in the first human hand allograft. *Transplantation.* 2003;76:688–693.
25. Banks AH. McIndoe's Lecture of 1941 on diagnosis and treatment of injuries of the middle third of the face. *British Dent J.* 1996;181 (9):346–347.
26. Case Report. *Plast Reconstr Surg.* March 1969;43(3): 231–4.
27. Nahai F. et al. Replantation of an entire scalp and ear by microvascular anastomoses of only one artery and one vein. *Br J Plast Surg.* October 1978;31(4):339–342.
28. Strauch B, et al. Replantation of amputated parts of the penis, nose, ear and scalp. *Clin Plat Surg.* Jan 1983; 10(1):115–124.
29. Morris PJ, Bradley JA, Boyal L, Earley M, Hagan P, Milling M, Rumsey N. Facial transplantation: a working party report from the Royal College of Surgeons of England. *Transplantation.* 2004;77:330–338. ComitèConsultatif National d'Ethique, C. C. N. E. (France) www.ccneethique.fr.
30. Wiggins O, Barker J, Cunningham M, Francois C, Grossi F, Kon M, Maldonado C, Martinez S, Perez-Abadia G, Vossen M, Banis J. On the ethics of facial transplant research. *AJOB.* 2004;4:1–12.
31. Yagi M, Ogua JH, Kawasaki M, Yagi M. Autogenous transplantation of the canine larynx. *Ann Otol Rhinol Laryngol.* 1966;75(3):849–864.
32. Takenouchi S, Ogura JH, Kawasaki M, Yagi M. Autogenous transplantation of the canine larynx. *Laryngoscope.* 1967;77(9):1644–1667.
33. Silver CE, Rosen RG, Dardik I, Eisen H, Schwibner BH, Som ML. Transplantation of the canine larynx. *Ann Surg.* 1970;172(1):142–150.
34. Kluyskens P, Ringoir S. Follow-up of a human larynx transplantation. *Laryngoscope.* 1970;80(8):1244–1250.
35. Strome M, Stein J, Esclamado R, Hicks D, Lorenz RR, Brawn W, et al. Laryngeal transplantation and 40-month follow-up. *N Engl J Med.* 2001;344(22):1676–1679.
36. Birchall MA, Lorenz RR, Berke GS, Genden EM, Haughey BH, Gilmionow M, Srome M. Laryngeal Transplantation in 2005: A review. *Am J Transplant.* 2005;6(1): 20–26.
37. Fageeh W, Raffa H, Jabbad H, Marzouki A. Transplantation of the human uterus. *Int J Gynecol Obstet.* 2002; 76:245–251.
38. Brannstrom M, Wranning CA, Racho El-Akouri R. Transplantation of the uterus. *Mol Cell Endocrinol.* 2003;202(2):177–184.
39. Bar Oz B, Hackman R, Einarson T, et al. Pregnancy outcome after cyclosporin therapy during pregnancy: a meta-analysis. *Transplantation.* 2001;71(8):1051–1055.
40. Schmid BP. Monitoring of organ formation in rat embryos after in vitro exposure to azathioprine, mercaptopurine, methotrexate or cyclosporin A. *Toxicology.* 1984;31(1):9–21.
41. Scott JR, Pitkin RM, Yannone ME. Transplantation of the primate uterus. *Surg Gynecol Obstet.* 1971;133:414–418.
42. Callaghan C, Ali A, Pettigrew G. Transplant surgery. *Br Med J.* 2004;329:23–25.
43. Stevenson AFG. Tissue engineering: in vitro embryonal nidation in a murine endometrial construct. *Indian J Exp Biol.* 2003;41(6):563–569.
44. Millesi H, et al. The interfascular nerve grafting of the median and ulnar nerves. *J Bone Joint Surgery.* 1972;54:727.
45. Taylor GI, Ham J. The Free vascularised nerve graft. *Plast Reconstr Surg.* 1976;57:413.
46. Bain JR. Peripheral nerve and neuromuscular allotransplantation: current status. *Microsurgery.* 2000;20: 384–388.
47. Mackinnon SE, Doolabh VB, Novak CB, Trulock EP. Clinical outcome following nerve allograft transplantation. *Plast Reconstr Surg.* 2001;107:1419–1429.
48. Russell RC, O'Brien BM, Morrison WA, Pamamull G, MacLeod A. The late functional results of upper limb revascularization and reimplantation. *J Hand Surg [Am].* 1984;9:623–633.
49. Owen ER, Dubernard JM, Lanzetta M, Kapila H, Martin X, Dawahra M, Hakim NS. Peripheral nerve regeneration in human hand transplants. *Transplant Proc.* 2001;33:1720–1721.
50. Dubernard JM, Owen ER, Lanzetta M, Hakim N. What is happening with hand transplants? *Lancet.* 2001;357: 1711–1712.
51. Midha R, Mackinnon SW, Becker LE. The fate of Schwann cells in peripheral nerve allografts. *J Neuropathol Exp Neurol.* 1994;53:316–322.
52. Morris PJ, Bradley JA, Boyal L, Earley M, Hagan P, Milling M, Rumsey N. Facial transplantation: a working party report from the Royal College of Surgeons of England. *Transplantation.* 2004;77:330–338. Comitè Consultatif National d'Ethique, C. C. N. E. (France) www.ccneethique.fr.
53. Hu, W., Lu, J., Zhang, L., et.al. " A preliminary report of penile transplantation". *European Urology.* 50:851–853. 2006.
54. Holmgren G. Some experiences in the surgery of otosclerosis. *Acta Otolaryng.* 1923;5:460–466.

Index

Note: The letter 't' following the locators refer to tables and letter 'f' following the locators refer to figure

A
Abel, J., 40, 49
ABS, see Artificial bowel sphincter (ABS)
ACLF, see Acute-on-chronic liver failure (ACLF)
Acute liver failure (ALF), 30, 57–62, 67–71
  indications of, 69
  pathophysiological basis of, 69
Acute lung injury
  definition, 5–6
  epidemiology, 6
  management of, 6
  pathogenesis of, 6
Acute-on-chronic liver failure (ACLF), 57–59, 67, 69, 70–71
Acute renal failure (ARF), 9–13, 16, 138, 140, 143
  epidemiology, 9–10
  optimization after implantation, 12–13
  pathophysiology, 11–12
  risk factors, 10–11
Albisser, A.M., 84
ALF, see Acute liver failure (ALF)
Alison, M.R., 146
Allograft rejection, 122
AMC-bioartificial liver, 61f
Andersson, L.C., 93
Andrus, F.C., 40
Anorectal transplantation, 120
  assessing feasibility of, 115–118
  description, 119
  indications, 121–123
  pre-operative preparation, 119
  recorded variables post transplantation, 120
  technological advances, 118–119
ARF, see Acute renal failure (ARF)
Arteriovenous fistula (AVF), 49, 50f
Artificial bowel sphincter (ABS)
  AMS 800, 123–124
  complications, 129–130
  contraindications, 127
  device activation/deactivation, 124–125
  functional outcome of, 125–127
  implantation of, 128–129
  indications, 127
  types, 127–128
Artificial circulatory support
  arterial line filters, 30–31
  CABG, 22–23
  cannulation for cardiopulmonary bypass, 24–26
  conduits, 23
  CPB safety features, 34–35
  cross-clamp fibrillation, 31
  direct gas interface oxygenators, 28
  heat exchangers, 30
  history, 21–22
  long-term circulatory support, 36–37
  membrane oxygenators, 29–30
  monitoring during CPB
    activated clotting time, 31–32
    arterial and venous saturations, 34
    arterial pressure, 32–33
    ECG, 34
    gas flows in flowmeter, 32
    'Tycos' pressure, 34
    urine output, 33–34
    venous pressure, 33
    venous reservoir level, 31
  non-physiological aspects of cardiopulmonary bypass, complications of
    bleeding, 35
    ECG complications, 36
    kidney dysfunction, 36
    low cardiac output, 36
    neurological events, 35
    pulmonary complications, 36
  open heart surgery, 22
  protecting myocardium, 31
  pump to substitute for heart
    centrifugal pump, 28
    roller pump, 27–28
  replicating lungs, 28
  of short-term CPB circuit, 26–27
  valve operations, 24
Artificial extracorporeal systems, 63–64
  albumin, importance of, 63–64
  devices, design of, 64–67
    MARS, 64
    prometheus, 65–67
    SPAD, 64–65
  MARS clinical trial, 67–69
  prometheus, 70
  safety profile of, 70
  SPAD clinical trial, 69–70
Artificial kidney
  access to blood stream, 48–49
  anticoagulation blood component, 48

179

Artificial kidney (cont.)
  basic components of, 42t
  blood component, 48–49
  capillary fiber membrane, 43f
  criteria for, 51t
  dialyzate, 49–50
    composition, 49–50
    Kolff Brigham dialyzer, 45, 46f
    water, 49–51
  future prospect of, 51–52
  introduction, 39
  membrane support structure of, 43–48
  semipermeable membrane, 39–42
  used on humans, 44f
Artificial pancreas (AP) Project, 90
Artificial urinary sphincter (AUS), 123
Auditory brain steam response (ABR), 135
AVF, see Arteriovenous fistula (AVF)

B
Banerjee, M., 144
Bellmann, R., 69
Bellomo, R., 13
Bilger, R.C., 133
Bournemouth's Education Resources for Training in Insulin and Eating (BERTIE), 81

C
CABG, see Coronary artery bypass grafting (CABG)
Cardiopulmonary bypass (CPB)
  circuit, 22, 25–27, 30, 31
  complications of non-physiological aspects, 35–36
  monitoring during, 31–34
  safety features, 34–35
Cardiovcar failure
  cardiogenic shock, 2–3
  classification of shock, 1
  distributive shock, 3–4
  hypovolemic shock, 1–2
  obstructive shock, 4
Central nervous system diseases, 150

Chamuleau, R.A., 60, 61
Chinzei, R., 145
Christensen, J.L., 127
Chronic renal failure (CRF), 138
Cochlear implant
  common indications, 134
  complications of, 136
  ethical issues of, 135
  past/present/future of, 133–134
  services of, 134
  suitability of, 135
  surgery, 135–136
Composite tissue allograft (CTA), see Composite tissue transplantation
Composite tissue transplantation
  face allograft of, 170–172
  first successful hand transplant of CTA, 166–169
  immunology of, 169–170
  laryngeal transplantation, 172–173
  penis transplantation, 175
  peripheral nerve transplantation, 173–174
  tongue transplantation, 174–175
  uterine, 173
Computed tomography (CT), 135
Constipation/fecal impaction, 130
Continuous glucose monitoring system (CGMS), 85–86, 86f
Continuous subcutaneous insulin infusion (CSII), 79
Continuous venovenous hemodiafiltration (CVVHDF), 15
Conventional insulin treatment, 77–79
  closed loop insulin pumps, 84–85
    glucose sensors, 85–87
    and JDRF artificial pancreas (AP) project, 90
    current state of play, 87
    control algorithms, 89–90
    pumps, 87
    sensors, 87–89
  need for closed loop system, 83
  open loop insulin pumps
    history of, 79–80
    intraportal insulin delivery, 83
    pros and cons of, 80–83
    transplants, 83–84

Coronary artery bypass grafting (CABG), 22–23
Cosgrove, D., 10
CPB, see Cardiopulmonary bypass (CPB)
Cultured autologous skin substitutes, 102
Cultured epidermal autografts (CEAs), 102
Cultured skin substitute (CASS), 102
Cuprophan, 41–42

D
Dawn phenomenon, 79
Dekel, B., 139
De Novo Kidney Creation, 142–143
Devesa, J.M., 125
Devile, M., 1
Diabetes Control and Complications Trial (DCCT), 83
Dimarakis, I., 137
Direkze, N.C., 140
Doria, C., 69
Dosage adjustment for normal eating (DAFNE), 81
Dynamic neo-sphincter
  abdomino-perineal excision of rectum, 110–111
  complications of, 111–112
  indications of, 110
  types of, 110

E
Elmiyeh, B., 137
Embryonic stem cells, 137–138
Ende, N., 144
Endogenous Albumin-Bound Toxins, 58t
Endothelium, 139–140
Epidermic grafts, 94
Epidermolysis bullosa (EB), 101
Experimental organ transplantation
  anorectal transplantation
    assessing feasibility of, 115–118
    description, 119
    indications, 121–123
    pre-operative preparation, 119
    recorded variables post transplantation, 120

technological advances of, 118–119
artificial bowel sphincter (ABS)
AMS 800, 123–124
complications, 129–130
contraindications, 127
device activation/deactivation, 124–125
functional outcome of, 125–127
implantation of, 128–129
indications, 127
types, 127–128
evolution for quality of life, 114–115
Extracorporeal liver assist device (ELAD), 59, 60f, 61–62
Extracorporeal membrane oxygenation (ECMO), 8, 21, 36

F
Face allograft, 170–172
Fayad, G., 137
Felldin, M., 68
Flores, C., 137
Frankel, A., 39
Fujikawa, T., 144
Full-thickness skin grafts (FTSGs), 101–102

G
Gerlach, J.C., 59
Glomerular filtration rate (GFR), 39
Glomeruli, 141–142
Gómez, C.M.H., 1
Gordon, M.Y., 137
Grompe, M., 145
Guo, J.K., 141

H
Habib, N.A., 137
Hand allografts, 169
Haemodialysis access system, 52f
Hakim, N.S., 165
Hepatoblastoma-based ELAD, 61–62
Hess, D., 144
Hoerstrup, S.P., 149
Human leucocyte antigens (HLA), 123
Humes, H.D., 143

I
Interstitium, 140
Ischemia, 112–114, 139, 141, 153–154

J
Juvenile Diabetes Research Foundation (JDRF), 90

K
Kang, E.M., 144
Kidney, functions of, 40t
Kirwan, C., 39
Kolff Brigham dialyzer, 45, 46f
Korbling, M., 146
Kratz, G., 93

L
Laryngeal transplantation, 172–173
Lechner, A., 144
Levičar, N., 137
Lin, F., 141, 148
Liver substitution
  artificial extracorporeal systems in
    albumin, importance of, 63–64
    devices, design of, 64–67
    MARS, 64
    MARS clinical trial, 67–69
    prometheus, 65–67, 66f, 70
    safety profile, 70
    SPAD, 64–65
    SPAD clinical trial, 69–70
  bioartificial systems, 59–63
    clinical trials of, 60–63
    design of devices, 59–60
    safety concerns, 63
  current liver support systems, assessment of, 58–59
  functions required of liver support system in, 58
Liver support system
  assessment of, 58–59
  functions required of, 58
Lung protective ventilation
  corticosteroids, 7
  extracorporeal support, 8
  fluid strategy, 7
  high-frequency oscillatory ventilation, 8
  inhaled pulmonary vasodilators, 7–8
  NIV, 9
  positive end expiratory pressure, 7
  prone ventilation, 8
  ventilation, disadvantages of, 8–9
  weaning, 9

M
Ma, N., 153
Macia, M., 69
Magnetic resonance image (MRI), 98, 135
Major histocompatibility complex (MHC), 118, 122–123
Major histocompatibility antigens (MHA), 170
Malignant disease, 127
Mallet, V.O., 146
MARS circuit, 65f
Mesenchymal stem cells (MSC), 138
Methicillin-resistant *Staphylococcus aureus* (MRSA), 99, 109
MHC, *see* Major Histocompatibility Complex (MHC)
Model Predictive Control (MPC), 89
Modern skin engineering
  concept of, 100
  future of, 102–103
  historical overview of, 93–94
  introduction to, 93
  skin substitutes in, 100
    characteristics and clinical use, 100
    types, 101–102
  structure of skin in, 93
  wound healing in, 95
    dermal, 96
    epidermal, 95–96
  wounds, clinical management of
    debridement, 98–99
    dressings, 99
    post-debridement treatment, 99
    pre-debridement assessment, 97–98
Molecular adsorbents recirculating system (MARS), 64
Mono-component insulins, 78
Mulholland, J., 21

Mullhaupt, B., 69
Multiorgan failure after artificial organ implantation
  acute lung injury
    definition, 5-6
    epidemiology, 6
    management, 6
    pathogenesis of, 6
  acute renal failure
    epidemiology, 9-10
    optimization after implantation, 12-13
    pathophysiology, 11-12
    risk factors, 10-11
  cardiovcar failure
    cardiogenic shock, 2-3
    classification of shock, 1
    distributive shock, 3-4
    hypovolemic shock, 1-2
    obstructive shock, 4
  current best practice guidelines, 17
  lung protective ventilation, 6-7
    corticosteroids, 7
    extracorporeal support, 8
    fluid strategy, 7
    high-frequency oscillatory ventilation, 8
    inhaled pulmonary vasodilators, 7-8
    NIV, 9
    positive end expiratory pressure, 7
    prone ventilation, 8
    ventilation, disadvantages of, 8-9
    weaning, 9
  optimization after implantation, 12-13
  respiratory failure
    causes of, 5
    definition of different, 4-5
    management of, 5
  RRT as, 13-16
Multiple daily injections (MDI), 80

N
Nephron, 39
Nerve growth factor (NGF), 118
Nettelblad, H.C., 93
Neuropetide-3 (NT-3), 118
Ng, I.O., 146
NIV, see Non-invasive ventilation (NIV)

Non-invasive ventilation (NIV), 9
Nyberg, S.L., 63

O
Obichere, Austin, 107
Oh, S.H., 145
Olanow, C.W., 153
Organ replacement, 137
  adult cell, 138
  artificial kidney, 143
  and cardiac-related bioengineering, 149-150
  central nervous system diseases, 150
  de novo kidney creation, 142-143
  diabetes, 143-144
  embryonic, 137-138
  endothelium, 139-140
  glomeruli, 141-142
  interstitium, 140
  for kidney diseases, 138-139
  Parkinson's disease, 150-151
  and pulmonary regeneration, 150
  stem cell therapy for diabetes, 144-145
    clinical studies, 145
    liver diseases, 145
  stem cell therapy for ischemic heart diseases, 147-149
    clinical studies, 148
    mechanisms of action, 148-149
  stem cell therapy for liver diseases, 145-147
    clinical studies, 146-147
    myocardial infarction/heart disease, 147
  stem cell therapy in stroke, 153-154
  stem cell therapy Parkinson's disease
    clinical studies, 152-153
    stroke, 153
  tubular epithelium, 140-141
Owen, E.R., 165

P
Parkinson's Disease, 150-151
Passive neo-sphincter, 108
  complications of, 109
  indications, 108-109
  types of, 109
Patel, P., 1

Penis transplantation, 175
Peripheral nerve transplantation, 173-174
Petersen, B.E., 145
Physiological neo-sphincter, 112-113
  complications of, 113-114
  indications of, 113
  types of, 113
Porcine Hepatocyte-Based BAL, 60-61
Press, M., 77
Prometheus, 65-67, 70
Proportional-integral-derivative (PID), 89
Prosthetic artificial sphincter (PAS), 127-128
Prosthetic bowel sphincter
  complications of, 129
  contraindications, 127
  functional outcome, 123-127
  implantation, 128
  indications, 127
  types, 127

R
Recombinant erythropoietin (r-epo), 39
Renal replacement therapy (RRT)
  adverse effects of, 15
  anticoagulation, 15
  choice of anticoagulation, 16
  CVVHDF, 15
  extracorporeal inflammatory mediator removal, 16
  indications for, 14
  optimal dose of hemofiltration, 16
  optimal treatment modalities for, 16
  physiological functions of kidney and clinical measurement, 13
  principle of hemofiltration, 15
  renal function, assessment of, 13-14
  vascular access, 15
Renal tubule cell assist device (RAD), 52, 143
Ross Basket, 24

S
Sakaida, I., 145
Sen, S., 57

Shape memory alloy (SMA), 127–128, 140
Sin, D.D., 5
Single-pass albumin dialysis (SPAD), 64–65, 66f
Skin
  structure of, 93
  substitute in, 100
    characteristics and clinical use, 100
    future of, 102–103
    types, 101–102
Soria, B., 144
Sphincters, artificial
  dynamic neo-sphincter, 109
    complications of, 111–112
    dynamic graciloplasty, functional outcome of, 111
    following abdomino-perineal excision of rectum, 110–111
    indications of, 110
    types of, 110
  origin of, 107
  passive neo-sphincter, 108
    complications, 109
    indications, 108–109
    types of, 109
  physiological neo-sphincter, 112–113
    complications, 113–114
    indications, 113
    types of, 113
  prosthetic bowel sphincter, 123
    complications of, 129
    contraindications, 127
    functional outcome, 123–127
    implantation, 128
    indications, 127
    types, 127
  surgically fashioned bowel, 108
Split-thickness skin grafts (STSGs), 101
Stem cell therapy, 138–139
  for diabetes, 144–145
  for ischemic heart diseases, 147–148
  for liver diseases, 145–146
  in stroke, 153–154
Suliman, I., 107

T
Tang, D.Q., 144
Theise, N.D., 146
Thompson, L., 152
Tongue transplantation, 174–175
Transforming growth factor (TGF), 58
Transplantation
  laryngeal, 172–173
  pennis, 175
  peripheral nerve, 173–174
  tongue, 174–175
Tubular epithelium, 140–141
'Tycos' pressure, 34

U
Ultrafiltration, 15, 39, 42, 45, 50

V
Vina, R., 145

W
Wei, H.J., 149
Williams, Roger, 57
Wong, W.D., 127

Y
Yamada, T., 145
Yamamoto, M., 138

Z
Zheng, F., 141